Biochemistry of Inflammation

IMMUNOLOGY AND MEDICINE SERIES

Immunology of Endocrine Diseases
Editor: A. M. McGregor

Clinical Transplantation: Current Practice and Future Prospects
Editor: G. R. D. Catto

Complement in Health and Disease
Editor: K. Whaley

Immunological Aspects of Oral Diseases
Editor: L. Ivanyi

Immunoglobulins in Health and Disease
Editor: M. A. H. French

Immunology of Malignant Diseases
Editors: V. S. Byers and R. W. Baldwin

Lymphoproliferative Diseases
Editors: D. B. Jones and D. H. Wright

Phagocytes and Disease
Editors: M. S. Klempner, B. Styrt and J. Ho

Immunology of Sexually Transmitted Diseases
Editor: D. J. M. Wright

Mast Cells, Mediators and Disease
Editor: S. T. Holgate

Immunodeficiency and Disease
Editor: A. D. B. Webster

Immunology of Pregnancy and its Disorders
Editor: C. M. M. Stern

Immunotherapy of Disease
Editor: T. J. Hamblin

Immunology of Prophylactic Immunization
Editor: A. J. Zuckerman

Immunology of Eye Disease
Editor: S. Lightman

Lymphoproliferative Diseases
Editors: D. B. Jones and D. H. Wright

Immunology of Renal Diseases
Editor: C. D. Pusey

Immunology of HIV Infection
Editor: A. G. Bird

Biochemistry of Inflammation
Editors: J. T. Whicher and S. W. Evans

Immunology of Gastrointestinal Diseases
Editor: T. T. MacDonald

Immunology of ENT Disorders
Editor: G. Scadding

Immunology of Infection
Editors: J. G. P. Sissons, J. Cohen and L. K. Borysiewicz

IMMUNOLOGY

SERIES · SERIES · SERIES · SERIES AND SERIES · SERIES · SERIES · SERIES

MEDICINE

Volume 18

Biochemistry of Inflammation

Edited by

J. T. Whicher and S. W. Evans

Department of Chemical
Pathology and Immunology
Old Medical School, Leeds, UK

Series Editor: K. Whaley

KLUWER ACADEMIC PUBLISHERS
DORDRECHT / BOSTON / LONDON

Distributors

for the United States and Canada: Kluwer Academic Publishers, PO Box 358, Accord Station, Hingham, MA 02018-0358, USA
for all other countries: Kluwer Academic Publishers, Distribution Center, PO Box 322, 3300 AH Dordrecht, The Netherlands

British Library Cataloguing in Publication Data

Biochemistry of inflammation. – (Immunology and medicine; 18)
I. Whicher, J. T. II. Evans, S. W. III. Series 616.072

ISBN 0792389859

Library of Congress Cataloging-in-Publication Data

Biochemistry of inflammation/edited by J. T. Whicher and S. W. Evans.
p. cm. — (Immunology and medicine series; v. 18)
Includes bibliographical references and index.
ISBN 0-7923-8985-9 (Casebound)
1. Inflammation—Pathophysiology. 2. Inflammation—Mediators.
I. Whicher, J. T. II. Evans, S. W. III. Series.
[DNLM: 1. Acute Phase Proteins—physiology. 2. Complement—physiology.
3. Complement Activation—physiology. 4. Cytokines—physiology.
5. Inflammation—immunology. 6. Inflammation—physiopathology.
W1 1M53BI v. 18]
RB131.B55 1992
616′.0473—dc20
DNLM/DLC
for Library of Congress 91-35351
CIP

Published in the United Kingdom by Kluwer Academic Publishers, PO Box 55, Lancaster, UK.

Kluwer Academic Publishers BV incorporates the publishing programmes of D. Reidel, Martinus Nijhoff, Dr W. Junk and MTP Press.

Typeset by Technical Keying Services, Manchester.
Printed in Great Britain by Hartnolls Limited, Bodmin, Cornwall.

Contents

Series Editor's Foreword

The interface between clinical immunology and other branches of medical practice is frequently blurred and the general physician is often faced with clinical problems with an immunological basis and is expected to diagnose and manage such patients. The rapid expansion of basic and clinical immunology over the past two decades has resulted in the appearance of increasing numbers of immunology journals and it is impossible for a non-specialist to keep apace with this information overload. The *Immunology and Medicine* series is designed to present individual topics of immunology in a condensed package of information which can be readily assimilated by the busy clinician or pathologist.

K. Whaley, Glasgow
August 1991

Preface

In the last 10 years our understanding of inflammation has increased dramatically. As with most other areas of medical science, this has in large part been due to the impact of molecular biology and to our ability to identify and clone the genes for many important intercellular mediators. It is evident that inflammation is a complex and concerted response of the organism to foreign bodies or tissue damage. Many cell types from the classical inflammatory cells to tissue cells are involved and they communicate via a multitude of different systems. The study of inflammation can be approached from many directions and it is the purpose of this book to bring together ideas from a number of different bichemical disciplines which are frequently not integrated. The first chapter describes visually the main issues addressed within the book and will, we hope, prove valuable as an overview of this complex subject. The remaining chapters have been organized into three themes: the affector molecules, the regulatory components and the processes of inflammation itself.

The affector molecules are epitomized by the complement system, now regarded as playing an essential role in inflammation, and from a biochemical standpoint one of the best understood mediator systems. The kinins, long known to induce vascular permeability in inflammation, have now become recognized as key effector molecules with the realization that they may be produced by kallikreins both in the plasma and from tissue cells, notably the polymorphonuclear leukocyte. This brings them into the family of mediators directly produced by the activity of inflammatory cells. A number of the mediator systems of inflammation such as complement and coagulation are comprised of cascades of proteolytic enzymes. They are thus highly susceptible to activation by proteases released from cells. These are present in the lysosomes and also in a complex array of granules in some inflammatory cell types. Much of the damage produced by inflammation and the remodelling which follows is dependent upon the release of proteolytic enzymes from both inflammatory cells and tissue cells. In addition, there is increasing evidence that proteases contribute to various intracellular control mechanisms. Not surprisingly in such a complex situation a bewildering array of inhibitors exists. The importance of these complex systems is only now beginning to be appreciated. The importance of locally produced prostaglandins in inflammation has been well recognized for many years and indeed has been the basis for much of the pharmacological intervention in the processes of inflammation. Recently, it has become clear that besides these classic mediators a number of other extremely important products of arachidonic acid metabolism, especially platelet activity factor, play a part in inflammation. Production of reactive oxygen species is the key process in the development of inflammatory damage. These molecules are necessary for bacteriological activity of phagocytic cells; however it is now recognized that oxygen-derived products, particularly in the joint, may be key mediators in the chronic damage which follows inflammation.

While many of the mediators and affector molecules of inflammation have been known about and investigated for many years, the regulatory molecules are only now being unravelled. It is clear that glucocorticoids, previously thought of as simple immunosupressive hormones, are intricately involved in the normal control mechanisms regulating inflammation and the response to trauma. Not only is the secretion of these hormones controlled by inflammatory products, such as interleukin 1 and interleukin 6, but they have complex functions in regulating the activity of immune and inflammatory cells. Platelet activating factor is a powerful endogenous mediator which not only behaves locally as an inflammatory mediator in a manner analogous to kinins and prostaglandins but also is increasingly being shown to act systematically with functions analogous to the cytokines. The cytokines primarily involved in inflammation, interleukin 1, tumour necrosis factor and interleukin 6, have both local effects in the control of inflammatory cells and post-inflammatory remodelling, and important systemic effects on the vascular, nervous and endocrine systems adjusting the 'milieu interieur' of the organism and optimizing the inflammatory process.

The last two chapters describe the process of inflammation. Whilst inflammation may be thought of as an essentially local process it is clear that systemic effects (often called the acute phase response) occur. These effects, including changes in body temperature, vascular permeability, circulating hormones, acute phase protein synthesis and leukocytosis, are considered in the penultimate chapter. All these processes alter local inflammation in a complex way but have probably evolved to optimize its function or more provocatively to minimize inflammatory damage. At the local level inflammation is based on complex patterns of cell recruitment and activation. This important basis of the local inflammatory response is described in the final chapter.

List of Contributors

D. R. BLAKE
Bone and Joint Research Unit
London Hospital Medical College
25–29 Ashfield Street
London E1 1AD
UK

P. BRAQUET
Institut Henri Beaufour
17, avenue Descartes
92350 Le Plessis Robinson
France

C. W. DENKO
Department of Medicine/Rheumatology
Case Western Reserve University
University Hospitals of Cleveland
Cleveland, OH 44106
USA

S. DION
Department of Pharmacology
Medical School
University of Sherbrooke
Sherbrooke J1H 5N4
Canada

G. DRAPEAU
Department of Pharmacology
Medical School
University of Sherbrooke
Sherbrooke J1H 5N4
Canada

G. W. DUFF
Section of Molecular Medicine
Department of Medicine and Pharmacology
University of Sheffield
Royal Hallamshire Hospital
Sheffield S10 2JF
UK

J. A. EASTGATE
Section of Molecular Medicine
Department of Medicine and Pharmacology
University of Sheffield
Royal Hallamshire Hospital
Sheffield S10 2JF
UK

S. W. EVANS
Department of Chemical Pathology
and Immunology
Old Medical School
University of Leeds
Leeds LS2 9JT
UK

G. HARRIS
Department of Immunology
London Hospital Medical College
Turner Street
London E1 2AD
UK

G. A. HIGGS
Celltech Ltd.
216 Bath Road
Slough, Berks. SL1 4EN
UK

D. HOSFORD
Institut Henri Beaufour
17, avenue Descartes
92350 Le Plessis Robinson
France

P. J. MCLAUGHLIN
Department of Immunology
University of Liverpool
PO Box 147
Liverpool L69 3BX
UK

LIST OF CONTRIBUTORS

A. R. McPHADEN
Department of Pathology
Western Infirmary
Glasgow
G11 6NT
UK

M. PAUBERT-BRAQUET
Institut Henri Beaufour
17, avenue Descartes
92350 Le Plessis Robinson
France

S. H. PEERS
Department of Biochemical Pharmacology
St Bartholomew's Hospital Medical College
Charterhouse Square
London EC1M 6QB
UK

D. PERRETT
Department of Medicine
St Bartholomew's Hospital Medical College
West Smithfield
London EC1A 7BE
UK

E. R. PETTIPHER
Department of Immunology and Infectious Diseases
Pfizer Central Research
Groton
Connecticut
USA

D. REGOLI
Department of Pharmacology
Medical School
University of Sherbrooke
Sherbrooke J1H 5N4
Canada

N.-E. RHALEB
Department of Pharmacology
Medical School
University of Sherbrooke
Sherbrooke J1H 5N4
Canada

A. ROT
Sandoz Forschungsinstitut
Vienna
Austria

J. A. SALMON
Department of Pharmacology
Wellcome Research Laboratories
Langley Court
Beckenham
Kent BR3 3BS
UK

J. A. SYMONS
Section of Molecular Medicine
Department of Medicine and Pharmacology
University of Sheffield
Royal Hallamshire Hospital
Sheffield S10 2JF
UK

C. I. WESTACOTT
Department of Chemical Pathology and Immunology
Old Medical School
University of Leeds
Leeds LS2 9JT
UK

K. WHALEY
Department of Pathology
Western Infirmary
Glasgow
G11 6NT
UK

J. T. WHICHER
Department of Chemical Pathology and Immunology
Old Medical School
University of Leeds
Leeds LS2 9JT
UK

P. G. WINYARD
Bone and Joint Research Unit
London Hospital Medical College
25–29 Ashfield Street
London E1 1AD
UK

J. F. WOESSNER, JR
Department of Biochemical and Molecular Biology
University of Miami School of Medicine
Miami
FL 33101
USA

1
An overview of the inflammatory response

S. W. EVANS and J. T. WHICHER

INTRODUCTION

Inflammation comprises a complex array of adaptive responses to tissue injury which are both local and systemic (Figure 1.1). The local responses result in recruitment of phagocytic cells and removal of endogenous or foreign material. The systemic responses may alter the 'milieu interior' to allow these processes to occur more efficiently. While such an overview is apparently extremely simple and attractive it belies the complexity of the biochemistry which underlies it. Perhaps because of the importance of inflammation to the survival of the organism there seems to be a great replication of functions amongst the biochemical mediators and regulators of this response, though they act through only a small number of cell types. A major challenge to the medical scientist is to unravel the relative importance of the different mediator systems so that therapeutic intervention can be achieved. The cellular processes of inflammation fall into four major groups: changes in blood flow caused by changes in smooth muscle cell function causing vasodilatation, alterations in vascular permeability engendered by cytoskeletal contraction in endothelial cells, migration of phagocytic leukocytes to the site of inflammation, and phagocytosis.

The molecules participating in the biochemical process can generally be considered to fall into one of three categories: mediators, inhibitors and regulatory molecules. Thus the chemical mediator systems such as complement and prostaglandins produce molecules which initiate pro-inflammatory cellular events. Inhibitory elements such as protease inhibitors may block the mediator system themselves or 'mop up' pro-inflammatory molecules such as proteinases released from leukocytes. Regulation may be achieved by molecules produced locally at the site of inflammation and which modulate cell function, such as TNF, or produced at a distant site such as glucocorticosteroids.

Inflammation may be initiated in very different ways and through different pathways. Simple trauma activates mast cells which release mediators which cause vasodilatation, vascular leakage and possibly proteolytic activation of biochemical mediator systems such as complement. Immune complexes may activate complement and interact directly with phagocytic cells. Bacterial products may activate macrophages to produce proteases. However inflammation is induced, the kinin, complement and clotting systems are all recruited and interact in what Oscar Ratnof called a 'tangled web'. Eicosanoids are also released from phagocytic and tumour cells. The response is thus stereotyped despite different mechanisms of initiation of acute inflammation. It is in the field of cytokine regulation, however, that fascinating clues suggesting possible mechanisms for curtailment or prolongation of inflammation are to be found. The progression of inflammation into the chronic phase is important, as it is this which damages the host tissues through the production of proteases and oxygen radicals from phagocytes.

In this chapter the biochemical systems discussed later in this book are brought together as a series of figures which summarize their key components.

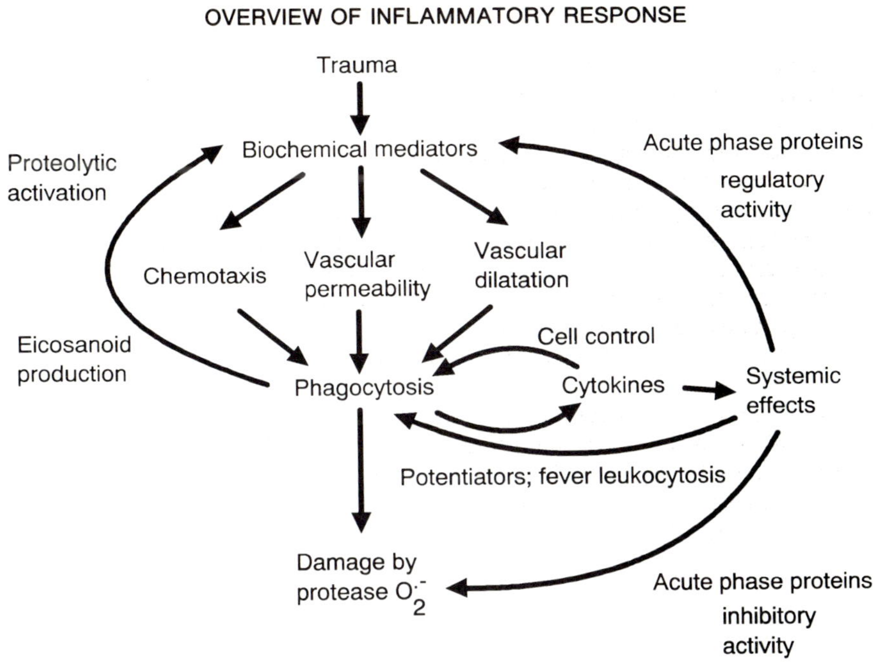

Figure 1.1 An overview of inflammation.

Legend for Figures 1.1 to 1.13

Cells		
Fibroblast	Fb	
Macrophage	Mϕ	
Polymorphonuclear leukocyte	PMN	
T helper cell	T_H	
Product		
Complement components	C	e.g. C1a
Interferon	IFN	
Interleukins	IL	e.g. IL 1
Leukotrienes	LT	e.g. LTD_4
Platelet activating factor	PAF	
Prostaglandins	PG	e.g. PGE_2
Superoxide anion radical	$O_2^{\cdot -}$	
Tumour necrosis factor	TNF	
Text and arrow styles		
Cell, cell product or target molecule	e.g. mast cell, histamine, elastin	
local physiological event	e.g. *chemotaxis*	
MAJOR PHYSIOLOGICAL EVENT	e.g. *PAIN* or *ACUTE PHASE RESPONSE*	

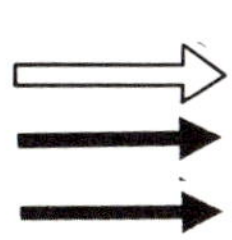

Product

Stimulation

Inhibition

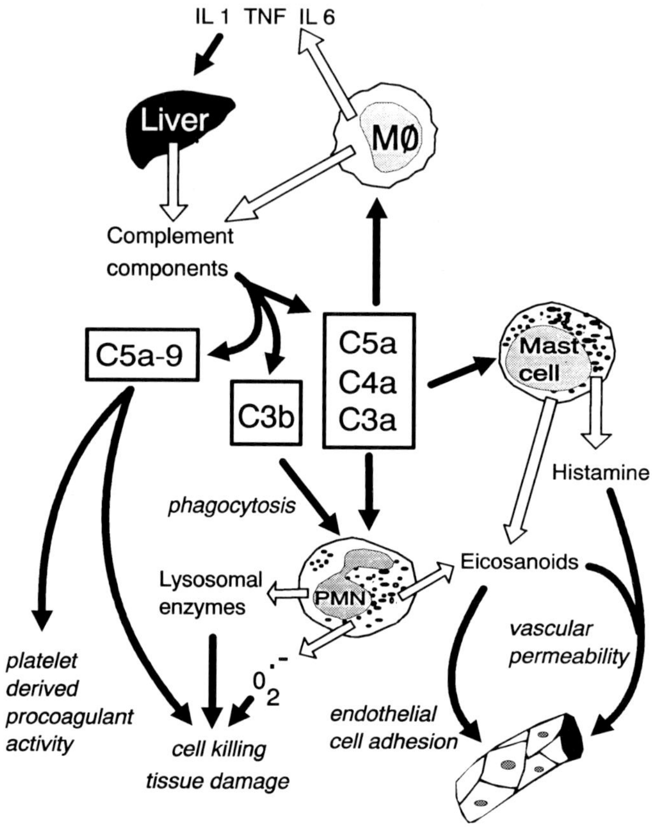

Figure 1.2 The majority of complement components are produced by the liver, although significant local production by macrophages also occurs. Control of hepatocyte-derived components is regulated in part by macrophage-derived cytokines. Inactive components are proteolytically activated in a cascade system to generate a number of key mediators. Three products of the activation cascade, C5a, C3a and C4a, mediate mast cell release of a variety of bioactive molecules including histamine which results in increased vascular permeability. C5a, and possibly C3a and C4a, also stimulate polymorphonuclear cells to release eicosanoids which in turn act to increase vasodilation (PGE_2), vascular permeability (LTD_4) and to induce expression of adhesion molecules involved in leukocyte–endothelial cell interaction. In addition PMN also release oxygen radicals and lysosomal enzymes following stimulation with C5a or certain microbial components and immune complexes incorporating C3b. C3a, C4a, C5a and C567 are also chemotactic for leukocytes. C3b receptors on phagocytes and other cell types mediate phagocytosis of bacteria, cell debris or immune complexes coated with C3b. Components 5a to 9 form the membrane attack complex responsible for cell lysis and platelet derived pro-coagulant activity.

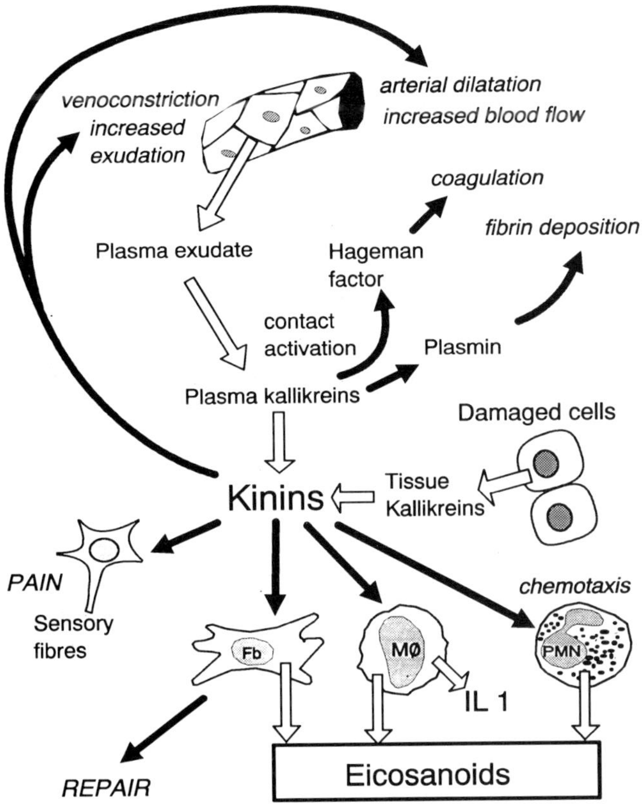

Figure 1.3 Kinins are generated from precursor molecules synthesized in the liver by a family of serine proteases called kallikreins. Kallikreins themselves are derived from PMN and damaged tissue cells (tissue kallikreins) and from blood (plasma kallikreins). Kinins have many potential activities associated with inflammation. Direct effects of kinins on the vascular system are mediated by receptors found on endothelial cells (vasodilatation, increased capillary permeability and endothelium-derived relaxing factor (EDRF) production) and smooth muscle cells (venoconstriction). Kinins stimulate fibroblasts to proliferate and to synthesize collagen and macrophages to produce cytokines such as IL 1. Many cells also produce eicosanoids when stimulated with kinins. The plasma kallikreins also play a role in blood clotting, cleaving plasmin and activating Hageman factor to trigger coagulation.

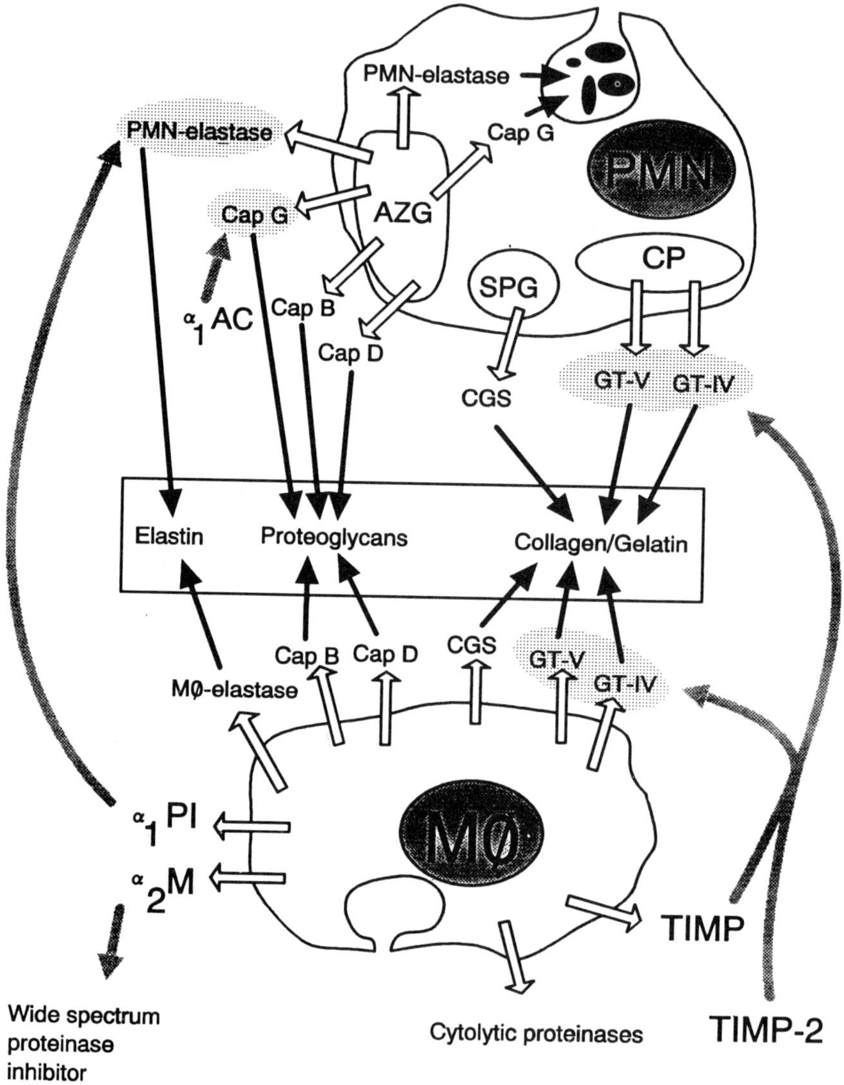
PMN-elastase
PMN-elastase
Cap G
Cap G
AZG
PMN
CP
SPG
α1 AC
Cap B
Cap D
CGS
GT-V
GT-IV
Elastin
Proteoglycans
Collagen/Gelatin
Cap B
Cap D
CGS
GT-V
GT-IV
MØ-elastase
α1 PI
α2M
MØ
TIMP
Wide spectrum
proteinase
inhibitor
Cytolytic proteinases
TIMP-2

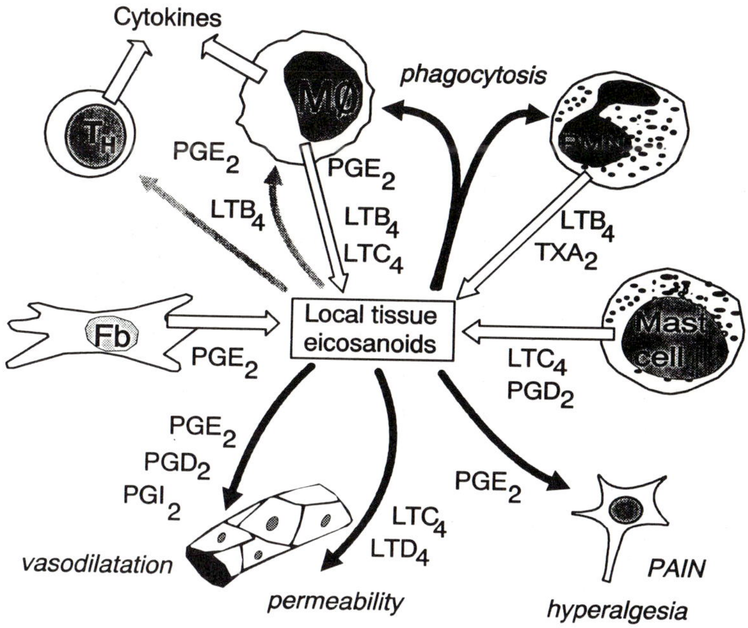

Figure 1.5 The lipid-derived eicosanoids are manufactured from arachidonic acid by a variety of different cells including: macrophages, PMN, mast cells, fibroblasts, eosinophils and endothelial cells. The importance of each cell in terms of eicosanoid production at a site of inflammation is not clear; however, some cells appear better at producing particular eicosanoids than others. Macrophages produce PGE_2, PGI_2, TXA_2, LTB_4 and to a lesser extent LTC_4; PMN produce TXA_2 and LTB_4; fibroblasts and chondrocytes produce PGE_2 and possibly PGI_2 while mast cells produce PGD_2 and LTC_4. Important pro-inflammatory activities of the eicosanoids include: stimulating vasodilatation (PGE_2, PGI_2 and PGD_2), increasing vascular permeability (LTC_4, LTD_4) and stimulating PMN mobility and adhesion (LTB_4). The eicosanoids also exhibit some anti-inflammatory activities; in particular PGE_2 and PGI_2 inhibit cytokine production by macrophages and inhibit T_H cell proliferation and cytokine production. A third property of some eicosanoids (PGE_2) is the ability to mediate pain, hyperalgesia.

Figure 1.4 (*Opposite*) Proteinases are released by many cells resident in or arriving at a site of inflammation. The PMN and the macrophage are important examples of cells which produce a variety of proteinases. In the PMN they are released from different granules including: PMN elastase, cathepsin G (Cap G), cathepsin B (Cap B) and cathepsin D (Cap D) from azurophilic granules (AZG), collagenase (CGS) from specific granules (SPG), and gelatinase type IV and type V (GT-IV, GT-V) from C particles (CP). PMN elastase and Cap G are thought to act as antimicrobial proteinases, while Cap B, Cap D, CGS, GT-IV and GT-V act to facilitate migration of PMN through the tissue. Macrophages produce many of the same proteinases as PMN, Cap B and D, CGS, GT-IV and GT-V. In addition they produce a set of poorly defined proteinases utilized in the cytolytic process. Macrophages also produce a distinct elastase, $M\phi$-elastase. A number of proteinase inhibitors have been described: α_2-macroglobulin (α_2-M) is a wide-spectrum relatively non-specific inhibitor produced by the liver and by macrophages; α_1-proteinase inhibitor (α_1-PI) and α_1-antichymotrypsin (α_1-AC) show more restricted specificity, inhibiting different subsets of serine proteinases, important substrates being PMN-elastase and Cap G respectively. GT-IV and GT-V are inhibited by highly specific, tissue inhibitors of metalloproteinase (TIMP) produced by macrophages and TIMP-2 by other tissue cells.

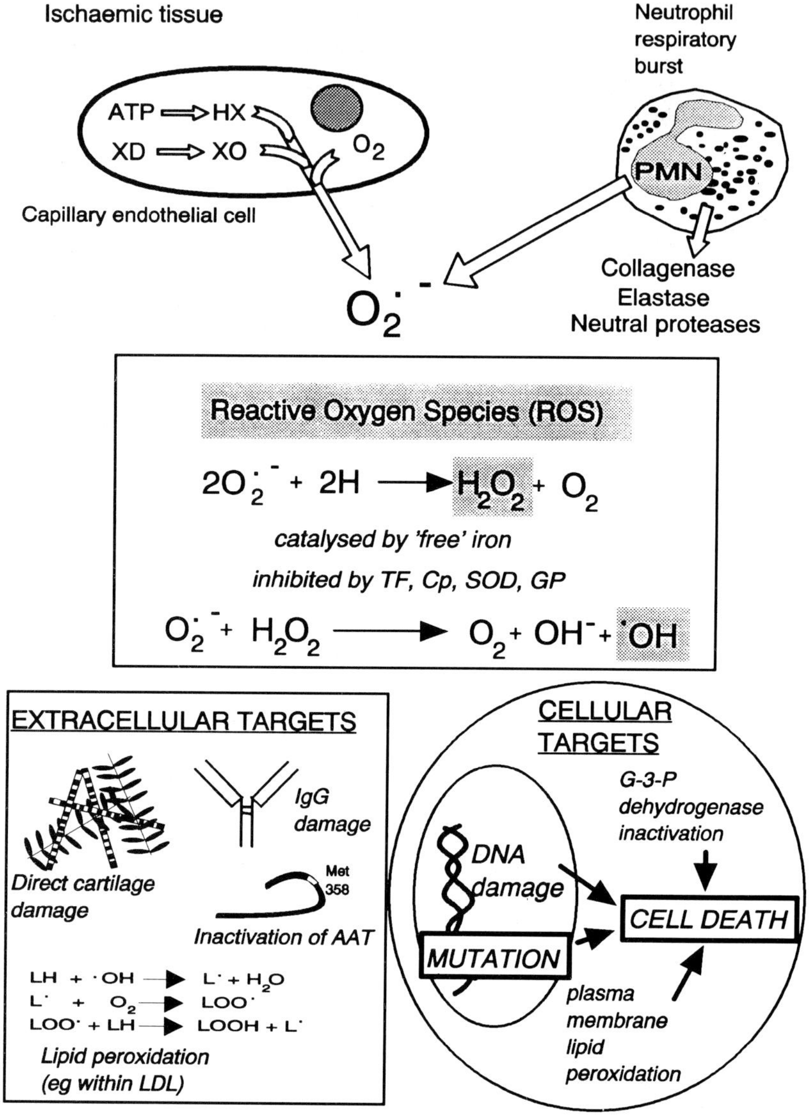

Figure 1.6 Toxic oxygen species are produced by two main pathways: (1) uncoupling of the xanthine dehydrogenase enzyme system in ischaemic tissue (endothelial cells) and (2) the linked NADPH oxidase and myeloperoxidase systems (respiratory burst) of PMN. The major toxic oxygen species generated by both pathways is the superoxide anion radical ($O_2^{\cdot -}$). $O_2^{\cdot -}$ is rapidly converted into H_2O_2, a powerful oxidant, and the highly reactive $^{\cdot}OH$ radical. Toxic oxygen species have been shown to act on a number of important cellular and extracellular targets including: glucose-3-phosphate (G-3-P) dehydrogenase, DNA, IgG, α_1-antitrypsin (AAT), cartilage and low-density lipoprotein (LDL).

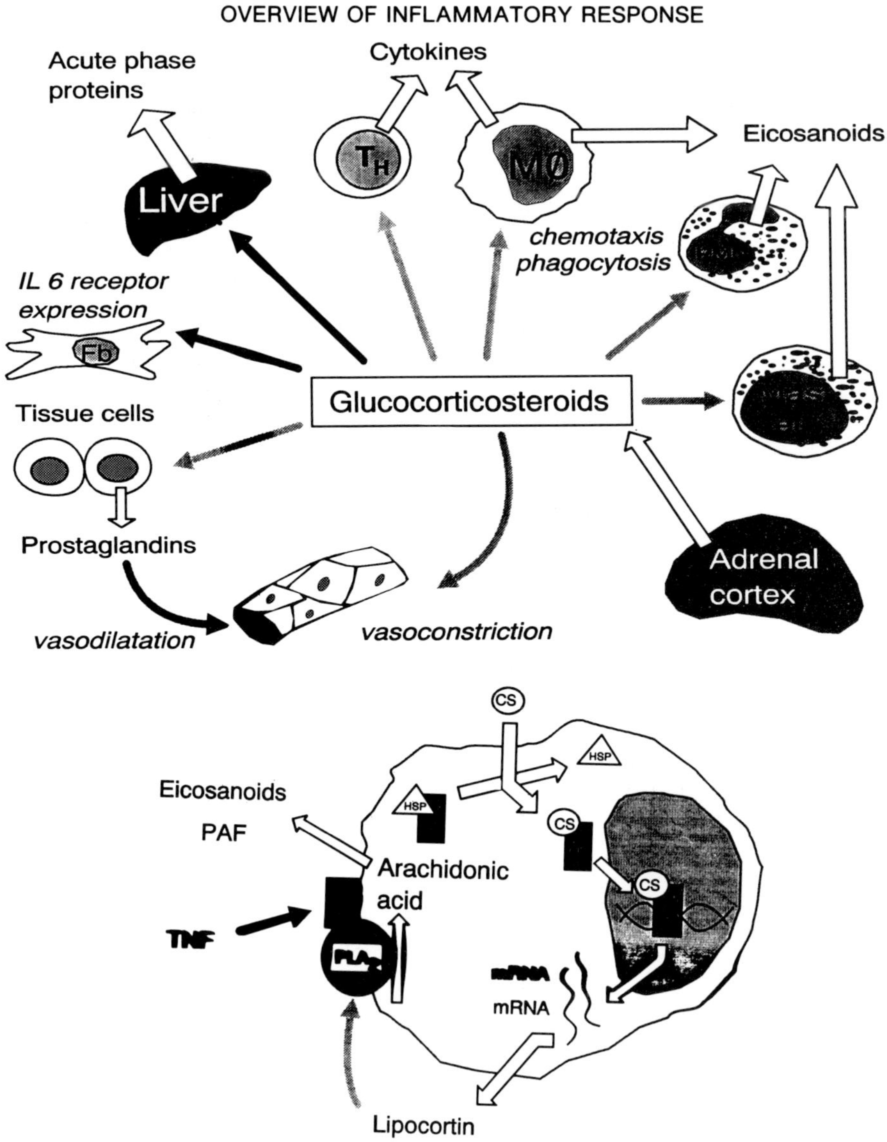

Figure 1.7 (**a**) One of the major responses to trauma is the production by the adrenal cortex of glucocorticosteroids. The actions of glucocorticosteroids are anti-inflammatory and include: (1) inhibition of oedema by stimulating vasoconstriction of small blood vessels and inhibiting the production of vasodilatory prostaglandins; (2) inhibiting the recruitment and activity of PMN, mast cells lymphocytes and monocytes; (3) IL 6 receptor induction on fibroblasts and hepatocytes. (**b**) Glucocorticosteroids (CS) bind to a cytosolic receptor after displacement of the 90 kD heat shock protein (HSP). Receptor bound CS is translocated to the nucleus where it associates with specific regions of DNA inducing the transcription of certain species of mRNA, including that coding for lipocortin, and inhibiting synthesis of others, especially for cytokines. One function of the translated lipocortin is to antagonize the action of TNF by inhibiting phospholipase A_2 (PLA_2) activity inhibiting the production of eicosanoids and platelet activating factor (PAF).

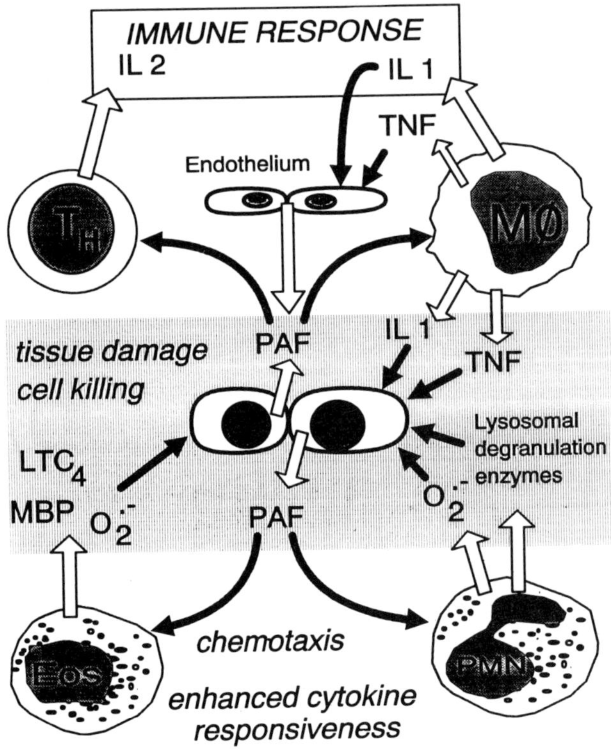

Figure 1.8 Platelet activating factor (PAF) is a phospholipid produced in a variety of cells, especially at the site of an inflammatory reaction, damaged by lysosomal enzymes, toxic oxygen species and the major basic protein (MBP). Endothelial cells and undamaged tissue cells in the vicinity of the inflammation can also be stimulated to release PAF by eicosanoids IL 1 and TNF. In a potential amplification loop PAF itself stimulates the production of IL 1 and TNF by macrophages. Other activities of PAF include activation of eosinophils and PMN enhancing their cytokine responsiveness. PAF may also inhibit or stimulate proliferation and IL 2 production by T lymphocytes.

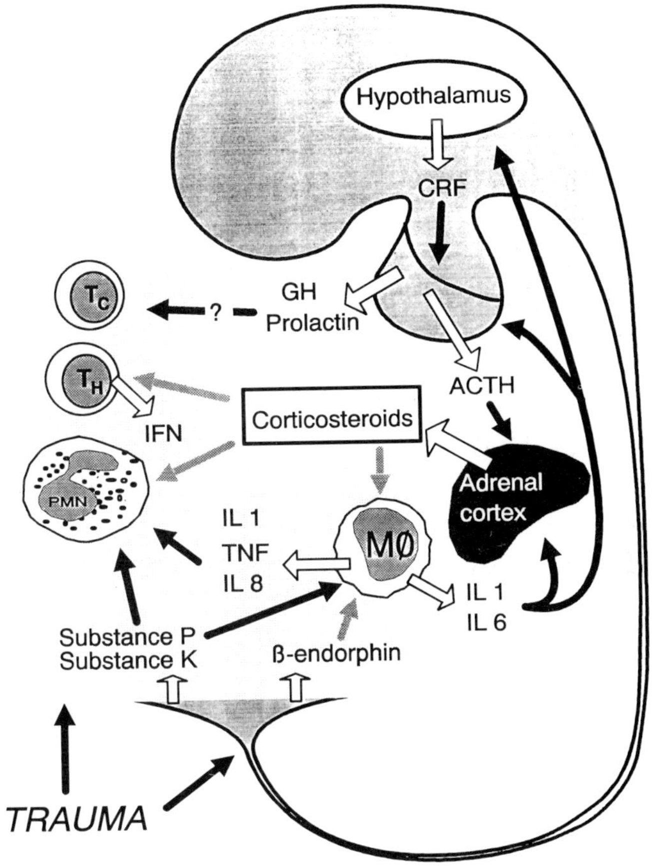

Figure 1.9 Interaction of the neurological, endocrine and immune systems has a potentially important role in the regulation of inflammation. The hypothalamic–pituitary–adrenal axis forms the basis of much of this interaction. Cytokine induction of corticotrophin releasing factor (CRF) by the hypothalamus mediates ACTH release. ACTH, together with cytokines such as IL-1 and IL-6, stimulates corticosteroid release by adrenal cells. Corticosteroids have a major anti-inflammatory action, inhibiting macrophage PMN and lymphocyte function. Other pituitary hormones, such as growth hormone and prolactin, may also have an important role in stimulating T lymphocyte development and differentiation. Peripheral nerves in traumatized tissue release a number of mediators with potential regulatory roles in inflammation. Substance P and substance K appear to be pro-inflammatory, stimulating macrophage and PMN activity. β-Endorphin, on the other hand, appears to act as an anti-inflammatory cytokine, possibly inhibiting macrophage function

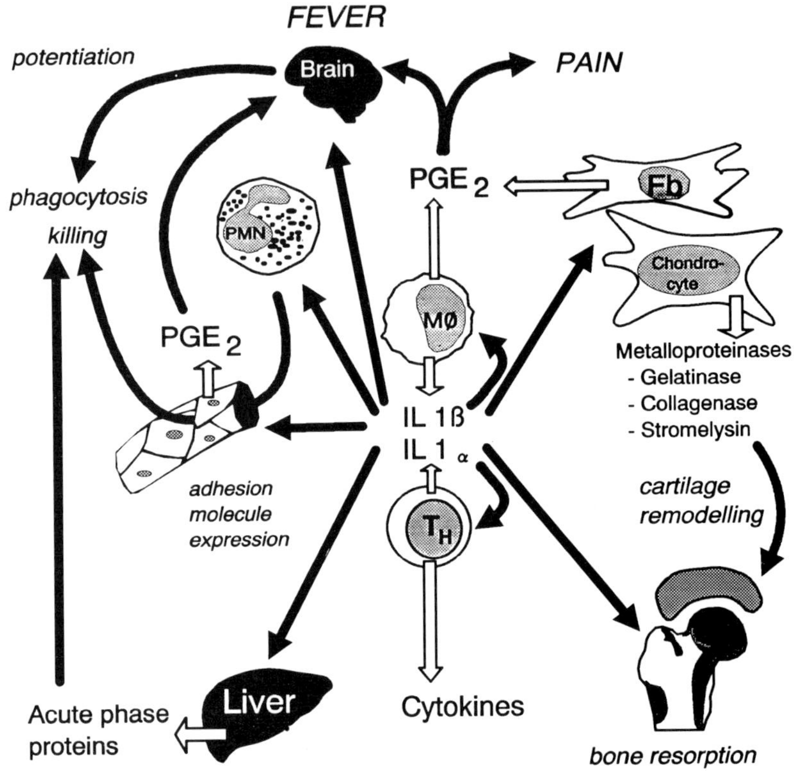

Figure 1.10 IL 1α and IL 1β are distinct molecules which act on the same receptors. Important pro-inflammatory activities of IL 1 include: induction of fever, activation of PMN, activation of epithelial cells leading to increased adhesion molecule expression and eicosanoid synthesis, stimulation of cytokine production by T lymphocytes and production of IL 1 itself, by a variety of cells including monocytes. Other biological activities associated with IL 1 are the stimulation of proteinases by tissue resident macrophages and chondrocytes, the activation of osteoblasts leading to bone resorption, and the induction of acute phase protein synthesis by the liver.

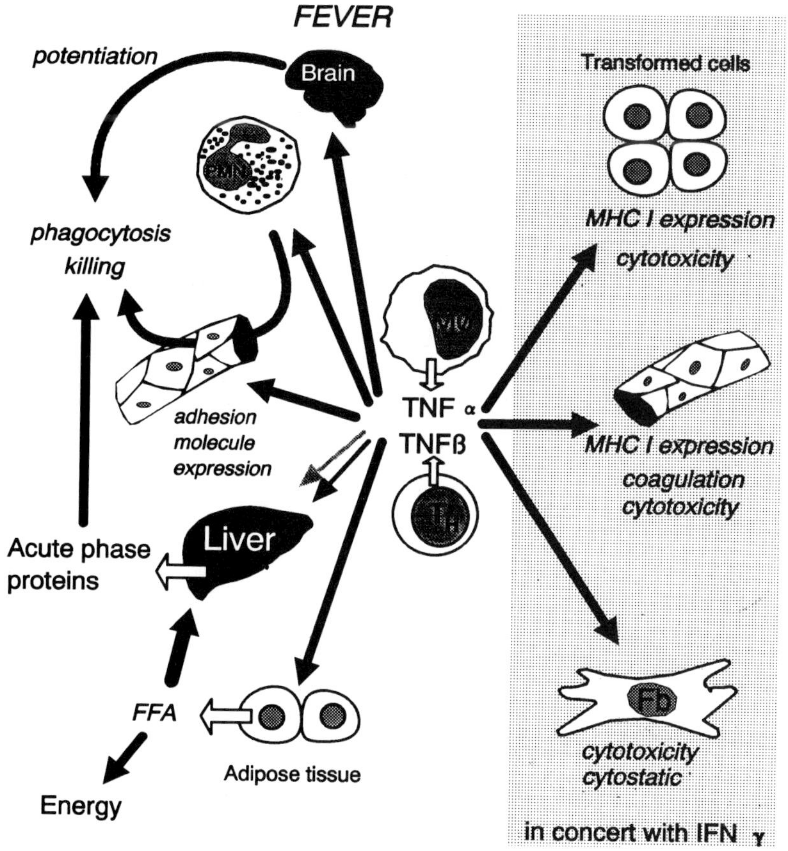

Figure 1.11 TNFα and TNFβ are distinct molecules, preferentially produced by different cells (TNFα by monocytes and TNFβ by lymphocytes) but which, *in vitro* at least, are biologically indistinguishable. Virtually all nucleated eukaryotic cells express receptors for TNF and these cytokines have a wide variety of biological activities *in vitro*; stimulation of acute phase protein synthesis, release of free fatty acids from adipose cells, enhanced expression of endothelial cell and PMN adhesion molecules, activation of PMN. Together with IFNγ, TNF enhances MHC class I antigen expression on a variety of cells, and is also cytotoxic for many cells expressing TNF receptors. *In vivo* TNF has been reported to mediate fever, cachexia and acute phase protein synthesis.

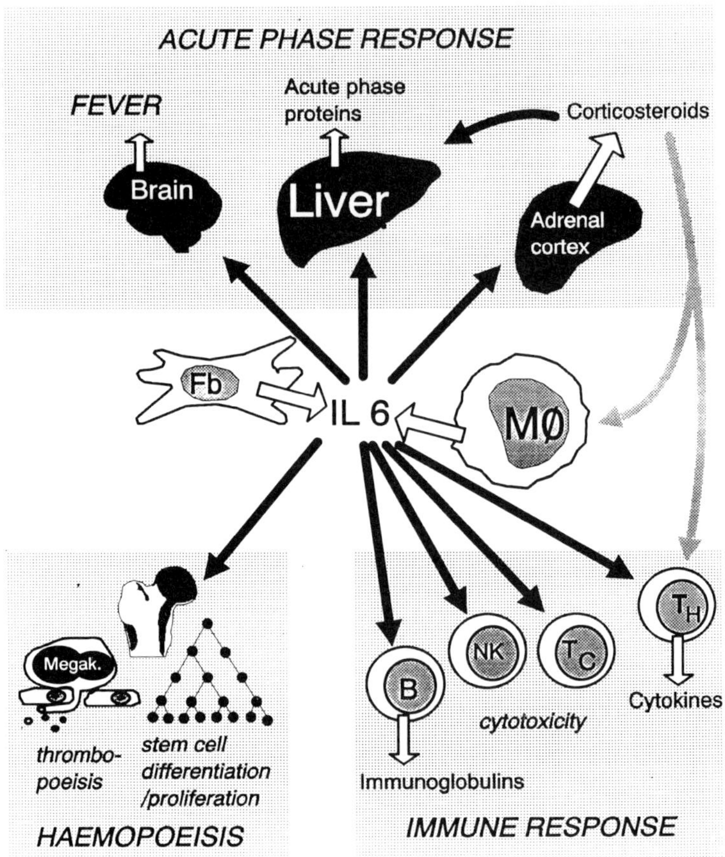

Figure 1.12 Interleukin 6 is a cytokine produced by many different cell types, although macrophages and fibroblasts are major sources of this cytokine. Important biological activities associated with the down-regulation of inflammation mediated by IL 6 include stimulation of acute phase protein synthesis by the liver, glucocorticosteroid release by the adrenal cortex and possibly the induction of fever. IL 6 also acts on the haemopoietic and immune systems. It stimulates thrombopoiesis and stem cell differentiation to replace cells utilized in the inflammatory response and activates lymphocytes to produce effector molecules such as cytokines and immunoglobulins or effector functions such as cytotoxicity.

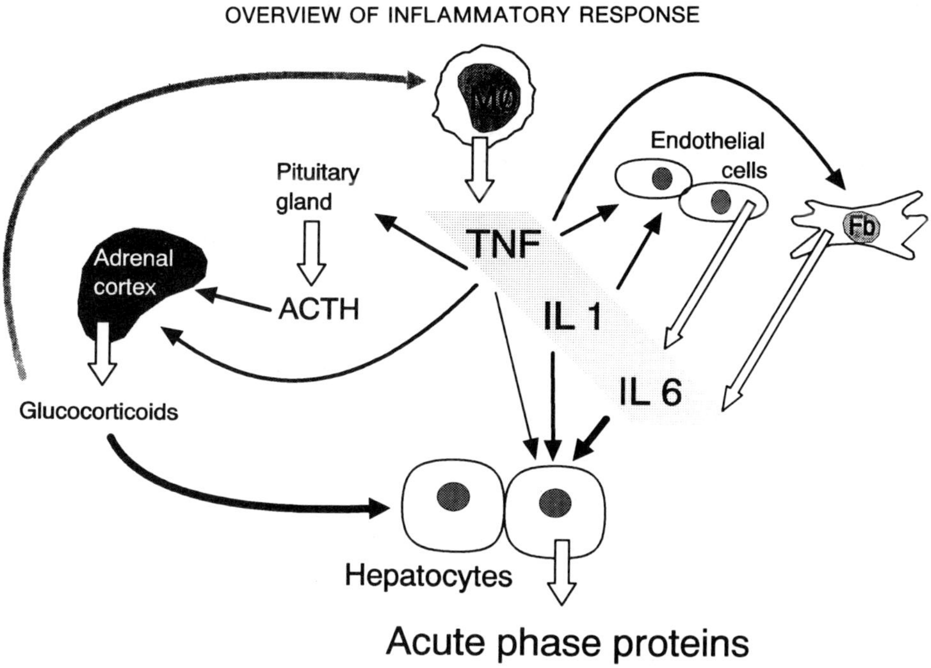

Figure 1.13 The acute phase proteins are a family of liver-derived plasma proteins which function in inflammation as mediators, as inhibitors of mediator pathways, as inhibitors of proteases released from phagocytosing leukocytes and as scavengers of the molecular debris of tissue damage. The response may serve to replenish proteins utilized performing their function in inflammation. A variety of cytokines induce synthesis of these proteins by the hepatocyte. Glucocorticosteroids which may themselves be induced by some of the same cytokines are necessary for maximum synthesis, though they have a negative feedback on cytokine synthesis by the macrophage. Endothelial cells, fibroblasts and macrophages produce the acute phase protein-inducing cytokines which may in some cases potentiate each others' production.

2
The complement system and inflammation

A. R. McPHADEN and K. WHALEY

THE COMPLEMENT SYSTEM

Introduction

The complement system comprises a group of about 20 distinct plasma proteins which have a key role to play in host defence against infection and in helping to mediate inflammation.

Historically the bactericidal activity of the complement system, termed alexin, was observed in the late nineteenth century[1]. Subsequently it became obvious that this bacteriolyis was dependent upon two distinct factors, namely alexin and a second, heat-stable, factor now known to be antibody[2]. At that stage it was thought that alexin itself was a single factor; however, work which took place in the early years of the twentieth century demonstrated that alexin, or complement as it is now called, was not a single plasma protein. Initially four factors were identified[3], but as the complexity of the system unfolded and improved methods of protein purification and fractionation became available and all 20 components have now been isolated and characterized[4]. These proteins can be divided into four main groups, namely the classical pathway components, the alternative pathway components, the terminal components and the control proteins (Table 2.1). The reaction mechanisms that occur between the different components are fairly well understood, although the fine details of certain of the molecular interactions still remain unresolved.

Complement activation

Activation of the complement system occurs in a cascade fashion similar to that observed for the coagulation and kinin mediator systems. At several points in the activation sequence an inactive precursor molecule or zymogen is activated, with the zymogen acquiring proteolytic activity specific for its substrate. This substrate is in turn activated ready to carry out its role in the cascade. One of the main consequences of such a cascade system is that stepwise amplification can occur at each activation step, since the newly generated proteolytic enzyme is able to activate a number of substrate molecules. For this reason tight control of the cascade has to be maintained.

The system can be activated by either the classical or alternative pathways. Classical pathway activation usually follows binding of antigen to antibody; however, alternative pathway activation is independent of antibody. The alternative pathway exists in a low-grade activated state which only becomes fully activated in the presence of a suitable activating substance or surface, as will be described later. Phylogenetically the alternative pathway probably represents a more ancient activation pathway which is independent of a specific immune response, namely antibody. In addition, because it is antibody-independent, it is able to react very quickly as a form of host defence.

Activation by either pathway results in the generation of target-cell bound enzymes which cleave and activate C3 and C5 (C3 convertase and C5 convertase respectively). Subsequent formation of the multimolecular membrane attack complex (MAC) from the terminal components C5–9 can then occur. The MAC can act to lyse the target cells or bacteria. In addition a number

Table 2.1 The complement system of proteins

Component	*Serum concentration* (μg/ml)	*Polypeptide chain structure*
Classical pathway		
C1q	250	18 (6 × 3)
C1r	100	1
C1s	80	1
C4	430	3
C2	20	1
Alternative pathway		
B	150	1
D	2	1
P	30	4
C3	1300	2
Terminal sequence		
C3	1300	2
C5	75	2
C6	60	1
C7	60	1
C8	80	3
C9	50	1
Control proteins		
C1 inhibitor	180	1
C4 binding protein	250	6–8
I (C3b/C4b inactivator)	50	2
H (β1H globulin)	300	1
S Protein	150	1
Carboxypeptidase N	?	?

of biologically active peptides not necessary for perpetuating the cascade are released during the activation sequence. A number of these peptides are active as inflammatory mediators and as such will be described later in detail.

Classical pathway

The classical pathway consists of six components, C1, C4, C2, C1 inhibitor (C1inh), C4 binding protein (C4bp) and C3b/C4b inactivator (I) which are necessary for the formation and regulation of the classical pathway C3 convertase C4b2a (Figure 2.1). The initial activation step *in vivo* is the interaction of C1 with antigen–antibody complexes which contain IgM or IgG antibody classes[5]. C1 itself is a calcium-dependent macromolecule comprising three glycoproteins, C1q, C1r and C1s, as two reversibly interacting subunits[6] C1q and $C1r_2s_2$. It is the C1q moiety which interacts with the immunoglobulin Fc region. Multivalent C1q attachment is required for C1q activation, meaning that one cell surface bound molecule of IgM is sufficient for activation, whereas two adjacent molecules of IgG are needed[7]. Immune complex interaction with C1q is not the only mechanism of classical pathway activation. A number of other substances such as the lipid A moiety

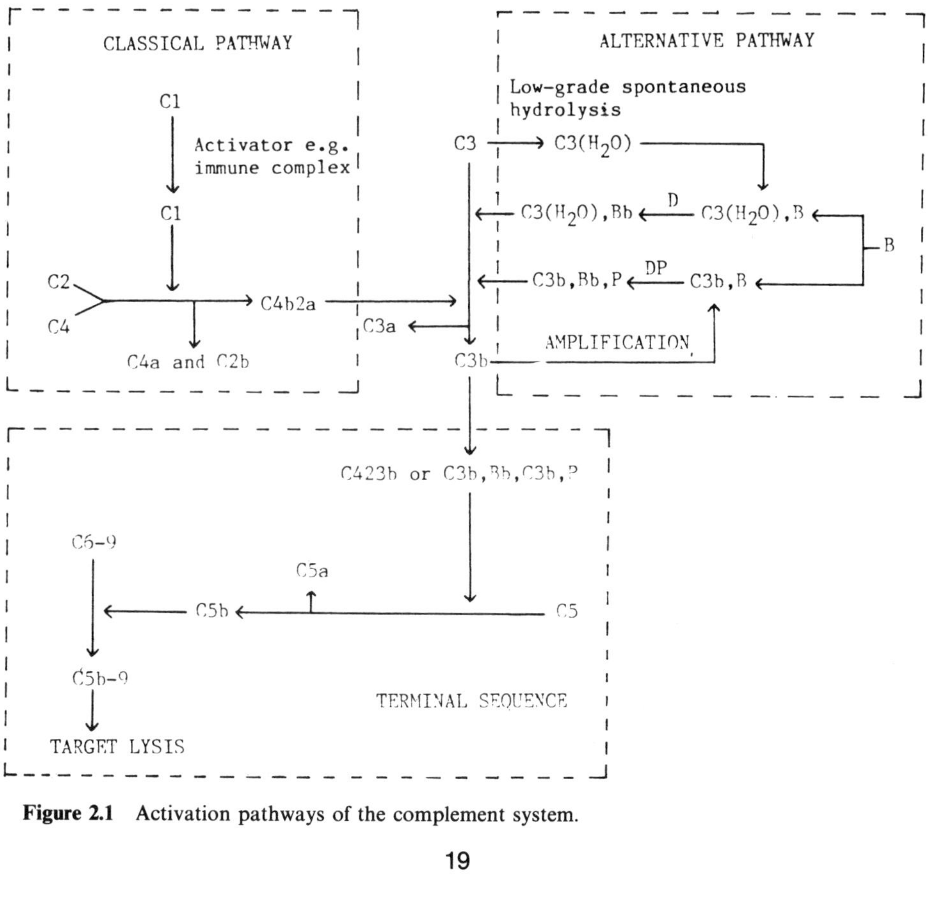

Figure 2.1 Activation pathways of the complement system.

of endotoxin, mitochondrial membranes, certain Gram-negative bacteria and complexes of C-reactive protein with pneumococcal polysaccharide can also produce C1 activation[8]. The relative importance of such activation *in vivo* is, however, unclear.

On binding to an activator of C1 a conformational change occurs in C1q which allows the autocatalytic activation of C1r. C1r produces a single proteolytic cleavage in C1s, its only natural substrate, to generate the active form of C1s[9]. C1s as part of the C1 macromolecule can then carry out proteolytic cleavage and activation of C4 and C2. C4 is cleaved into C4b and C4a with the small peptide C4a being released as one of the anaphylatoxins[10]. Newly generated C4b has two important abilities. Firstly it is able to bind to immune complexes or other acceptor molecules on the surface of activating surfaces, this being a very short-lived ability, and secondly it possesses a stable magnesium ion-dependent binding site for C2 or more specifically the C2b fragment of C2[11]. C2 can therefore become bound to C4b to form the proconvertase C4bC2 which is activated by C1s cleaving C2 into C2a and C2b[12]. Thereafter C2a remains held to C2b only by non-covalent bonding. It is this C2a fragment which possesses the enzymatic site of the classical pathway C3 convertase C4b2a[13,14]. This C3 convertase is, however, inherently unstable, with C2a rapidly decaying off the complex, although it can be reconstituted with fresh cleavage of C2 by C1s[11]. This inherent instability helps prevent the generation of excessive classical pathway C3 convertase activity.

Rigid control of classical pathway activation is largely maintained by C1inh, C4bp and I. Activated C1 has a half-life of only 13 seconds, since C1 inhibitor covalently binds to the C1s moiety of C1 abrogating its enzymatic activity and so preventing C1 cleavage of C4 and C2[15]. C1 inhibitor also interacts with activated C1r leading to the release of two molecules of C1r C1s $(C1inh)_2$ from the activated C1 complex[16,17]. C4bp and I control the availability of C4b and so control assembly of the classical pathway C3 convertase C4b2a. I achieves this by degrading C4b in the presence of its co-factor C4bp[18]. Spontaneous decay/dissociation of C4b2a also appears to be enhanced by C4bp[19].

Alternative pathway

Six components, namely C3, factor B (B), factor D (D), properdin (P), β1H globulin (H) and I are involved in the initiation, generation and maintenance of the alternative pathway C3 and C5 convertases C3bBbP and C3bBbC3bP respectively. The activation mechanisms are complex and are summarized in Figure 2.1.

Initiation occurs through low-grade hydrolysis of fluid phase C3 to give $C3(H_2O)$[20]. In the presence of magnesium ions $C3(H_2O)$ can bind B which is then cleaved by D which is normally present in plasma in its activated form. Ba is released leaving $C3(H_2O)Bb$ as the initial C3 convertase[21]. This convertase is, however, confined to the fluid phase and has only a weak C3 cleaving activity. The initial C3 convertase now functions to cleave C3 into C3a, an anaphylatoxin, and metastable C3b, the latter being deposited on and covalently binding to the surfaces of surrounding particles[22]. The

C3b-dependent positive feedback or amplification loop can now operate (Figure 2.1) since each newly generated C3b molecule has the potential to form the more efficient C3 convertase C3bBb in the presence of B, D and magnesium ions, both in the fluid phase and on the surface of nearby particles. Properdin has a stabilizing effect on C3bBb since it retards the decay of Bb from C3bBb and hence prolongs the half-life of the alternative pathway C3 convertase[23].

Control of alternative pathway amplification is carried out by H and I both in the fluid phase and on non-activating surfaces. I in the presence of H as a co-factor degrades C3b to iC3b which can no longer bind B to generate the C3 convertase[18]. In addition H alone acts both to restrict the formation of, and also to accelerate the rate of decay of, C3bBb[24]. It is worth mentioning at this point that certain widely distributed cell-associated proteins serve a regulatory role. Decay acceleration factor (DAF), membrane co-factor protein (MCP) and complement receptor type 1 (CR1) are thought to be important[25]. DAF prevents C3 convertase assembly and mediates convertase dissociation, an effect which is also observed for the classical pathway C3 convertase. MCP has co-factor activity for I-mediated degradation of C3b to iC3b. CR1 has both DAF and MCP activity.

Overall it is thought that prevention of C3b deposition on host cells by the actions of these proteins stops damage occurring to host tissues during episodes of complement activation[25]. This tight regulation of alternative pathway activation is certainly valid for fluid phase and non-activating surfaces. However, substances which activate the alternative pathway do so through the fact that their surfaces provide a sanctuary for the C3b generated by C3(H_2O)Bb. This surface bound C3b is protected from the control proteins H and I but is still able to bind B and P to form C3bBbP[26,27]. Alternative pathway activators therefore allow a shift from low-grade fluid phase activation to efficient solid phase turnover. Such activators have surfaces which are low in sialic acid[28,29], the net effect of which appears to be to reduce the number of regulatory protein binding sites on C3b without affecting factor B binding sites[30].

Terminal sequence

The common pathway that leads to completion of the complement activation cascade irrespective of whether initial activation occurs via the classical or alternative pathways is the terminal sequence (Figure 2.1). One molecule of C5, C6, C7 and C8 plus up to 18 C9 molecules constitute the terminal sequence proteins whose highly ordered interactions result in the formation of the membrane attack complex (MAC) C5b–9. When assembled this macromolecular complex has a hydrophobic outer layer which allows insertion into biological membranes and a hydrophilic core that creates a transmembrane channel through which water and ions can pass. Insertion of sufficient numbers of MACs into a target cell membrane can therefore lead to the membrane becoming 'leaky' with resulting osmotic lysis and target cell death. The terminal sequence represents a mechanism by which the complement system can mediate cell injury or lyse susceptible bacteria.

Activation of the terminal sequence follows formation of C5 convertase activity. This is dependent upon covalent binding of C3b immediately adjacent to the cell surface or activating surface bound classical and alternative pathway C3 convertases C4b2a and C3bBb respectively[31]. Each of the C5 convertases is therefore designated C4b2a3b and C3bBbC3b. This newly bound C3b acts as a binding site for native C5 and renders it susceptible to cleavage into C5a and C5b by the C2a or Bb moiety of each convertase. Each C3 convertase therefore generates the C3b necessary to convert its specificity to a C5 convertase.

Assembly of the membrane attack complex follows C5 cleavage. C5a, the third anaphylatoxin, is released leaving C5b which has a metastable binding site for C6. Bimolecular C5b6 remains loosely bound to C3b on the target cell surface until interaction with C7 occurs, at which time the C5b67 complex undergoes a hydrophilic–amphiphilic transition and binds to lipid membranes in its immediate vicinity[32]. The lipid membranes may belong to nucleated cells, erythrocytes, bacteria or viruses and the insertion event commits MAC assembly to a specific site. The inserted C5b67 now acts as a membrane-bound C8 'receptor', C8 binds and the C5b–8 complex penetrates deeper into the hydrophobic bilayer creating a 30 Å diameter transmembrane channel[33]. Subsequent binding of C9 occurs, initially as a single C9 molecule; however, as increasing numbers are incorporated (C9 polymerization) the channel structure increases its size up to a 100 Å diameter pore in the membrane[34,35]. Significant water and ion fluxes can then occur with possible lysis of the target[36]. Not surprisingly inhibitors of MAC channel formation exist as a defence measure against bystander host cell lysis at sites of complement activation. Plasma S protein and very low-density lipoprotein (VLDL) inhibit the binding of C5b–7 complexes to membranes[37]. In addition S protein prevents C9 polymerization[38]. Two widely distributed plasma membrane-associated C8 and C9 binding glycoproteins also exist and act to inhibit MAC-mediated pore formation[39,40]. Their importance is demonstrated by the fact that deficiency states can lead to inappropriate red cell lysis and the disease paroxysmal nocturnal haemoglobinuria[41]. There will be further discussion of the role of these proteins, later in this chapter.

Complement biosynthesis

Brief mention will be made of this topic in order to highlight features relevant to a discussion of complement and inflammation. Two main cell types appear to be responsible for the synthesis of the vast majority of the complement components in most animals including humans, namely hepatocytes and mononuclear phagocytes (monocytes, macrophages and Kupffer cells)[42]. The hepatocyte is responsible for maintaining the plasma levels of most components, as shown by studies in those patients who have undergone orthotopic liver transplantation and a change in component allotype[43,44]. As such the liver is therefore the largest producer of complement proteins in the body. Mononuclear phagocytes, however, also have a very important role to play. They are present in virtually all tissues where they act as a local source of components[45,46]. In the tissues the concentration of complement components is likely to be relatively low compared with plasma, so local synthesis is essential to the host in order to ensure that the vital role played by complement in mediating early host defence, including mounting an effective inflammatory response, is maintained[47]. *In vivo* confirmation of this is provided by studies of patients with rheumatoid arthritis, where it has been shown that up to 50% of the C3 in inflamed joints is synthesized locally[48]. Also of importance is the fact that recruitment of substantial numbers of mononuclear phagocytes into the tissues can occur fairly rapidly, so markedly increasing local complement component biosynthetic capacity when needed for the maintenance of effective host defences at that site. Further overall biosynthetic versatility results from the fact that both hepatocyte and mononuclear phagocyte complement production can be up-regulated or down-regulated depending on the stimulus. Indeed the production of individual components can be differentially modulated by a single stimulus. Experimentally these stimuli have been shown to include gamma-interferon, immune complexes, prostaglandin E_2, the anaphylatoxins and interleukin 1, all agents which are often found in inflammatory exudates. Overall the maintenance of an appropriate supply of complement components to the tissues is assured, thereby allowing the host to cope with the wide spectrum of physiological and potentially pathological events encountered *in vivo*.

A rapid and marked increase in plasma C3 concentration by up to 50% is seen as a response to a number of stimuli such as infection by bacteria, viruses or parasites, chemical or physical insult, radiation or neoplasia. C3 is therefore included among a group of plasma proteins collectively called the acute phase reactants (APRs)[49]. Also included are C-reactive protein, fibrinogen, alpha-1-antitrypsin, alpha-2-macroglobulin and serum amyloid A protein, all of which increase by variable amounts under the influence of identical stimuli to those described for C3. The biological functions of these APRs are varied, but overall their actions appear to be directed towards the modulation of the inflammatory response, limiting tissue damage and possibly promoting the restoration of tissue homeostasis after inflammatory and immune reactions.

In the foregoing description the main emphasis was placed on describing the individual components, their activation and their subsequent role in generating and maintaining the macromolecular enzymes which are essential to the complement activation cascade. At a number of the activation steps small peptides or fragments such as the anaphylatoxins C4a, C3a and C5a are released. It is these peptides which are now known to be central to the contribution that the complement system makes to the inflammatory response. The remainder of this chapter is therefore devoted to a detailed description of this contribution.

THE COMPLEMENT SYSTEM AND INFLAMMATION

Introduction

The role of the complement system as an inflammatory mediator is complex, with a number of the interactions at a biochemical level being as yet only partly understood. Despite this there are defined areas in which the complement system makes a significant contribution as follows: (1) increasing blood vessel permeability; (2) producing vasodilatation; (3) promoting oedema formation; (4) increasing neutrophil adhesiveness; (5) stimulating inflammatory cell chemotaxis; (6) inducing release of toxic oxygen species and lysosomal enzymes from phagocytic cells; (7) MAC-induced ion fluxes and inflammation.

As each of these effects is described in detail below it will become apparent that no unique single biological event is produced by a particular complement component or peptide fragment. A fair degree of overlap exists, with the relative potency of producing a certain effect often being the important observation. This reflects the fact that the inflammatory response is not a set of individual, temporally well-defined events, rather it is a complex interplay of changes whose occurrence can be simultaneous and whose separation into a set of separate events is often inappropriate. In this chapter such a division will be made for ease of description; however, the simultaneous and sometimes mutually interdependent nature of a number of the changes will become obvious. It is important to remember at this point that although the complement system is one of the most potent mediator systems *in vivo* that promotes and perpetuates inflammation, it is not the only one. Discussion of the other systems such as the kinin system, cyclooxygenase/lipoxygenase products and the coagulation system is outwith the scope of this chapter; however, where important interactions exist these will be mentioned.

Vascular changes

It is convenient to group together blood vessel permeability, vasodilatation and oedema formation under the heading of vascular changes. The main complement peptides which mediate these changes are the anaphylatoxins C4a, C3a and C5a. In Figure 2.1 it can be seen that these represent cleavage products of C4, C3 and C5 respectively. They do not form part of the activation cascade convertases but are released into the fluid phase to mediate other effector functions.

Experimentally it was initially shown that C4a, C3a and C5a can increase vascular permeability with C5a being the most potent and C4a the least effective[50]. Mediation of this effect appeared to be through the binding of these peptides to specific surface receptors on mast cells which thus stimulated released histamine, the histamine then producing much of the increase in vascular permeability[51]. Evidence is now accumulating, however, indicating that this is an oversimplification, and that the vascular changes occurring at sites of complement-induced inflammation have a more complex pathogenesis. Histamine-dependent mechanisms may make a more significant contribution to the immediate and often shorter-lived vascular alterations seen following mild physical trauma or in classical type I hypersensitivity reactions, but this does not seem to be the case for the more prolonged vascular responses in many complement-induced inflammatory situations[52]. It is now recognized that increased vascular permeability and vasodilatation are two separately controlled components of the inflammatory response with synergism being needed between them to produce significant and prolonged tissue oedema[53,54]. Experiments using intradermal injection of C5a as the inflammatory challenge, and producing a classical wheal-and-flare reaction, have shown that often within as little as 2 minutes of its administration there is an increased adherence of neutrophils to the endothelium of small blood vessels in the area of the C5a injection site. This accumulation of neutrophils seems to be a pivotal occurrence for subsequent alterations in blood vessel permeability, vasodilatation and oedema formation[55]. It is proposed that the neutrophils induce increased blood vessel permeability by direct production of, as yet, poorly defined 'permeability factors', or else induce the endothelial cells to which they are attached to elicit such factors[56]; leukotrienes, D series prostaglandins and toxic oxygen radicals have all been implicated. Vasodilatation appears to be mediated by prostaglandins which are produced by the neutrophils or endothelial cells with prostaglandin E_2 being one of the best characterized and studied. Induction of vasodilatation alone by the administration of prostaglandin E_2 is insufficient to produce tissue oedema[53]; neutrophil margination and vessel permeability alterations are essential. Support for the central role played by the neutrophil in regulating the inflammatory vascular changes was obtained by studying patients with neutropenia due to bone marrow failure[56]. These patients have a very much reduced vascular response to an inflammatory challenge with C5a, a response which virtually returned to normal when an infusion of neutrophils was given. In these same individuals mast cell degranulation and histamine release are normal, so underlining the relatively minor role that histamine plays in this form of complement induced inflammation. Indeed in normal individuals challenged with C5a, antihistamines have little effect in abrogating the vascular inflammatory reactions that occur. The use of prostaglandin synthetase and lipoxygenase inhibitors supports a role for prostaglandins as chemical mediators of complement-induced vascular responses; however, uncertainty still exists regarding their exact sites of action and relative potency. Certain leukotrienes such as B4 may also have a role to play in helping to mediate neutrophil adherence to endothelial cells, although this is, as yet, rather less well defined[57].

In most of the experimental systems used to study the inflammatory reactions induced by C5a very low doses of around 1 ng of C5a were effective at producing a marked response[58]. This amount is thought to be physiologically attainable at sites of complement activation, and therefore gains *in vivo* credibility. Furthermore, repeated exposure to it appeared not to produce significant desensitization. The relative effectiveness of C3a and particularly C4a need greater study before their *in vivo* contribution can be better assessed.

At this stage mention has to be made of the specific degradation that the anaphylatoxins undergo *in vivo*. They are all acted upon by plasma carboxypeptidase N[59], originally called anaphylatoxin inactivator, which removes the C-terminal arginine residue from each of them, giving C4 des-Arg, C3a des-Arg and C5a des-Arg[60]. The relevance of this event is that it proceeds very rapidly to completion, particularly for C3a, with the newly generated des-Arg products actually mediating the *in vivo* biological effects[61]. It is now widely accepted that the des-Arg derivatives of all the anaphylatoxins produce no histamine release from mast cells[60]. When injected into the skin, however, they trigger an inflammatory wheal-and-flare reaction, macroscopically and microscopically indistinguishable from the one caused by the native anaphylatoxin[58]. This evidence therefore lends further support to the fact that histamine has little role to play in anaphylatoxin-induced inflammatory reactions *in vivo*. Attention will be drawn where relevant to important differences in the degree of biological effectiveness of des-Arg products in subsequent sections of this chapter.

Neutrophil adhesiveness

As described earlier, the neutrophil is now considered to play a crucial role in achieving an optimal vascular inflammatory response, a vital prerequisite for which is adhesion to vascular endothelium at sites of developing inflammation. The concept of modulation of neutrophil adhesiveness therefore becomes a critical issue. *In vitro* studies using purified C5a showed that binding to the neutrophil C5a receptor promotes the ability of neutrophils to bind to endothelial cells but not to smooth muscle cells or fibroblasts[62]. Both C5a and C5a des-Arg seem equipotent in this respect. In addition, neutrophil aggregation and up-regulation of cell surface C3 receptor numbers is induced[63,64]. The relevance of the latter finding to adhesiveness becomes obvious when it is realized that certain neutrophil surface adhesion molecules called MAC1 and p150, 95 appear to be identical to CR3 and CR4 respectively, both of which are types of neutrophil cell surface C3 receptors whose production is enhanced by C5a/C5a des-Arg[64,65]. No alterations in endothelial 'stickiness' have been detected after exposure to C5a or C5a des-Arg. The situation is now created whereby complement-induced changes have promoted neutrophil margination so facilitating subsequent vasodilatation as described above. Vascular stasis resultant upon vasodilatation will then encourage neutrophil aggregation and further margination; a positive feedback situation has been created.

Chemotaxis

One of the best-known biological and pro-inflammatory activities mediated by the complement system is chemotaxis. Measurable chemotactic responses are seen for neutrophils, basophils, eosinophils and monocytes with C5a being the most potent chemotactic agent[66,67]. In experimental systems C5a is up to 1000 times more potent than C3a, with C4a being less active than C3a[61]. *In vitro* comparisons of C5a versus C5a des-Arg chemotactic activity for neutrophils have shown on average a 10-fold greater potency in favour of C5a. Doubt exists, however, as to whether this is a genuine reflection of the situation *in vivo*. Evidence exists suggesting that C5a des-Arg may be at least as chemotactically active *in vivo* as C5a[68]. In the rabbit it has been shown that aerosol administration of human C5a des-Arg produces a more marked intrapulmonary accumulation of neutrophils compared with an equal dose of C5a. Since C5a des-Arg is the predominant species present *in vivo*, due to the action of carboxypeptidase N, this potency of action compared with the *in vitro* situation is not totally unexpected. Possible origins for the *in vitro/in vivo* discrepancy may be as follows:

1. Evidence exists for there being a greater resistance of C5a des-Arg compared with C5a to further proteolytic degradation[61]. The des-Arg species therefore displays enhanced biological availability and effect in an *in vivo* model where the route of administration, such as by aerosol, limits carboxypeptidase N access to the C5a.
2. More importantly, the full expression of human C5a des-Arg chemotactic activity requires the presence of a plasma co-factor or co-chemotaxin, a factor which is not necessary for C5a to achieve its full potential[69].

In vitro experimentation may therefore be an inaccurate representation of the *in vivo* situation should it be deficient in this co-factor if, for example, the culture conditions lack serum or contain too low a serum concentration. Inclusion of whole serum at an optimal concentration for *in vitro* chemotactic assay mixes is now part of most standard experimental protocols. The proposed mechanism of action of the co-factor is interesting. Human C5a and C5a des-Arg have an oligosaccharide moiety attached to them. The plasma co-factor has strong carbohydrate binding properties so it is thought that the co-factor is acting to overcome any possible inhibitory steric or charge effects caused by the oligosaccharide during receptor binding by the C5a des-Arg[70]. Native C5a, however, binds so avidly to its receptor that the oligosaccharide moiety has little inhibitory effect and a co-factor is therefore unnecessary. Comparison with porcine C5a des-Arg which lacks the oligosaccharide unit shows that no co-factor is required for it to elicit a chemotactic response. Indeed it has been shown that removal of the carbohydrate from human C5a des-Arg increases its chemotactic activity markedly. No similar increase is seen for C5a following identical treatment.

The importance of C5a and C5a des-Arg as potent inflammatory mediators is emphasized by a recent study from the field of microbiology. It showed that group B streptococci, when present in the tissues of a host, produced a minimal acute inflammatory reaction and little in the way of neutrophil accumulation. This phenomenon seems to be due to the fact that this group of streptococci produce a specific enzyme which degrades C5a and C5a des-Arg, thereby abrogating their biological actions[71]. For the bacterial species it represents a virulence factor; for the complementologist it demonstrates the important role C5a and C5a des-Arg play in the inflammatory response. Group A streptococci appear to produce a not-dissimilar factor.

As stated above, mononuclear phagocytes, namely monocytes and macrophages, are chemotactically responsive to the anaphylatoxins. For macrophages it appears that the degree of responsiveness is closely tied in with their tissue of origin. This is demonstrated by the fact that alveolar-derived macrophages are poorly responsive to C5a whereas peritoneal macrophages are very responsive[61]. The cellular mechanism operating to create this differential reactivity is unclear; however, it may reflect important differences in expected function of the two cell populations. Monocytes, the precursors of tissue macrophages, seem uniformly chemotactically responsive, indicating that the programming occurs after arrival at the 'end-organ'.

Chemotaxis *in vivo* involves the directed migration of cells into the tissues from the intravascular compartment. Maintenance of a good supply of these cells is therefore of vital importance, and complement-derived peptides appear to have a role to play for neutrophils in this capacity. These peptides are derived from C3, namely C3e and C3d-K[72,73]. They both induce a leukocytosis by causing the release of neutrophils from the bone marrow into the peripheral blood ready for use at sites of inflammation. The exact molecular mechanisms which govern the neutrophil release are, however, unclear.

Toxic oxygen radical and lysosomal enzyme release from phagocytic cells

It is thought that a significant pro-inflammatory contribution may be made by neutrophils releasing toxic oxygen radicals and lysosomal enzymes into their immediate environment. *In vitro* and *in vivo* studies of the former have shown that a number of biological stimuli, including C5a treatment of neutrophils, induce the production and release of significant amounts of the toxic oxygen species superoxide anion and hydrogen peroxide[74]. Thereafter, despite defence measures in the form of the enzymes superoxide dismutase and catalase, damage particularly to endothelial cells can occur with resulting increased permeability and leakage of a protein-rich oedema fluid[75]. These oxygen species may therefore represent one of the neutrophil-derived permeability factors mentioned earlier. More work is required before the importance of their contribution is fully understood.

At sites of inflammation the release of lysosomal enzymes by phagocytic cells probably directly contributes to the tissue damage which occurs[76]. In addition to this lysosomal enzymes are also known to be able to activate C1 and factor B *in vitro*, so potentially increasing the level of complement activation. Again a positive feedback loop could operate; it is not known, however, if this actually occurs *in vivo*. The enzyme release is stimulated by C5a, C5a des-Arg, C3e and by crosslinking of CR1 (complement receptor type 1) on the surface of phagocytic cells[77–79]. This crosslinking is likely at sites of complement activation where C3b becomes bound to the activating surface such as microorganisms and antigen–antibody complexes, and is then able to crosslink the CR1 receptors. Interestingly, recent work has shown that not all immune complexes with incorporated C3b are equally effective at inducing enzyme release. Complexes containing IgG induce lysosomal enzyme release from neutrophils; however, IgM-containing complexes produce only a very small effect[80].

Membrane attack complex involvement in inflammation

It was formerly thought that the vast majority of complement system-derived pro-inflammatory mediation was through the actions of the anaphylatoxins and C3b, as described in the preceding pages. Recent work has shown, however, that the membrane attack complex C5b–9 may have a role to play in certain situations. Seeger *et al.*, in a rabbit model of complement-induced inflammatory lung disease, showed that terminal complement activation in the lungs led to local prostanoid generation and an increase in permeability of the small pulmonary blood vessels[81]. They suggested that MAC formation in cell membranes at the site of complement activation led to calcium ion influx through the transmembrane pore that was formed. This ion influx then triggered the arachidonate cascade. Inhibition of these biological effects by calcium ion antagonists helped to support this theory. Care must be taken when interpreting these results, since it may represent a species-specific reaction. Confirmation in other animal models is required.

Also of relevance to MAC-mediated events that can occur at inflammatory sites is the platelet release reaction. It has been shown that treating platelets with C5b–9 leads to alpha granule and dense body release reactions[82]. In addition the platelets release microvesicles which are coated with C5b–9 and which have membrane receptor sites for coagulation factor Va. Again calcium ion influx with secondary activation of platelet protein kinases is thought to be responsible for the C5b–9 effects. Overall, therefore, C5b–9 is generating platelet-derived pro-coagulant activity, and is possibly helping to explain why activation of the coagulation system is a not-uncommon accompaniment of certain acute inflammatory states.

Human neutrophils also show the phenomenon of microvesicle shedding. It has been shown that when treated with purified MACs these cells protect themselves by aggregating the MACs then releasing them on the surface of microvesicles[83]. In addition, a degree of specific MAC protein degradation by the neutrophil has been observbed.

Overall, therefore, terminal sequence activation with MAC formation and membrane insertion can represent a lethal cell lytic event, or else may result in specific alterations of cell function, some of which appear to be pro-inflammatory. The *in vivo* MAC control measures described above, and the C8 and C9 binding glycoproteins mentioned earlier, act to ensure the maintenance of a balanced state by not only minimizing potentially damaging bystander cell lysis but at the same time facilitating the more biologically beneficial effects. It is likely that this subtle balance will be disrupted in certain disease states or during episodes of intense complement activation such that important, sometimes detrimental, effects on the host will result.

THE COMPLEMENT SYSTEM AND DISEASE

The complement system is now known to play an important role in the pathogenesis of a number of human diseases. Many of these diseases have a prominent inflammatory component, the creation of which is often strongly associated with complement activation. Immune complex diseases, certain complement deficiency syndromes and the adult respiratory distress syndrome (ARDS) will be examined in turn to illustrate this concept.

Complement and immune complex disease

Antigen–antibody complexes or immune complexes are constantly being formed in the body as the end-result of the specific humoral immune response. In most situations their formation produces no detrimental effects on the host, and indeed is often beneficial in that it 'neutralizes' the antigen. It is now widely accepted, however, that the deposition or formation of immune complexes in the tissues can be associated with tissue damage and immune complex disease in certain situations[84]. Complement can play a major role in the generation of such diseases by virtue of the fact that the complexes, once formed, cause activation of the system with resultant inflammation and oedema formation as described in the preceding pages. Human diseases where this mechanism occurs include:

1. Extrinsic allergic alveolitis where acute respiratory problems and even respiratory failure follows inhalation of an antigen in a presensitized host. Good examples of this condition include farmer's lung, pigeon-fancier's lung or mushroom-picker's lung.
2. Rheumatoid arthritis, where a marked inflammatory reaction occurs in the synovial lining of many joints due to the formation of antigen–antibody complexes at these sites.
3. The Jarisch–Herxheimer reaction which follows penicillin treatment of syphilitics who have high specific antibody levels. The resultant antigen release from the killed causative treponemes allows marked antigen–antibody interaction.
4. Glomerulonephritis, where in certain types there seems to be intraglomerular formation or trapping of antigen–antibody complexes with resultant glomerular inflammation, dysfunction and renal impairment.

Interestingly, the result of complement activation by immune complexes *in vivo* is not purely detrimental to the host. In addition to significantly contributing to the pathogenesis of the disease states described above, complement activation can also have an important protective role to play. It is now known that complement activation acts to prevent both the formation and persistence of large insoluble immune complexes in the circulation and tissues. These actions, which are principally mediated by the classical pathway and alternative pathway respectively, help to prevent the development of, and reduce the severity of, the injurious effects of immune complexes in the tissues. Complement activation can therefore have divergent or differing effects with the exact outcome being dependent upon the nature of the immune complex, its location, the rate of formation and the degree and type of complement activation produced. Much work is required before it will be possible to predict and hopefully modulate the biological consequences of the presence of immune complexes in certain disease states.

Inherited complement deficiency syndromes and disease

Inherited human complement deficiency states are not common conditions; however, they provide an informative insight into the important biological functions carried out by, or significantly contributed to by, the complement system *in vivo*. Inherited deficiency states of the majority of the complement components have now been documented with certain shared biological effects and disease states being seen[85]. The commonest clinical abnormalities associated with homozygous genetic deficiency states are: (a) immune complex diseases including glomerulonephritis, various arthritides and systemic lupus erythematosus; and (b) recurrent, sometimes life-threatening infections, particularly respiratory infections and neisserial infections including meningitis. This emphasizes the vital role played by the complement system in ensuring both proper handling of immune complexes by the host as described earlier, and in facilitating opsonization, phagocytosis and lysis of potentially pathogenic bacteria. It is important to remember to test for complement deficiency states in patients with recurrent infections or immune complex diseases when the more common aetiologies have been excluded.

An interesting form of inflammatory reaction is seen in hereditary C1 inhibitor deficiency (hereditary angioedema, HAE)[86]. In this disease there is a genetically determined deficiency or dysfunction of the C1 inhibitor protein due, it is now known, to structural abnormalities in the patient's C1 inhibitor gene. The net effect is to allow excessive activation of C1 and so excessive activation of the classical complement pathway with depletion of C4 and C2. Clinically the patient experiences distressing episodes of acute tissue swelling or oedema affecting particularly the hands, feet, face and gastrointestinal tract. If the larynx is affected then stridor and asphyxiation can result, a mode of death which formerly befell up to one-third of HAE patients before the advent of modern therapy. Microscopic examination of the oedematous tissues shows capillary and venular dilatation with marked extracellular oedema due to increased vascular permeability. A rather surprising finding which is, as yet, poorly understood is an almost complete lack of an acute inflammatory cell infiltrate in the affected tissues. In this disease oedema formation is therefore entirely independent of neutrophil involvement. Defining the chemical mediators responsible for these tissue changes has been difficult and controversial. Initially a peptide, C2-kinin, released from C2 by the action of C1s, was blamed. Opinion, however, changed, with bradykinin becoming the front-runner. New evidence has now brought the investigation full circle with a C2-derived peptide again being favoured[87].

Complement and the adult respiratory distress syndrome (ARDS)

This syndrome is a well-characterized and potentially lethal complication of clinical shock, the initial shocked state being most often due to sepsis, severe trauma or acute pancreatitis[88]. Indeed ARDS is often called 'shock lung'. It has been shown that complement activation with anaphylatoxin generation, particularly C5a/C5a des-Arg, is a critical factor in the development of ARDS[89]. Examination of lungs from patients with the condition reveals microvascular leukostasis and plugging, along with leakage of a protein-rich oedema fluid from the small blood vessels, all changes which have been tied in to the effects of the anaphylatoxins described earlier in this chapter. In animal models complement or neutrophil depletion prevents the development of ARDS, so adding to the evidence that supports an interdependent role for complement and neutrophils in the pathogenesis of this condition. Currently high doses of corticosteroids, if administered early enough, are effective at preventing the development of ARDS in 'at-risk' patients[88]. Their action appears to be due to their ability to significantly reduce neutrophil aggregation and accumulation in the lungs, so abrogating the subseqeunt release of toxic metabolites by these cells therein.

CONCLUSIONS

The inflammatory response is one of the most universal and essential biological responses encountered in most species. The complement system of proteins, in addition to its many other roles, contributes significantly to the development and maintenance of the inflammatory response in a large number of animals, including humans. Most important amongst the pro-inflammatory mediators are the anaphylatoxins, with C5a and C5a des-Arg having the greatest diversity of biological action and potency of effect. Vascular inflammatory changes, neutrophil adhesion, chemotaxis and release of toxic ions and enzymes from inflammatory cells are included in the range of complement-induced inflammatory effects.

Recognition of the important role that the complement system plays in the inflammatory response, a response which can sometimes be detrimental to the host, has stimulated a search for specific inhibitors of complement activation. Formerly general protease inhibitors were available; however, their range of enzyme inhibition was wide and so they were highly toxic to the host if administered *in vivo*. Recently a far more specific inhibitor called rosmarinic acid has been isolated from the bacterium *Melissa officinalis*. Its successful use *in vivo* to inhibit complement-induced inflammatory reactions has now been documented[90]. This possibly heralds the advent of more specific therapy for inflammatory diseases such as immune complex diseases and the adult respiratory distress syndrome whose molecular pathogenesis is so closely linked to complement activation.

References

1. Buchner, H. (1889). Uber die nahere natur der bakteri-entodtenden substanz in blutserum. *Zbl. Bakt.* (*Naturwiss.*), **6**, 561–5
2. Bordet, J. (1898). Sur l'agglutination et la dissolution des globules rouge par le sérum d'animaux injecties de sang defibriné. *Ann. Inst. Pasteur* (*Paris*), **12**, 688–95
3. Rapp, H. J. and Borsos, T. (1970). *Molecular Basis of Complement Action* (New York: Appleton-Century-Crofts)
4. Whaley, K. (1987). The complement system. In Whaley, K. (ed.), *Complement in Health and Disease*, pp. 1–35 (Lancaster: MTP Press)
5. Doods, A. W., Sim, R. B., Porter, R. R. and Kerr, M. A. (1978). Activation of the first component of human complement (C1) by antigen–antibody complexes. *Biochem. J.*, **175**, 383–90
6. Ziccardi, R. J. (1983). Nature of the metal ion requirements for assembly and function of the first component of human complement. *J. Biol. Chem.*, **258**, 6187–92
7. Borsos, T. and Rapp, H. J. (1965). Complement fixation on cell surfaces by 19S and 7S

antibodies. *Science*, **150**, 505–7
8. Colomb, M. G., Arland, G. J. and Villiers, C. L. (1984). Activation of C1. *Phil. Trans. R. Soc. Lond.*, **306**, 283–92
9. Henson, D. C., Siegel, R. C. and Schumaker, V. N. (1985). Segmental flexibility of the C1q subcomponent of human complement and its possible role in the immune response. *J. Biol. Chem.*, **260**, 3576–83
10. Schreiber, R. D. and Müller-Eberhard, H. J. (1974). Fourth component of human complement: description of a three poly-peptide chain structure. *J. Exp. Med.*, **140**, 1324–35
11. Kerr, M. A. (1980). The human complement system: assembly of the classical pathway C3 convertase. *Biochem. J.*, **189**, 173–81
12. Polley, H. J. and Müller-Eberhard, H. J. (1968). The second component of human complement: its isolation, fragmentation by C1 esterase and incorporation into C3 convertase. *J. Exp. Med.*, **130**, 533–51
13. Nagasawa, S. and Stroud, R. M. (1977). Cleavage of C2 by C1s into the antigenically distinct fragments C2a and C2b: demonstration of binding of C2b to C4b. *Proc. Natl. Acad. Sci. USA*, **74**, 2998–3000
14. Kerr, M. A. and Porter, R. R. (1978). The purification and the properties of the second component of human complement. *Biochem. J.*, **171**, 99–107
15. Harpel, P. C. and Cooper, N. R. (1975). Studies on human plasma C1/inactivator–enzyme interactions. I, Mechanisms of interaction with C1s, plasmin and trypsin. *J. Clin. Invest.*, **55**, 593–604
16. Sim, R. B., Arland, G. J. and Colomb, M. G. (1979). C1-inhibitor dependent dissociation of human complement component C1 bound to immune complexes. *Biochem. J.*, **179**, 449–57
17. Ziccardi, R. J. and Cooper, N. R. (1979). Active disassembly of the first complement component C1 by C1-inactivator. *J. Immunol.*, **123**, 788–92
18. Fujita, T. and Nussenzweig, V. (1979). The role of C4-binding protein and β1H in proteolysis of C4b and C3b. *J. Exp. Med.*, **150**, 267–76
19. Gigli, I., Fujita, T. and Nussenzweig, V. (1980). Modulation of the classical pathway C3 convertase by the plasma proteins C4-BP and C3bINA. *J. Immunol.*, **124**, 1521 (abstract)
20. Tack, B. F., Harrison, R. A., Janatova, J., Thomas, M. L. and Prahl, J. W. (1980). Evidence for the presence of an internal thiolester bond in the third component of human complement. *Proc. Natl. Acad. Sci. USA*, **77**, 5764–8
21. Isenman, D., Kells, D. I. C., Cooper, N. R., Müller-Eberhard, H. J. and Pangburn, M. K. (1981). Nucleophilic modification of human complement protein C3: correlation of conformational changes with acquisition of C3b-like functional properties. *Biochemistry*, **19**, 4458–67
22. Fearon, D. T., Austen, K. F. and Ruddy, S. (1973). Formation of a haemolytically active cellular intermediate by the interaction between properdin factors B and D and the activated third component of complement. *J. Exp. Med.*, **138**, 1305–13
23. Fearon, D. T. and Austen, K. F. (1975). Properdin: binding to C3b and stabilisation of the C3b-dependent C3 convertase. *J. Exp. Med.*, **142**, 856–63
24. Weiler, J. M., Daha, M. R., Austen, K. F. and Fearon, D. T. (1976). Control of the amplification convertase of complement by the plasma protein β1H. *Proc. Natl. Acad. Sci. USA*, **73**, 3268–72
25. Sim, R. B., Malhotra, V., Ripoche, J., Day, A. J., Micklem, K. J. and Sim, E. (1986). Complement receptors and related complement control proteins. *Biochem. Soc. Symp.*, **51**, 83–96
26. Fearon, D. T. and Austen, K. F. (1977). Activation of the alternative complement pathway due to resistance of zymosan-bound amplification convertase to endogenous regulatory mechanisms. *Proc. Natl. Acad. Sci. USA*, **74**, 1683–7
27. Fearon, D. T. and Austen, K. F. (1977). Activation of the alternative complement pathway by rabbit erythrocytes by circumvention of the regulatory action of endogenous control proteins. *J. Exp. Med.*, **146**, 22–33
28. Fearon, D. T. (1978). Regulation by membrane sialic acid of β1H-dependent decay-dissociation of the amplification C3 convertase of the alternative complement pathway. *Proc. Natl. Acad. Sci. USA*, **75**, 1971–6
29. Pangburn, M. K. and Muller-Eberhard, H. J. (1978). Complement C3 convertase: cell surface restriction of B1H control and generation of restriction neuraminidase-treated cells. *Proc. Natl. Acad. Sci. USA*, **75**, 2416–20

30. Kazatchkine, M. D., Fearon, D. T. and Austen, K. F. (1979). Human alternative complement pathway: membrane associated sialic acid regulates the competition between B and B1H for cell-bound C3b. *J. Immunol.*, **122**, 75–81
31. Vogt, W., Schmidt, G., Buttlar, B. V. and Deiminger, L. (1978). A new function of the activated third component of complement: binding to C5, an essential step for C5 activation. *Immunology*, **34**, 29–40
32. Hammer, C. A., Abramovitz, A. S. and Mayer, M. M. (1976). A new activity of complement component C3: cell-bound C3b potentiates lysis of erythrocytes by C5b,6 and terminal components. *J. Immunol.*, **117**, 830–4
33. Mayer, M. M., Hammer, C. H., Michaels, D. W. and Shin, M. L. (1978). Immunologically-mediated membrane damage. The mechanism of complement action and the similarity to lymphocyte-mediated cytotoxicity. *Immunochemistry*, **15**, 813–31
34. Tschopp, J. (1984). Ultrastructure of the membrane attack complex of complement. Heterogeneity of the complex caused by different degrees of C9 polymerisation. *J. Biol. Chem.*, **259**, 7857–63
35. Tschopp, J., Engel, A. and Podack, E. R. (1984). Molecular weight of poly (C9): 12–18 molecules form the trans-membrane channel of complement. *J. Biol. Chem.*, **259**, 1922–8
36. Mayer, M. M. (1972). Mechanism of cytolysis by complement. *Proc. Natl. Acad. Sci. USA*, **69**, 2954–8
37. Podack, E. R., Kolb, W. P. and Müller-Eberhard, H. J. (1979). The C5b–6 complex: formation, isolation and inhibition of its activity by lipoprotein and the S-protein of human serum. *J. Immunol.*, **120**, 1841–8
38. Dahlbach, B. and Podack, E. R. (1985). Characterisation of human S protein, an inhibitor of the membrane attack complex of complement. Demonstration of a free reactive thiol group. *Biochemistry*, **24**, 2368–74
39. Hansch, G. M., Schonermark, S., Rauterberg, E. W., Roelke, D. and Shin, M. L. (1985). Homologous species restriction in C5-9 mediated lysis of human erythrocytes: inhibition of lysis by a membrane protein with C8 binding capacity. *Complement*, **2**, 33 (abstract)
40. Zalman, L. S. and Müller-Eberhard, H. J. (1985). Purification of a human erythrocyte membrane protein capable of inhibiting C5b-9 and poly C9 channels. *Complement*, **2**, 90–1 (abstract)
41. Müller-Eberhard, H. J. (1988). Molecular organisation and function of the complement system. In Richardson, C. C., Boyer, P. D., Dawid, I. B. and Meister, A. (eds), *Annual Review of Biochemistry*, pp. 321–47 (Palo Alto: Annual Reviews)
42. Colten, H. R. (1976). Biosynthesis of complement. *Adv. Immunol.*, **22**, 67–118
43. Alper, C. A. and Rosen, F. S. (1976). Genetics of the complement system. In Harris, H. and Hirschorn, K. (eds), *Advances in Human Genetics*, pp. 141–88 (New York and London: Plenum Press)
44. Hobart, M. J., Lachmann, P. J. and Calne, R. Y. (1977). C6: Synthesis by the liver *in vivo*. *J. Exp. Med.*, **140**, 629–30
45. Hume, D. A., Robinson, A. P., MacPherson, G. C. and Gordon, S. (1983). The mononuclear phagocyte system of the mouse defined by immuno-histochemical localisation of antigen F4/80. Relationship between macrophages, Langerhans cells, reticular cells and dendritic cells in lymphoid and haematopoietic organs. *J. Exp. Med.*, **158**, 1522–36
46. Whaley, K. (1980). Biosynthesis of complement components and the regulatory proteins of the alternative complement pathway by human peripheral blood monocytes. *J. Exp. Med.*, **151**, 501–16
47. De Ceulaer, C., Papazoglou, S. and Whaley, K. (1980). Increased synthesis of complement component by monocytes, synovial fluid macrophages and synovial membrane cells from patients with rheumatoid arthritis. *Immunology*, **41**, 37–43
48. Ruddy, S. and Colten, H. R. (1974). Rheumatoid arthritis. Biosynthesis of complement proteins by synovial tissues. *N. Eng. J. Med.*, **290**, 1284–5
49. Fey, G. H. and Fuller, G. M. (1987). Regulation of acute phase gene expression by inflammatory mediators. *Mol. Biol. Med.*, **4**, 323–8
50. Williams, T. J. and Jose, P. J. (1981). Mediation of increased vascular permeability after complement activation. Histamine independent action of rabbit C5a. *J. Exp. Med.*, **153**, 136–53
51. Johnson, A. R., Hugli, T. E. and Müller-Eberhard, H. J. (1975). Release of histamine from rat mast cells by the complement peptides C3a and C5a. *Immunology*, **28**, 1067–80

52. Issekutz, A. C. (1984). Role of polymorphonuclear leukocytes in the vascular responses of acute inflammation. *Lab. Invest.*, **50**, 605–7
53. Wedmore, C. V. and Williams, T. J. (1981). Control of vascular permeability by polymorphonuclear leukocytes in inflammation. *Nature*, **289**, 646–50
54. Jose, P. J., Forrest, M. J. and Williams, T. J. (1981). Human C5a des Arg increases vascular permeability. *J. Immunol.*, **127**, 2376–80
55. Yancey, K. B., Hammer, C. H., Harvath, L., Renfer, L., Frank, M. M. and Lawley, T. J. (1985). Studies of C5a as a mediator of inflammation in normal human skin. *J. Clin. Invest.*, **75**, 486–95
56. Yancey, K. B., Bielory, L., Wright, R., Young, N., Frank, M. M. and Lawley, T. J. (1986). Patients with bone marrow failure demonstrate decreased cutaneous reactivity to human C5a. *J. Invest. Dermatol.*, **88**, 388–92
57. Buchanan, M. R., Vazquez, M. J. and Gimbrone, M. A. (1983). Arachidonic acid metabolism and the adhesion of human polymorphonuclear leukocytes to cultured vascular endothelial cells. *Blood*, **62**, 889–95
58. Swerlick, R. A., Yancey, K. B. and Lawley, T. J. (1988). A direct in vivo comparison of the inflammatory properties of human C5a and C5a des Arg in human skin. *J. Immunol.*, **140**, 2376–81
59. Bokisch, V. A. and Müller-Eberhard, H. J. (1970). Anaphylatoxin inactivator of human plasma: its isolation and characterisation as a carboxypeptidase. *J. Clin. Invest.*, **49**, 2427–36
60. Damerau, B., Zimmermann, B., Grunefeld, E., Czorniak, K. and Vogt, W. (1980). Biological activities of C5a and C5a des Arg from hog serum. *Int. Arch. Allergy. Appl. Immunol.*, **63**, 408–14
61. Hugli, T. E. (1979). The structural basis for anaphylatoxin and chemotactic functions of C3a, C4a and C5a. *CRC Crit. Rev. Immunol.*, **1**, 321–66
62. Tonnesen, M. G., Smedly, L. A. and Henson, P. M. (1984). Neutrophil-endothelial cell interactions. Modulation of neutrophil adhesiveness induced by complement fragments C5a and C5a des Arg and formyl-methionyl-leucyl-phenylalanine *in vitro*. *J. Clin. Invest.*, **74**, 1581–92
63. Craddock, P. R., Hammerschmidt, D. E., White, J. G., Dalmasso, P. and Jacob, H. S. (1977). Complement (C5a)-induced granulocyte aggregation *in vitro*: a possible mechanism of complement-mediated leukostasis and leukopenia. *J. Clin. Invest.*, **60**, 261–4
64. Ross, G. D. and Medof, M. E. (1985). Membrane complement receptors specific for bound fragments of C3. *Adv. Immunol.*, **37**, 217–67
65. Springer, T. A. and Anderson, D. C. (1986). The importance of the MAC-1, LFA-1 glycoprotein family in monocyte and granulocyte adherence, chemotaxis and migration into inflammatory sites: insights from an experiment of nature. In Evered, D., Nugent, J. and O'Connor, M. (eds), *Ciba Foundation Symposium 118, Biochemistry of Macrophages*, pp. 102–26 (London: Pitman)
66. Damerau, B., Grunefeld, E. and Vogt, W. (1978). Chemotactic effects of the complement-derived peptides C3a, C5ai and C5a (classical anaphylatoxin) on rabbit and guinea pig polymorphonuclear leukocytes. *Arch. Pharmacol.*, **305**, 181–4
67. Fernandez, H. N., Henson, P. M., Otani, A. and Hugli, T. E. (1978). Chemotactic response to human C3a and C5a anaphylatoxins. I. Evaluation of C3a and C5a leukotaxis *in vitro* and under simulated *in vivo* conditions. *J. Immunol.*, **120**, 109–14
68. Stimler, N. P., Hugli, T. E. and Bloor, C. M. (1980). Pulmonary injury induced by C3a and C5a anaphylatoxins. *Am. J. Pathol.*, **100**, 327–48
69. Perez, H. D., Goldstein, I. M., Webster, R. O. and Henson, P. M. (1981). Enhancement of the chemotactic activity of human C5a des Arg by an anionic polypeptide (co-chemotaxin) in normal human serum and plasma. *J. Immunol.*, **126**, 800–4
70. Gerard, C., Chenoweth, D. E. and Hugli, T. E. (1981). Response of human neutrophils to C5a: a role for the oligo-saccharide moiety of human C5a des Arg-74 but not of C5a in biologic activity. *J. Immunol.*, **127**, 1978–82
71. Hill, H. R., Bohnsack, J. F., Morris, E. Z., Augustine, N. H., Parker, C. J., Cleary, P. P. and Wu, J. T. (1988). Group B streptococci inhibit the chemotactic activity of the fifth component of complement. *J. Immunol.*, **141**, 3551–6
72. Ghebrehiwet, B. and Müller-Eberhard, H. J. (1979). C3e: an acidic fragment of human C3 with leukocytosis inducing activity. *J. Immunol.*, **123**, 616–21
73. Meuth, J. L., Morgan, E. L., Di Scipio, R. G. and Hugli, T. E. (1983). Suppression of T lymphocyte functions by human C3 fragments. I. Inhibition of human T cell proliferative

responses by a kallikrein cleavage fragment of human iC3b. *J. Immunol.*, **130**, 2605–11
74. Sacks, T., Moldow, C. F., Craddock, P. R., Bowers, T. K. and Jacob, H. S. (1978). Oxygen radicles mediate endothelial cell damage by complement-stimulated granulocytes. An *in vitro* model of immune vascular damage. *J. Clin. Invest.*, **61**, 1161–7
75. Yamada, Y., Moldow, C. F., Sacks, T., Craddock, P. R., Boogaerts, M. A. and Jacob, H. S. (1981). Deleterious effects of endotoxin on cultured endothelial cells: an *in vitro* model of vascular injury. *Inflammation*, **5**, 115–26
76. Harlan, J. M., Killen, P. D., Harker, L. A., Striker, G. E. and Wright, D. G. (1981). Neutrophil-mediated endothelial injury *in vitro*: mechanisms of cell detachment. *J. Clin. Invest.*, **68**, 1394–403
77. Chenoweth, D. E. and Hugli, T. E. (1980). Human C5a and C5a analogs as probes of the neutrophil C5a receptor. *Mol. Immunol.*, **17**, 151–61
78. Ghebrehiwet, B. (1984). The release of lysosomal enzymes from human polymorphonuclear leukocytes by human C3e. *Clin. Immunol. Immunopathol.*, **30**, 321–9
79. Sim, R. B. and Walport, M. J. (1987). C3 receptors. In Whaley, K. (ed.), *Complement in Health and Disease*, pp. 125–61 (Lancaster: MTP Press)
80. Lucisano, Y. M. and Mantovani, B. (1988). The role of complement in the stimulation of lysosomal enzyme release by polymorphonuclear leukocytes induced by immune complexes of IgG and IgM. *Immunology*, **65**, 171–5
81. Seeger, W., Hartmann, R., Neuhoff, H. and Bhakdi, S. (1989). Local complement activation, thromboxane mediated vaso-constriction and vascular leakage in isolated lungs. *Am. Rev. Resp. Dis.*, **139**, 88–99
82. Sims, P. J., Faioni, E. M., Wiedmer, T. and Shattil, S. J. (1988). Complement proteins C5b-9 cause release of membrane vesicles from the platelet surface that are enriched in the membrane receptor for coagulation factor Va and express prothrombinase activity. *J. Biol. Chem.*, **263**, 18205–12
83. Morgan, B. P., Dankert, J. P. and Esser, A. F. (1985). Recovery of human neutrophils from complement attack: production of membrane vesicles bearing the membrane attack complex. *Complement*, **2**, 56 (abstract)
84. Whaley, K. (1987). Complement and immune complex diseases. In Whaley, K. (ed.), *Complement in Health and Disease*, pp. 163–83 (Lancaster: MTP Press)
85. Thomson, R. A. (1987). Inherited complement deficiencies. In Whaley, K. (ed.), *Complement in Health and Disease*, pp. 37–51 (Lancaster: MTP Press)
86. Kerr, M. A. and Yeung-Laiwah, A. A. C. (1987). C1-inhibitor deficiency and angio-oedema. In Whaley, K. (ed.), *Complement in Health and Disease*, pp. 53–78 (Lancaster: MTP Press)
87. Strang, C. J., Cholin, S., Spragg, J., Davis, A. E., Schneeberger, E. E., Donaldson, V. H. and Rosen, F. S. (1988). Angio-oedema induced by a peptide derived from complement component C2. *J. Exp. Med.*, **168**, 1685–98
88. Hammerschmidt, D. E. (1987). Activation of complement and granulocytes in shock. In Whaley, K. (ed.), *Complement in Health and Disease*, pp. 267–87 (Lancaster: MTP Press)
89. Jacob, H. S. (1983). Complement-mediated leucoembolisation: a mechanism of tissue damage during extracorporeal perfusions, myocardial infarction and in shock – a review. *Q. J. Med.*, **207**, 289–96
90. Engelberger, W., Hadding, U., Etschenberg, E., Graf, E., Leyck, S., Winkelmann, J. and Parnham, M. J. (1988). Rosmarinic acid: a new inhibitor of complement C3-convertase with anti-inflammatory activity. *Int. J. Immunopharmacol.*, **10**, 729–37

3
The kinin system: current concepts and perspectives

D. REGOLI, N.-E. RHALEB, G. DRAPEAU and S. DION

INTRODUCTION

The participation of kinins in the initiation and maintenance of the inflammatory process has been repeatedly affirmed and analysed[1,2]. Indeed, generation of kinins is increased in the initial phase of the inflammatory process both in experimental animals[3,4] and in humans[5]. Despite their rapid inactivation by a variety of peptidases, a local generation of kinins may be maintained during the subacute and chronic phase of inflammation by the continuous release of kallikreins from neutrophils and other blood cells[6,7]. Thus, the initial activation of local kallikreins is followed by a multiplicative cascade of events which accentuate the release of other endogenous mediators such as histamine, prostaglandins and the sensory neuropeptides which take part in the inflammatory reaction. No wonder that various groups of scientists are working towards the identification and development of inhibitors of kallikreins or antagonists of kinin receptors, since these agents could moderate the excessive reaction of animal tissues to noxious stimuli.

THE KALLIKREIN–KININ SYSTEM

The various components of the kallikrein-kinin system are illustrated in Figure 3.1. Kinins (bradykinin and kallidin) are derived from larger proteins, the kininogens, which are synthesized primarily in the liver and possibly in other tissues. Kininogens have been intensively studied in recent years and their genetics, structure and functions have been identified and carefully reviewed by Müller-Esterl *et al.*[8]. Two types of kininogens, the high molecular weight kininogen (H-kininogen 88 000–114 000 D) and the low molecular weight kininogen (L-kininogen 50 000–68 000 D) have been found to:

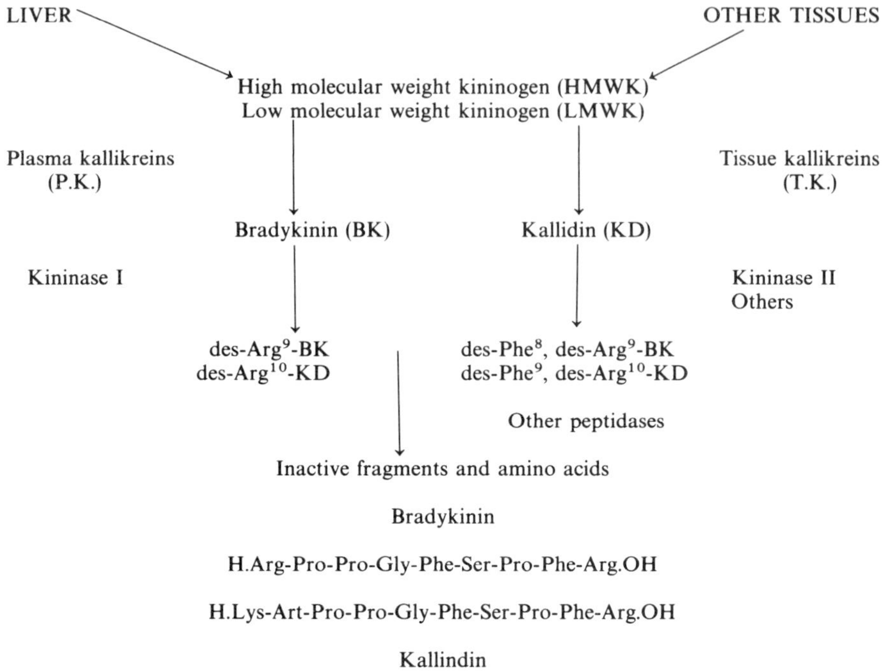

Figure 3.1 The kallikrein–kinin system and the primary structures of the kinins.

1. provide substrates for kallikreins,
2. inhibit cystein proteinases,
3. bind to subendothelial surfaces and then attract coagulation proenzymes for initiating the contact phase of coagulation[8,9].

H-kininogen has all three functions and possesses a histidine-reach region which allows for binding to subendothelial surfaces (Figure 3.2), while L-kininogen has only functions (1) and (2). The general structures of human kininogens and the various functional domains are illustrated in Figure 3.2. According to Müller-Esterl *et al.*[8] 'only one kininogen gene is present in the human genome ... the high molecular weight and low molecular weight kininogen mRNAs are encoded by a single gene, and the use of different polyadenylation sites in combination with alternative RNA splicing is responsible for the generation of two distinct types of mRNA'.

A special type of kininogen, the T-kininogen, has been identified in the rat. T-kininogen has a molecular weight of 68 000 and it is a substrate for trypsin and cathepsin C, but not for kallikreins. The T-kininogen has been found to increase during peripheral inflammation induced experimentally in the rat[10]: T-kininogen contains the sequence of T-kinin, the undecapeptide Ile-Ser-bradykinin.

H- and L-kininogens are hydrolysed by a group of trypsin-like enzymes,

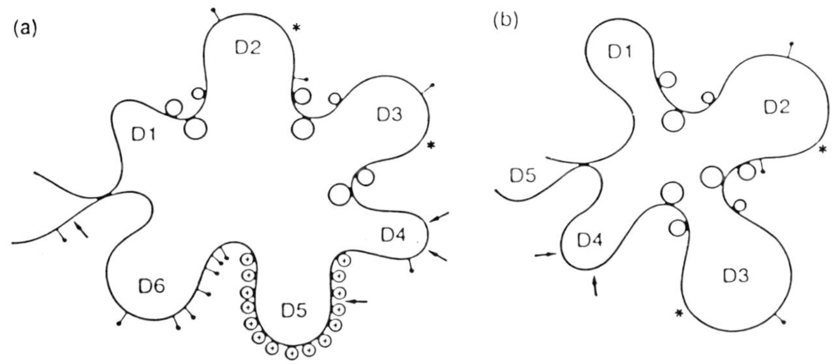

Figure 3.2 The general structure of human kininogens is represented as comprising multiple domains. Assignment of the domains is based on structural, functional and evolutionary evidence, the boundaries between the single domains are somewhat arbitrary. (**a**) HMW kininogen has six domains (D1–D6) and (**b**) LMW kininogens has five (D1–D5). *, Putative reactive site: ○, potential disulfide loop; ⧫ carbohydrate attachment site; ⊕, histidine-rich region; ↓, cleavage site for kallikrein. Similar domain structures are found for bovine and rat kinonogens including T-kininogen. Reproduced from Müller-Esterl *et al.*[8] with permission.

the kallikreins, which act on two basic amino acid residues within the kininogen molecules to release bradykinin or kallidin, whose primary structures are shown in Figure 3.1.

Kallikreins are present in plasma and in various organs (the kidney, some exocrine glands) and in various cell types, such as human polymorphonuclear leukocytes[6,7]. The kallikreins are divided into two main groups: tissue and plasma kallikreins, which differ in the molecular weight, isoelectric point, substrate specificity and type of kinin released. The kallikrein gene family is composed of closely related units, with genes varying greatly in number among different mammalian species. Humans have 24 genes, the rat 10–17 and the hamster 3 or 4[11]. These genes encode homologous trypsin-like serine proteases with a variety of natural substrates. Members of the kallikrein gene family include epidermal growth factor binding proteins A, B and C which convert epidermal growth factor precursor to the active form, and a subunit of nerve growth factor with protease activity responsible for cleavage and activation of another subunit of the molecule[12].

The role of these kallikreins in conversion of kininogens is uncertain. On the other hand plasma kallikrein would appear to be of major importance as a physiological kininogase. It is synthesized in the liver, it circulates as an inactive molecule in the plasma and is activated by Hageman factor. The activation of the plasma kallikrein system thus depends on contact with negatively charged Hageman factor. Activated kallikrein converts plasminogen to plasmin, and may be involved in the autoactivation of the Hageman factor. It is thus important in the clotting and fibrinolysis system in addition to generating kinins. Other roles in inflammation such as chemotaxis for plasmatic polymorphonuclear leukocytes may be important (see ref. 71). In plasma and tissues, kallikreins are generally present as large inactive precursors constituted of the active kallikrein moiety and of a short heptapeptide, Ala-Pro-Pro-Ile-Gln-Ser-Arg[13]. According to McDonald *et al.*[12], 'the activation process of tissue kallikreins may be similar to that of other serine-proteases, such as chymotrypsin, where the newly formed N-terminal Ile^{+1} links up via an ionic bond with Asp 194[14], altering the three dimensional structure to expose the active site'[12]. Activation of kallikreins under pathological conditions is brought about by a variety of stimuli such as extremes of temperature, strong acids and bases, all kind of pro-inflammatory agents as well as a variety of proteolytic enzymes including trypsin, kallikreins themselves (autocatalysis) and products of bacteria, such as thermolysin[13].

Activation of kallikreins leads to release of kinins, which are rapidly broken down by a variety of proteolytic enzymes, acting at the kinin C-terminal or somewhere in the middle of the peptide sequence. The most important peptidases involved in this process are (a) carboxypeptidase N (EC 3.4.17.3), (b) a carboxydipeptidase called kininase II (EC 3.4.15.1), (c) some chymotrypsin-like enzymes that may be present in blood and biological fluids[15], including the recently identified neutral endopeptidase (EC 3.4.24.11)[16]. Aminopeptidase N (EC 3.4.11.2) removes the first residue (Lys) from kallidin and thus releases bradykinin[15]. The nonapeptide bradykinin and the decapeptide kallidin (Lys-bradykinin) are converted into des-Arg^9-BK and des-Arg^{10}-KD by kininase I and into des-phe^8-des-Arg^9-BK and des-phe^9-des-Arg^{10}-KD by kininase II (see Figure 3.1). The products of the degradation by kininase I maintain some biological activities (see below), while those of kininase II appear to be completely inactive. Both these pairs of peptides are further broken down to inactive fragments by a variety of peptidases which are present in blood and tissues.

The most important sites of kinin degradation are the lung and the kidney; 90–95% of bradykinin is inactivated in a single passage through the lung[17] by kininase II, which is abundant in the pulmonary endothelium. The kinins that pass through the glomerular filter into the urine are rapidly inactivated by the kininase II and other enzymes of the brush border of the renal convoluted tubule[18,19] and by the newly identified neutral endopeptidase[16]. Inactivation of kinins may also occur rapidly in the extracellular fluid and in inflamed tissues. Because of rapid inactivation by the lung and the tissues, the concentration of kinins in circulating blood is very low, in the order of pg (see review article by Regoli and Barabé[20]). Kinins are therefore present in concentrations large enough to exert biological effects only in the proximity of the site of release: they should therefore be considered as autacoids. Bradykinin, kallidin and some of their metabolites exert a variety of biological effects through the activation of at least two different receptor types, and possibly by non-receptor mechanisms.

KININ RECEPTORS: PHARMACOLOGICAL CHARACTERIZATION

The existence of specific receptors for kinins has been demonstrated with pharmacological and biochemical assays.

Pharmacological assays on kinins have been performed in a variety of isolated organs. Such studies began in 1949, when Rocha e Silva *et al.*[21] identified a new activity in the snake venom which induced a slow (compared to that of histamine) contraction of the guinea pig ileum. Because of such an effect the principle was named bradykinin. This preparation has been extensively used, even recently by Vavrek and Stewart[22]. Assays were also performed on the rat uterus[22,23] and the rat duodenum, a preparation in which kinins induce relaxation[24]. Other tissues, used for measuring the *in vitro* biological effects of kinins until 1976, have been reviewed by Bertaccini[25]. During the past 15 years a few isolated vessels that appear to be suitable for pharmacological studies on kinins have been used in our laboratory, including the rabbit aorta and jugular vein[26,27] and dog carotid and renal arteries[28,29]. Examples of tracings obtained in the four preparations are shown in Figure 3.3. The rabbit's tissues respond to kinins by contraction, while the dog's tissues respond by relaxation. Rabbit aorta is particularly sensitive to des-Arg^9-BK, while the other three vessels show high sensitivity to BK and the dog renal artery also to des-Arg^9-BK. The effects of kinins in the four vessels appear to be due to activation of specific receptors, and two types of receptors have been characterized using agonists and antagonists[29,30]. Data obtained with nine peptides related to bradykinin or kallidin, namely the two naturally occuring kinins, their metabolites released by kininase I, the metabolites of kininase II and 3 analogues designed to improve the affinity and selectivity for the B_2 receptor types, are shown in Table 3.1.

In the two vessels of the dog, bradykinin and kallidin are more active than their metabolites; des-Arg^9-BK and des-Arg^{10}-KD. Both des-Arg^9-BK and des-Arg^{10}-BK are inactive on the dog carotid artery, but maintain 4–5% of their activity on the dog renal artery. Metabolites released by kininase II are inactive on both vessels. The three shown at the bottom of Table 3.1 are very active in both vessels.

In the other two preparations, the rabbit jugular vein and the rabbit aorta, different patterns of biological activities are observed. Bradykinin, kallidin and the three analogues (bottom of Table 3.1) show very high activities on the rabbit jugular vein while the kinin metabolites are inactive. On the contrary, some metabolites, des-Arg^9-BK and des-Arg^{10}-KD are potent stimulants of the rabbit aorta, being more active than the kinins. [Tyr(Me)^8]-BK and [Hyp^3,Tyr(Me)^8]-BK are inactive.

Based on these data, two orders of potency of kinins have been described as follows:

on the rabbit jugular vein:
[Hyp^3,Tyr(Me)^8]-BK > [Tyr(Me)^8]-BK > BK > des-Arg^9-BK = des-Arg^{10}-KD

on the rabbit aorta:
des-Arg^{10}-KD > des-Arg^9-BK > BK $\gg$ [Tyr(Me)^8]-BK = [Hyp^3,Tyr(Me)^8]-BK.

Thus, [Tyr(Me)^8]-BK and [Hyp^3,Tyr(Me)^8]-BK are pure B_2 receptor agonists, active on the rabbit jugular vein and inactive in the rabbit aorta, while des-Arg^9-BK has the opposite effect – it is active on the rabbit aorta and

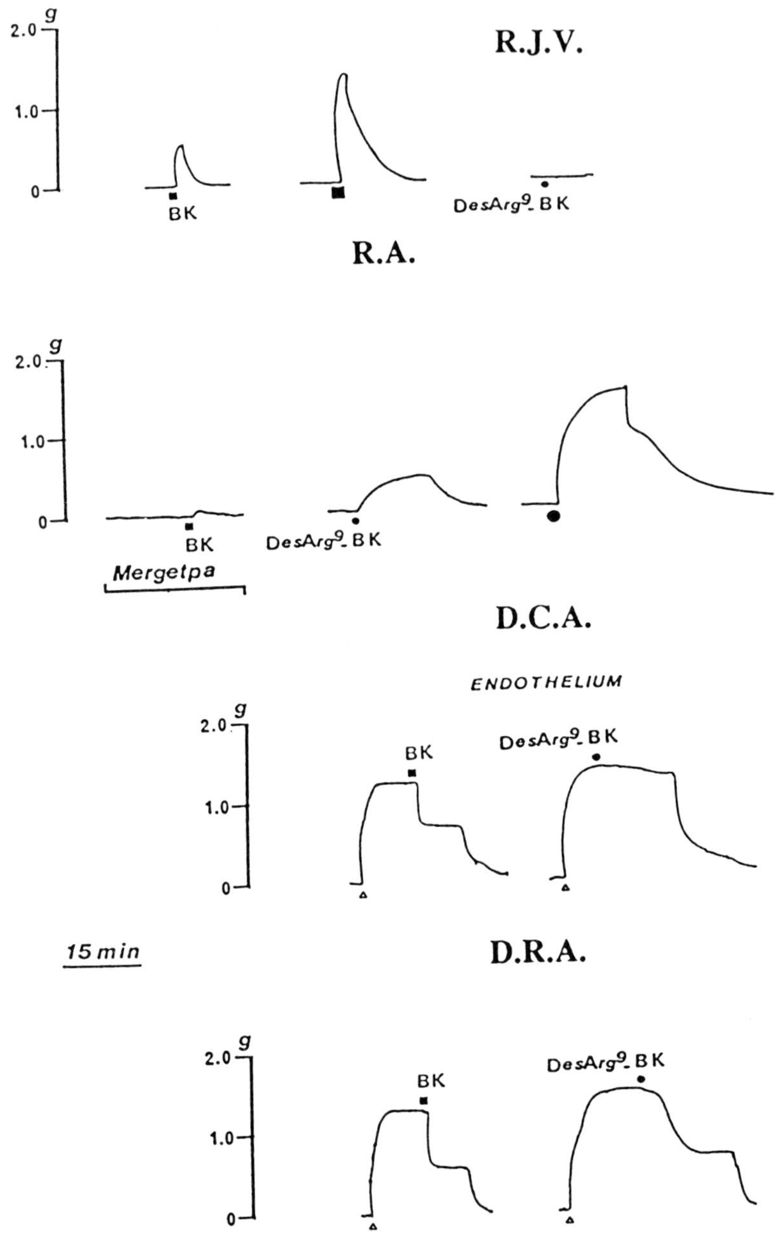

Figure 3.3 Tracings showing the effects of kinins (bradykinin (BK) and des-Arg^9-BK) on isolated vessels. R.J.V.: rabbit jugular vein (B_2); R.A.: rabbit aorta (B_1); D.C.A.: dog carotid artery (B_2), D.R.A.: dog renal artery (B_2, B_2, B_1). Peptide concentrations: R.J.V. BK 4.0×10^{-10} mol/L and 2.0×10^{-9} mol/L; des-Arg^9-BK 1.0×10^{-5} mol/L; R.A. BK 1.0×10^{-5} mol/L; des-Arg^9-BK 8.6×10^{-9} mol/L and 2.1×10^{-7} mol/L. D.C.A. NA 2.0×10^{-8} mol/L. BK 2.0×10^{-9} mol/L, des-Arg^9-BK 1.0×10^{-5} mol/L. D.R.A. NA 2.0×10^{-8} mol/L. BK 4.0×10^{-10} mol/L, des-Arg^9-BK 4.3×10^{-8} mol/L. Abscissa: time. Ordinate: tension in g.

Table 3.1 Pharmacological characterization of kinin receptors. Order of potency of agonists

Compound	*Preparation*							
	Dog carotid artery		*Dog renal artery*		*Rabbit jugular vein*		*Rabbit aorta*	
	pD_2	*RA*	*pD_2*	*RA*	*pD_2*	*RA*	*pD_2*	*RA*
Bradykinin (BK)	8.64	100	9.85	100	8.48	100	6.22	9
Kallidin (KD)	8.44	63	9.70	71	8.63	141	7.27	95
des-Arg^9-BK		<0.01	8.41	4		<0.1	7.29	100
des-Arg^{10}-KD		<0.01	8.57	5		<0.1	8.60	2042
des-Phe^8,des-Arg^9-BK	Inac.		–			<0.01		<0.1
des-Phe^9,des-Arg^{10}-KD	5.32	0.05	–		4.78	0.02		<0.1
[Tyr(Me)^8]-BK	8.64	100	9.89	110	8.59	129	Inac.	
[Hyp^3]-BK	8.63	98	10.14	195	8.88	254	6.17	8
[Hyp^3,Tyr(Me)^8]-BK	9.07	270	10.22	234	8.56	120	Inac.	

pD_2: −log of the concentration of agonist producing 50% of the maximum effect. RA: apparent affinity expressed as a percentage of that of the reference agonist, BK for D.C.A., R.J.V. and D.R.A. and des-Arg^9-BK for R.A.
Inac.: inactive at 10^{-5} mol/L.

inactive on the rabbit jugular vein. The receptor of the rabbit aorta, the first to be characterized[26], was named B_1 and that of the rabbit jugular vein was named B_2[20]. The other two vessels from the dog, when used with intact endothelium as in the experiments reported in Table 3.1, appear to contain B_2 receptors since they show the same order of potency of agonist as the rabbit jugular vein. Because of the residual activities by des-Arg^9-BK and des-Arg^{10}-KD, the dog renal artery was further investigated and the effects of bradykinin and its kininase I metabolite were measured *in arteries without endothelium* and after treatment with either B_2 or B_1 receptor antagonists. As shown in Table 3.2, des-Arg^9-BK is more potent than BK: moreover, the effect of bradykinin is blocked by a B_2 receptor antagonist, [Thi^{5,8},D-Phe^7]-BK, while that of des-Arg^9-BK is prevented by the B_1 receptor antagonist

Table 3.2 Pharmacological activities of bradykinin and analogues on the *dog renal artery without endothelium*

Peptide	*pD_2*	*R.A.*	*pA_2 against BK*	*pA_2 against des-Arg^9-BK*
BK	8.25	100	–	–
des-Arg^9-BK	8.60	224	–	–
[Thi^{5,8},D-Phe^7]-BK			6.63	Inac.
[Leu^8]des-Arg^9-BK			Inac.	7.81
Indomethacin (7.0×10^{-6} mol/L)	–	–	Inh.	Inh.

pD_2: R.A. as in Table 1.
pA_2: −log of the concentration of antagonist that reduces the effect of a double dose of agonist to that of a single dose[31].
Inac.: inactive; Inh.: inhibition.

[Leu^8]des-Arg^9-BK. These results indicate that, *in the absence of endothelium*, kinins are still able to relax the dog renal artery by activating B_2 or B_1 receptors, presumably localized on the smooth muscle membrane. Both receptors appear to act by promoting the release of prostaglandins, since the effects of kinins are abolished by indomethacin[29]. It is also worthy of mention that the dog renal artery without endothelium shows high sensitivity to des-Arg^9-BK from the beginning of the *in vitro* incubation, and does not manifest the progressive increase of sensitivity that is found in the rabbit aorta[26]. It therefore appears that the B_1 receptor of the dog renal artery is a stable component of the plasma membrane[29].

Kinin receptors were further characterized with antagonists, by evaluating the pA_2 (see definition at the bottom of Table 3.2) of several compounds, as shown in Table 3.3. The first two compounds are active on the rabbit aorta and inactive on the rabbit jugular vein: they are potent selective and specific B_1 receptor antagonists. The other two compounds ([$Thi^{5,8}$,D-Phe^7]-BK and [$Thi^{6,9}$,D-Phe^8]-KD are active on both preparations and show slightly higher affinity on the rabbit jugular vein than on the rabbit aorta. They are therefore weak, non-selective antagonists which show affinities for the two receptors at least one log unit lower than the respective agonists.

Some recent results obtained with other kinin antagonists are summarized in the second part of Table 3.3. [D-Phe^7]-BK is an agonist on the rabbit jugular vein and a weak antagonist on the rabbit aorta. Antagonist activity on B_2 receptor identified and analysed with [$Thi^{5,8}$,D-Phe^7]-BK is increased by the addition of a Hyp in position 3: the compound (no. 6 of Table 3.3) is more selective for B_2 receptors than [$Thi^{5,8}$,D-Phe^7]-BK, since it maintains a good affinity on the B_2 but is less active on the B_1 receptor. Antagonist affinity is further increased by the extension of the chain at the *N*-terminal

Table 3.3 Apparent affinities (pA_2) of kinin antagonists in the rabbit jugular vein (R.J.V.) and the rabbit aorta (R.A.)

Compound	*R.J.V.*		*R.A.*	
	pA_2	*Activity**	*pA_2*	*Activity*
[Leu^8]des-Arg^9-BK	Inac.	–	7.3	–
[Leu^9]des-Arg^{10}-KD	Inac.	–	8.4	–
[$Thi^{5,8}$,D-Phe^7]-BK	6.7	+	6.2	–
[$Thi^{6,9}$,D-Phe^8]-KD	6.9	+	6.4	–
[D-Phe^7]-BK	Inac.	+	5.9	–
[Hyp^3,$Thi^{5,8}$,D-Phe^7]-BK	7.0	+	5.6	–
D-Arg[Hyp^3,$Thi^{5,8}$,D-Phe^7]-BK	7.9	+	6.2	–
N.Ac-D-Arg[Hyp^3,$Thi^{5,8}$,D-Phe^7]-BK	7.5	–	5.5	–
D-Arg[Hyp^3,D-Phe^7]-BK	8.0	+	6.4	–
D-Arg[Phe^2,Hyp^3,D-Phe^7]-BK	6.9	+	5.4	–
[D-$Phe^{2,7}$]-BK	5.7	–	<5.0	–
[D-Phe^7,Hyp^8]-BK	6.1	–	<5.0	–

* Residual agonistic activity, +, present, –, absent.
Inac.: the compound is not an antagonist.

with a D-Arg: however, this change brings back activity on the B_1 receptor. Recent findings by Devillier *et al.*[32] (1988) have shown that B_2 receptor antagonists are potent histamine releasers, more active even than bradykinin. Histamine release by kinins can be prevented by acetylation of the N-terminal NH_2. When acetylated, D-Arg[Hyp^3,Thi^{5,8},D-Phe^7]-BK was found to maintain a fairly good affinity for the B_2 receptor and to be less active on the B_1 receptor. *N*-acetyl-D-Arg[Hyp^3,Thi^{5,8},D-Phe^7]-BK is almost inactive as histamine releasers and appears to be a fairly selective B_2 receptor antagonist.

Since Thi is an expensive and unnatural amino acid with potential toxic effects[22], some compounds not containing Thi[33] were prepared and tested: D-Arg[Hyp^3,D-Phe^7]-BK was found to be very active as an antagonist of B_2, while maintaining a fairly good affinity also on the B_1 receptor. Further modifications such as the replacement of Pro^2 with Phe or the elimination of D-Arg and Hyp^3 as in [D-Phe^{2,7}]-BK[33] were accompanied by drastic reductions of affinities on both B_2 and B_1 receptors. The last compound, [D-Phe^7,Hyp^8]-BK[33], was also found to be weak on both receptor systems. These compounds did not show any selectivity, when tested *in vivo* and in other preparations such as the guinea pig ileum, in contrast with recent reports by Stewart and Vavrek[33].

The results detailed above indicate that fairly active B_2 receptor antagonists, showing pA_2 around 8.0, can be obtained by replacing Pro^7 with D-Phe and by improving the affinity for the B_2 receptors with a Hyp in position 3 and an extension of the chain at the *N*-terminal with a D-Arg. D-Arg[Hyp^3,D-Phe^7]-BK can be acetylated to reduce or eliminate the histamine-releasing activity; moreover, the peptide bond between Phe^8 and Arg^9 can be replaced by CH_2–NH in order to protect the antagonist from degradation by kininases[34]: in this way a fairly selective B_2 receptor antagonist is obtained. Thus the data summarized in Table 3.3 indicate that pure antagonist for B_1 and B_2 receptors have been found and shown to be active only on their respective receptor, thus providing the best evidence for the existence and differentiation of two receptors for the kinins.

Pure B_1 antagonists were tested against angiotensin and noradrenaline on the rabbit aorta and against neurokinin on the rabbit pulmonary artery. When the effects of the various agents were blocked by the respective antagonists, namely [Sar^1,Leu^8]AT_{II}, prazosin and R.396, a NK-2 antagonist recently identified in our laboratory (Regoli, Drapeau, Dion, Rhaleb, Rouissi, unpublished), these agents had no effect on the responses of the preparations to des-Arg^9-BK. On the other hand, [Leu^8]-des-Arg^9-BK reduced the effect of des-Arg^9-BK without having any influence on the myotropic effects of AT_{II} and NA on the rabbit aorta, and the effect of NKA on the rabbit pulmonary artery. Similarly, a B_2 selective receptor antagonist gave identical results, when tested against BK, SP and acetylcholine in the dog carotid artery. The antagonist was found to be active only against BK. Atropine and a neurokinin receptor antagonists [D-Pro^4,D-Trp^{7,9}]SP (4–11) blocked respectively the effects of Ach and SP without modifying that of BK. Together with a definite proof of the existence of two different receptors for the kinins, the results described provide the essential tools for receptor characterization in terms of pure B_1 and B_2 receptor agonists and antagonists.

KININ RECEPTORS: BIOCHEMICAL STUDIES

Binding assays with kinins have been performed on a variety of preparations. Data obtained in various studies are summarized in Table 3.4. Both tritiated BK and iodinated analogues of BK, ([Tyr^{1}]-KD, [Tyr^{8}]-BK) have been used. Specific binding of BK to plasma membranes of rat uterus was reported by Reissman *et al.*[35], with tritiated BK. Three years later, Odya *et al.*[36] measured specific binding of BK on bovine uterus using various iodinated peptides, of which the most suitable was [^{125}I-Tyr^{1}]-KD. In the two studies, only the association constant was estimated and found to be around 10^{-10}M. A few years later, Fredrick *et al.*[37] estimated the K_d of [^{125}I-Tyr^{1}]-KD to be

Table 3.4 Kinin pharmacology: radioreceptor assays

Tissue	*Label (specific activity)*	K_{assoc} *(mol/l)*$^{-1}$	IC_{50} *(nmol/l)*	K_d *(nmol/l)*	B_{max} *(fmol/mg protein)*	*Reference*
Rat uterus	[^{3}H]BK (2 Ci/mmol)	3.6×10^{9} 2.2×10^{10}				35
Bovine myometrium	[^{125}I]Tyr^{1}-KD (1–2 Ci/μmol)	10^{10}			160	36
Human fibroblasts	[^{3}H]BK (52 Ci/nmol)			4.6	230	38
Bovine myometrium solubilized	[^{125}I]Tyr^{1}-KD (1–2 Ci/μmol)			0.16		37
Kidney						
medulla	[^{3}H]BK				59.4	39
cortex	(42 Ci/mmol)				13.3	39
CCT				8.9	68	39
Renomedullary interstitial cells	[^{125}I]Tyr^{1}-KD (1–2 Ci/μmol)	1.3×10^{9}				40
Guinea pig ileum	[^{3}H]BK (12.2 Ci/mmol)		1.9	5.0	25	41
Rabbit mesenteric vein	[^{3}H]des-Arg^{9}-BK (10 Ci/mmol)			104	0.06*	42
Rat jejunum (epithelial membranes)	[^{125}I]-[Tyr^{8}]-BK (1.8 Ci/μg)			0.69	332.8	44
Bovine pulmonary artery (endothelial cells)	[^{3}H]BK (61.7 Ci/mmol)			1.28	111.1	46
Calf pulmonary artery	[^{3}H]BK					
(endothelial cells)	(55 Ci/mmol)			2.1	47.9†	47
(smooth muscle cells)				4.9	17.3†	47
(adventitia fibroblasts)				7.9	26.3†	47
Rat brain	[^{125}I]-Tyr-BK			0.5	72	43
(cells in culture)	(500–800 Ci/mmol)			21	1193	
Guinea pig brain	[^{3}H]-BK			0.1	8.4	45
(synaptosomes)	(61.7 bi/mmol)					

* pmol/g of wet tissue.
† fmol/10^{6} cells.

approximately 0.16 nmol/L using a similar preparation. Using human fibroblasts, Roscher *et al.*[38] estimated at 4.6 nmol/L the K_d of [^{3}H]-BK and at 230 fmol/mg of protein the number of binding sites. Roscher *et al.*[38] also demonstrated the existence of a good correlation between the relative potency of several BK analogues to compete with [^{3}H]-BK for the binding and release of prostacyclin from human fibroblasts. A good correlation between binding and biological activities (on the rat uterus) has also been demonstrated by other authors[37]. Intense binding of [^{3}H]-BK to cortical and outer medullary collecting tubules of the rabbit kidney was demonstrated by Tomita and Pisano[39]. BK binding correlated fairly well with the concentration of kallikreins. Specific binding sites for bradykinin were also found by Fredrick *et al.*[40] in a particular fraction from cultured renal medullary interstitial cells of the rat. The characterization of kinin receptor using binding assays and agonists was attempted by Innis *et al.*[41] using [^{3}H]BK on guinea pig ileum membranes. The following order of potency for displacing [^{3}H]-BK was determined: BK > [Thi^{5,8}]-BK > KD > [Hyp^3]-BK $\gg$ des-Arg^9-BK, the last compound being very weak. The authors suggested that the ileum binding sites have the characteristics of a B_2 receptor type.

B_1 receptor sites were studied by Barabé *et al.*[42] using [^{3}H]-des-Arg^9-BK on strips of the rabbit mesenteric vein. A dissociation constant of 104 nM which corresponded to the ED_{50} of the biological assays was measured after 6 h of incubation *in vitro*. The number of sites (B_{max}) could not be estimated, since it increases continuously because of the novel formation of receptors[26].

In the first study describing the binding of [^{125}I]-Tyr-BK to rat brain cell in a primary culture, the presence of two high-affinity binding sites was recognized having dissociation constants of 0.5 nM and 21 nM, and with B_{max} of 1193 and 72 fmol/mg of protein, respectively[43]. By comparing the potency of various kinins the authors came to the conclusion that the sites have the characteristics of the B_2 receptor type. Binding of kinins in rat intestine, jejunum and descending colon (epithelia) were investigated by Cox *et al.*[44] using [^{125}I-Tyr^8]-BK. K_d values lower than 1 nmol were found, and the relative affinities of various kinins were compatible with the presence of a B_2 receptor site. In another study, Fujimara *et al.*[45] found a high-affinity site for [^{3}H]-BK on membranes of guinea pig brain: this site showed a K_d of 0.1 nM and a B_{max} of 8.4 fmol/mg of proteins. [^{3}H]-BK was well displaced by [D-Phe^7]-BK, a B_2 antagonist, while low displacement was observed with 1 μmol of [Leu^8]-des-Arg^9-BK, the selective B_1 receptor antagonist.

A very recent study by Sung *et al.*[46], performed with [^{3}H]-BK on endothelial cells of bovine pulmonary arteries maintained in culture, has resulted in the identification of two different binding sites with K_d of approximately 1 nmol/L and 0.5 μmol/L. Using agonists and antagonists, the high affinity site showed the typical characteristics of a B_2 receptor site, while the low affinity sites showed high affinity for des-Arg^9-BK and [Leu^8]des-Arg^9-BK, suggesting that it might be a B_1 receptor site. The same year, a study on endothelial cells, smooth muscle cells and adventitia fibroblasts of calf pulmonary artery demonstrated K_d values of 2.1–7.9 nmol/L and B_{max} of 17.3 and 47.9 nmol/L for [^{3}H]-BK and no displacement was seen with des-Arg^9-BK and [Leu^8]-des-Arg^9-BK. Cahill *et al.*[47] have reported that BK and des-Arg^9-BK stimulate prostacyclin production, suggesting again that B_1 and B_2 receptors may be present on endothelial cells in culture.

KININ RECEPTOR FUNCTIONS

Kinins exert a variety of biological effects both *in vivo* and *in vitro*. From *in vivo* studies it is known that kinins are potent hypotensive agents, that increase plasma extravasation and produce pain[48,20]. These effects have been attributed to activation of receptors which bring about the stimulation of various cell functions that can be evaluated and measured by *in vitro* assays. Some of these effects are summarized in Table 3.5. The most relevant pharmacological effects of kinins are on the cardiovascular system, and in particular on peripheral vessels. First of all, kinins act on endothelia promoting the release of endothelium-derived relaxing factor(s) (EDRF) and prostacyclin, two potent vasodilators which relax the arterial smooth muscles. In some peripheral vessels, for instance in the kidney, kinins act directly on the arterial smooth muscles and promote the release of prostaglandins that inhibit smooth muscle tone. Both B_1 and B_2 receptors are involved in renal arterial relaxation and appear to act by the same mechanism[29]. Thus, kinins induce relaxation of arterial vessels and lead to an increase of peripheral blood flow through indirect (via EDRF, PI_2, PG_s) or direct mechanisms (via smooth muscle receptors). Kinins are active also on the capillary endothelium, where they reduce the size of the endothelial cells and open holes in the capillary wall[49,50]. In this way kinins increase capillary permeability and favour extravasation of fluid from the blood to the intestinal fluid, through a B_2 receptor mechanism. Kinins also act directly on venous smooth muscle. Rabbit jugular veins contract in response to kinins even if the endothelium is removed. Venoconstriction may contribute to increase intracapillary pressure and plasma extravasation and may be brought about by either B_2 or B_1 receptors (Table 3.5). Kinins are the most active endogenous agents for producing pain, by acting on peripheral nerve endings of sensory fibres[48]. This action is mediated by B_2 receptors and is inhibited by B_2 antagonists in various animal models[51,52]. Any B_1 receptor participation in pain induction should be excluded, since B_1 receptor antagonists are inactive in

Table 3.5 Physiological actions of kinins and their receptors

Action	*Tissue (cell)*	*Receptor*
Vasodilatation	Endothelium, smooth muscle	B_2,B_1
Capillary permeability	Endothelium	B_2
Venoconstriction	Smooth muscle	B_2,B_1
Pain	Sensory fibres	B_2
Release of histamine	Mastocytes	*
Release of catecholamines	Sympathetic terminals	B_2
Release of prostaglandins	Various tissues	B_2,B_1*
Release of EDRF	Endothelia	B_2
Synthesis of collagen	Fibroblasts	B_1
Cell multiplication	Fibroblasts	B_1

* Non-receptor mechanism.

preventing pain evoked by kinins[52].

Similar to other peptides, kinins are potent releasers of endogenous agents, including histamine, catecholamines, prostaglandins, EDRF and leukotrienes[53–56]. These actions are extremely important in considering the possible contribution of kinins to the initiation and maintenance of the various phases of the inflammatory process. In fact, the activation of local kallikreins and the continuous supply of kallikreins from blood cells (e.g. polymorphonuclear neutrophils) generate large amounts of kinins in inflamed tissues[3,4] which persist for hours or days, because of the relatively long half-life of kallikreins[57] and the large supply of kininogens. Kinins act on their own (see Table 3.5) or by other intermediary endogenous agents (histamine, prostaglandins, leukotrienes), all of which contribute to the basic symptoms of inflammation. In this way a potent, persistent and multiplicative circle is established that can maintain the various phases of inflammation and continue to act also during the tissue repair phase. Indeed, kinins appear to be involved in the activation of fibroblasts, in cell multiplication and collagen secretion, according to Goldstein and Wall[58]. Both B_1 and B_2 receptors appear to be involved in this tissue repairing process.

MECHANISM OF ACTION OF KININS AT THE CELLULAR LEVEL

Kinin biological effects are determined by their interactions with various components of plasma membranes such as peptidases, receptors and possibly post-receptor proteins (for instance G proteins, phospholipases and protein-kinases). Through such interactions, kinins may induce changes of smooth muscle tone, or promote the release of hormones, neurotransmitters and autacoids, or stimulate ion transport in excitable tissues, including epithelia. Indirect actions are obtained through mediators (EDRF, prostaglandins, histamine, noradrenaline, etc.), while the direct ones, occurring in the same cell as the kinin receptors, are brought about by second messengers, as shown in Table 3.6.

Thus, some excitatory phenomena produced by bradykinin, such as the mobilization of Ca^{2+} and the activation of cGMP, observed in PC_{12} cells[59], the stimulation of C1 transport in rat colon[60], some effects (still not precisely identified) that may occur in rat fibroblasts[61] and possibly the contraction of the rabbit jugular vein and of other smooth muscle[62], as well as the potentiation of the electrical stimulation in the rat vas deferens[63], are presumably obtained by the following sequence of events:

$$[\text{BK-receptor}] \rightarrow \text{G-protein} \rightarrow PI_3 \rightarrow Ca^{2+} \text{ mobilization}$$

Worthy of notice is the fact that all these biological effects are mediated by B_2 receptors.

Some inhibitory effects of the kinins, such as the relaxation of the dog carotid artery, the dog renal artery, or the guinea pig trachea are indirect, since they are produced by mediators such as EDRF (dog carotid artery), prostacyclin and/or prostaglandins (dog renal artery) or by prostaglandins

Table 3.6

Tissue/cell	*Receptor*	*Biological effect*	*Mediator*	*Second messenger*	*Reference*
Neuroblastoma	B_2	Ca^{2+}	–	PI_3	59
Fibroblast (mice)	B_2	?	–	PI_3	61
Rabbit jugular vein	B_2	Contraction	–	PI_3	27
Rat colon	B_2	Cl-transport	–	PI_3	60
Rat vas deferens	B_2	Noradrenaline release	NA	PI_3	63
Dog carotid artery	B_2	Relaxation	EDRF	cGMP	28
Dog renal artery	B_2	Relaxation	PG_S	cAMP	29
Rat duodenum	B_2	Relaxation	–	cAMP	64
Guinea pig trachea	?	Relaxation	PG_S	?	65
Rat fibroblast	B_2	Release of PG_S	pG_S	cAMP	66
Sensory fibres	B_2	Stimulation	–	?	48
(a, b, c)	B_2	Stimulation	–	?	67
Rabbit aorta	B_1	Contraction	–	PI_3	26
Dog renal artery	B_1	Relaxation	PG_S	cAMP	29
Fibroblasts (man)	B_1	Collagen synthesis	–	?	58
Endothelial cells	B_1	EDRF, PGI_2 release	EDRF, PGI_2	–	46 68
Mastocytes (rat)	?	Histamine release	Hist	–	32,53

(guinea pig trachea), while the relaxation of the rat duodenum appears to be due to a direct action mediated by B_2 receptors via cAMP[64]. These inhibitory effects, including the release of prostaglandins from rat mastocytes[64], appear to be mediated also by B_2 receptors[61] with the following mechanism, exemplified for prostaglandins:

$$[\text{BK-receptor}] \rightarrow \text{Phospholipase } A_2 \rightarrow \text{Arachidonic acid} \rightarrow \text{prostaglandins}$$

B_2 receptors are therefore able to utilize a variety of mechanisms, both in terms of mediators (EDRF, PG_s, NA, etc.) or of second messengers (cAMP, cGMP, PI_3, ions). Because of this complex situation, classification of receptors should be based on classical pharmacological criteria such as the determination of the order of potency of agonists and the estimation of the apparent affinity of antagonists, two parameters that can be easily measured with biochemical and pharmacological assays.

A similar situation (multiple second messengers activated by the same receptor) appears to exist for B_1 receptors that mediate (a) the contractions of arterial and venous smooth muscle[26] (possibly through PI_3), and (b) the relaxation of arterial smooth muscle by the intermediary of prostaglandins[29]. B_1 receptors in limited numbers have been identified in endothelial cells in culture[46,47], and appear to promote the release of EDRF and prostacyclin.

B_1 receptors appear also to be involved in slow processes, such as collagen synthesis by fibroblasts and *cell multiplication*, as well as the release of interleukin 1 by macrophages[58,69]. Nothing is known, however, about the second messengers involved in these effects.

Not all effects of kinins appear to be mediated by specific receptors: for instance the release of histamine from rat peritoneal mast cells and the relaxation of the guinea pig trachea remain to be characterized: in fact, in both systems, BK, KD and some B_2 selective agonists are more active than des-Arg^9-BK: the order of potency of agonists therefore shows a typical B_2 receptor pattern. However, B_2 receptor antagonists are inactive on the trachea[65] or they act as full agonists (even more active than the kinins) on the rat peritoneal mast cells. Similar findings have been interpreted by Farmer *et al.*[70] as indicative of the existence of a B_3 receptor: Rhaleb *et al.*[65] have instead suggested that kinins may interact directly with phospholipases and promote the release of prostaglandins through a non-receptor mechanism. A similar interpretation has also been contemplated by Devillier *et al.*[32], when they suggested that BK stimulates the release of histamine from the rat peritoneal mast cells by interacting directly with protein kinase C. Future studies are needed to substantiate either the existence of a B_3 receptor type or the direct interaction by the kinins with post-receptor proteins.

PERSPECTIVES

A body of evidence supports the interpretation that the kallikrein–kinin system plays a major role in the inflammatory process. In fact, large amounts of kinins appear to be produced during the acute and chronic phases of inflammation. Kinins may be the only endogenous system which is continuously present and active at the site of inflammation. Indeed, kinins may undergo a prolonged release because of the continuous and consistent local liberation of active kallikreins (from neutrophils) which, in the inflammatory exudate, find perhaps the most favourable environment for remaining in active form. After intensive work, the methods for estimating kinins in biological fluid have become reliable and precise: numerous recent reports have established that kinin concentrations in circulating blood are extremely low, while they are high in inflammatory exudates. These peptides may therefore be considered as autacoids. At the concentrations found in inflammatory exudates, kinins are able to promote a complex and multiplicative cascade of biological effects which contribute to the rapid, exaggerated and prolonged inflammatory reaction. The contribution of the kallikrein–kinin system can be schematically presented as shown below.

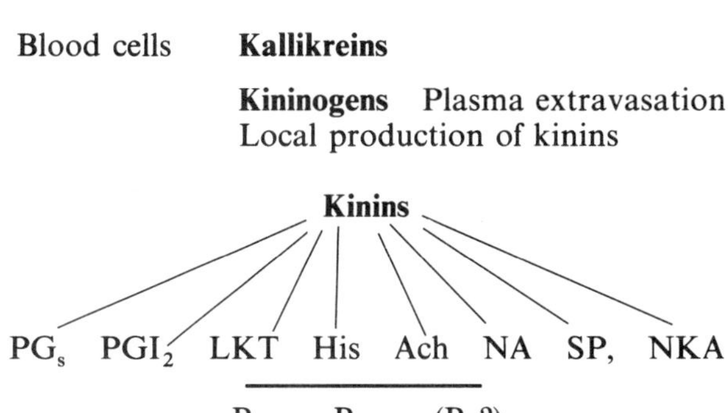

Once released, kinins exert indirect and direct effects: the former by the intermediary of other endogenous agents and the latter through direct actions on specific receptors. It does appear that kinins may play a key role in the inflammatory process, and prevention of their effects could provide an efficient means to reduce inflammatory reactions. In fact, the inhibition of kallikreins or the antagonism of kinin receptors will probably interrupt the vicious circle which initiates and maintains the activation of the numerous endogenous agents participating in the inflammatory reaction. Until now, antagonists of prostaglandins, leukotrienes, histamine, acetylcholine and neurokinins have failed to provide efficient anti-inflammatory agents, probably because the inactivation of one system is easily overcome by the others. It is hoped that the blocking of kallikreins or of kinin receptors will be more efficient because it might inactivate the 'primum movens' of the inflammatory process.

References

1. Garcia-Leme, J. (1978). Bradykinin system. *Handbook Exp. Pharmacol.*, **50(1)**, 464–522
2. Marceau, F., Lussier, A., Regoli, D. and Giroud, J. P. (1983). Pharmacology of kinins: their relevance to tissue injury and inflammation. A review. *Gen. Pharmacol.*, **14**, 209–29
3. Hori, Y., Jyoyama, H., Yamada, K., Takagi, M., Hirose, K. and Katori, M. (1988). Time course analyses of kinins and other mediators in plasma exudation of rat kaolin-induced pleurisy. *Eur. J. Pharmacol.*, **152**, 235–45
4. Tissot, M., Regoli, D. and Giroud, J. P. (1985). Bradykinin levels in inflammatory exudates. *Inflammation*, **9**, 419–24
5. Melmon, K. L., Webster, M. E., Goldfinger, S. E. and Seegmiller, J. E. (1967). The presence of a kinin in inflammatory synovial effusion from arthritides of varying etiologies. *Arthritis Rheum.*, **10**, 13–20
6. Wedmore, C. V. and Williams, T. J. (1981). Control of vascular permeability by polymorphonuclear leukocytes in inflammation. *Nature*, **289**, 646–50
7. Figueroa, C. D., McIver, A. G., Hotton, C., McKenzie, C., Dieppe, P., Whicher, J. T. and Bhoola, K. D. (1989). Presence of immunoreactive tissue kallikrein in human polymorphonuclear (PMN) leucocytes. In Moriya, H. (ed.), *Kinins V*, V247B, pp. 207–10 (New York: Plenum Press)
8. Müller-Esterl, W., Iwanaga, S. and Nakanishi, S. (1986). Kininogen revisited. *Trends Biochem. Sci.*, **11**, 336–9
9. Matheson, R. T., Miller, D. R., Lacombe, M., Han, Y. N., Iwanaga, S., Kato, H. and Wuepper, K. D. (1976). Flaujeac Factor Deficiency. Reconstitution with highly purified bovine high molecular weight kininogen and delineation of a new permeability-enhancing peptide released by plasma kallikrein from bovine high molecular weight kininogen. *J. Clin. Invest.*, **58**, 1395–406
10. Okamoto, H. and Greenbaum, L. M. (1983). Isolation and structure of T-kinin. *Biochem. Biophys. Res. Commun.*, **112**, 701–8
11. Fukushima, D., Kitamura, N. and Nakanishi, S. (1985). Nucleotide sequence of cloned cDNA for human pancreatic kallikrein. *Biochemistry*, **24**, 8037–43
12. MacDonald, R. J., Margolius, H. S. and Erdös, E. G. (1988). Molecular biology of tissue kallikreins. *Biochem. J.*, **253**, 313–21
13. Takada, Y., Skidgel, R. A. and Erdös, E. G. (1985). Purification of human urinary prokallikrein. Identification of the site of activation by the metallo-proteinase thermolysin. *Biochem. J.*, **232**, 851–8
14. Kraut, J. (1971). *Enzymes*, 3rd edn., vol. 3, pp. 165–83
15. Erdös, E. G. (1979). Kininases. *Handbook Exp. Pharmacol.*, **25**, (Suppl.), 427–48
16. Turner, A. J., Matsas, R. and Kenny, A. J. (1985). Are there neuropeptide-specific peptidases? *Biochem. Pharmacol.*, **34**, 1347–56
17. Ferreira, S. H. and Vane, J. R. (1967). The disappearance of bradykinin and eledoisin in the cirulation and vascular beds of the cat. *Br. J. Pharmacol.*, **30**, 417–24

18. Nasjletti, A., Colina-Chourio, J. and McGiff, J. C. (1975). Disappearance of bradykinin in the renal circulation of dogs. Effects of kininase inhibition. *Circ. Res.*, **37**, 59–65
19. Ward, P. E., Schultz, W., Reynolds, R. C. and Erdös, E. G. (1977). Metabolism of kinins and angiotensins in the isolated glomerulus and brush border of rat kidney. *Lab. Invest.*, 36, 599–606
20. Regoli, D. and Barabé, J. (1980). Pharmacology of bradykinin and related kinins. *Pharmacol. Rev.*, 32, 1–46
21. Rocha e Silva, M., Beraldo, W. T. and Rosenfeld, G. (1949). Bradykinin, a hypotensive and smooth muscle stimulating factor released from plasma globulin by snake venom and by trypsin. *Am. J. Physiol.*, **156**, 261–73
22. Vavrek, R. J. and Stewart, J. M. (1985). Competitive antagonists of bradykinin. *Peptides*, **6**, 161–4
23. Trautschold, I. (1970). Assay methods in the kinin system. *Handbook Exp. Pharmacol.*, **25**, 52–81
24. Horton, E. W. (1970). The estimation of urinary kallikrein. *J. Physiol.*, **148**, 267–82
25. Bertaccini, G. (1976). Active polypeptides of nonmammalian origin. *Pharmacol. Rev.*, **28**, 121–77
26. Regoli, D., Barabé, J. and Park, W. K. (1977). Receptors for bradykinin in rabbit aortae. *Can. J. Physiol. Pharmacol.*, **55**, 855–67
27. Guadreau, P., Barabé, J., St-Pierre, S. and Regoli, D. (1981). Pharmacological studies of kinins on venous smooth muscles. *Can. J. Physiol. Pharmacol.*, **59**, 371–9
28. Couture, R., Gaudreau, P., St-Pierre, S. and Regoli, D. (1980). The dog common carotid artery: a sensitive bioassay for studying vasodilator effects of substance P and of kinins. *Can. J. Physiol. Pharmacol.*, **58**, 1234–44
29. Rhaleb, N.-E., Dion, S., Barabé, J., Rouissi, N., Drapeau, G. and Regoli, D. (1989). Receptors for kinins in dog arterial vessels. *Eur. J. Pharmacol.*, **162**, 419–27
30. Regoli, D., Rhaleb, N.-E., Drapeau, G., Dion, S., Tousignant, C. and D'Orléans-Juste, P. (1988). Basic pharmacology of kinins. Pharmacologic receptors and other mechanisms. In Moriya, H. (ed), *Kinin V*, V247A, pp. 399–407 (New York: Plenum Press)
31. Schild, H. O. (1947). pA, a new scale for the measurement of drug antagonism. *Br. J. Pharmacol.*, **2**, 189–206
32. Devillier, P., Renoux, M., Drapeau, G. and Regoli, D. (1988). Histmaine release from rat peritoneal mast cells by kinin antagonists. *Eur. J. Pharmacol.*, **149**, 137–40
33. Stewart, J. M. and Vavrek, R. J. (1988). Design of bradykinin antagonists. In Marshall, G. R. (ed.), *Peptides: Chemistry and Biology*, pp. 433–7 (Leiden: Escorn)
34. Drapeau, G., Rhaleb, N.-E., Dion, S., Jukic, D. and Regoli, D. (1988). [Phe^8(CH_2-NH)Arg^9]-bradykinin, a B_2 receptor selective agonist which is not broken down by either kininase I or kininase II. *Eur. J. Pharmacol.*, **155**, 193–5
35. Reissman, S., Paegelow, I., Liebmann, C., Steinmetzger, H., Jankova, T. and Arold, H. (1977). In Papasova, M. and Atanassova, E. (eds), *Physiology and Pharmacology of Smooth Muscle*, pp. 208–17 (Sofia: Bulgarian Academy of Sciences)
36. Odya, C. E., Goodfriend, T. L. and Pena, C. (1980). Bradykinin receptor-like binding studies with iodinated analogues. *Biochem. Pharmacol.*, **29**, 175–85
37. Fredrick, M. J., Vavrek, R. J., Stewart, J. M. and Odya, C. E. (1984). Further studies of myometrial bradykinin receptor-like binding. *Biochem. Pharmacol.*, **33**, 2887–92
38. Roscher, A. A., Manganiello, V. C., Jelsema, C. L. and Moss, J. (1983). Receptors for bradykinin in intact cultured human fibroblasts. Identification and characterization by direct binding study. *J. Clin. Invest.*, **72**, 626–35
39. Tomita, K. and Pisano, I. (1984). Binding of [^{3}H]-bradykinin in isolated nephron segments of the rabbit. *Am. J. Physiol.*, **246**, F732–7
40. Fredrick, M. J., Abel, F. C., Rightsel, W. A., Muirhead, E. E. and Odya, C. E. (1985). B_2 bradykinin receptor-like binding in rat renomedullary interstitial cells. *Life Sci.*, **37**, 331–8
41. Innis, R. B., Manning, D. C., Stewart, J. M. and Snyder, S. H. (1981). [^{3}H]-Bradykinin receptor binding in mammalian tissue membranes. *Proc. Natl. Acad. Sci.*, **78**, 2630–4
42. Barabé, J., Babiuk, C. and Regoli, D. (1982). Binding of [^{3}H]-desArg^9-BK to rabbit anterior mesenteric vein. *Can. J. Physiol. Pharmacol.*, **60**, 1551–5
43. Lewis, R. E., Childers, S. R. and Phillips, M. I. (1985). [^{125}I]-Tyr-Bradykinin binding in primary rat brain cultures. *Brain Res.*, **346**, 263–72
44. Cox, H. M., Munday, K. A. and Post, J. A. (1986). Identification of selective, high affinity [^{125}I]-angiotensin and [^{125}I]-bradykinin binding sites in rat intestinal epithelia. *Br. J. Pharmacol.*, **87**, 201–9

45. Fujimara, Y., Mantione, C. R. and Yamamura, H. I. (1988). Identification of B_2 bradykinin binding sites in guinea pig brain. *Eur. J. Pharmacol.*, **147**, 487–8
46. Sung, C. P., Arleth, A. J., Kazuhisa, S. and Berkowitz, B. A. (1988). Characterization and function of bradykinin receptors in vascular endothelial cells. *J. Pharmacol. Exp. Ther.*, **247**, 8–13
47. Cahill, M., Fishman, J. B. and Olgar, P. (1988). Effect of des-arginine^9-bradykinin and other bradykinin fragments on the synthesis of prostacyclin and the binding of bradykinin by vascular cells in culture. *Agents Actions*, **24**, 224–31
48. Armstrong, D. (1970). Pain. *Handbook Exp. Pharmacol.*, **25**, 434–81
49. Gabbiani, G., Badonnel, M. C. and Majna, G. (1970). Intraarterial injections of histamine, serotonin or bradykinin: a topographic study of vascular leakage. *Proc. Soc. Exp. Biol. Med.*, **135**, 447–52
50. Roch-Arveiller, M., Giroud, J. P. and Regoli, D. (1985). Kinins and inflammation: emphasis on interactions of kinins with various cell types. In Keller, H. (ed) *Progress in Applied Microcirculation*, Vol. 7, pp. 81–95 (Basel: Karger)
51. Griesbacher, T. and Lembeck, F. (1987). Effect of bradykinin antagonists on bradykinin-induced plasma extravasation venoconstriction, prostaglandin E_2 release, nociceptor stimulation and contraction of the iris sphincter muscle in the rabbit. *Br. J. Pharmacol.*, **92**, 333–40
52. Steranka, L. R., Manning, D. C., Dehaas, C. J., Ferkany, J. W., Borosky, S. A., Connor, J. R., Vavrek, R. J., Stewart, J. M. and Snyder, S. H. (1988). Bradykinin as a pain mediator: receptors are localised to sensory neurons, and antagonists have analgesic actions. *Proc. Natl. Acad. Sci.*, **85**, 3245–9
53. Devillier, P., Renoux, M., Giroud, J. P. and Regoli, D. (1985). Peptides and histamine release from rat peritoneal mast cells. *Eur. J. Pharmacol.*, **117**, 89–96
54. Starke, K., Peskar, B. A., Schumaker, K. A. and Taube, H. D. (1977). Bradykinin and postgangliamic sympathetic transmission. *N.S. Arch. Pharmacol.*, **299**, 23–32
55. Nasjletti, A. and Malik, K. U. (1979). Relationships between the kallikrein–kinin and prostaglandin systems. *Life Sci.*, **25**, 99–110
56. D'Orléans-Juste, P., Dion, S., Mizrahi, J. and Regoli, D. (1985). Effects of peptides and nonpeptides on isolated arterial smooth muscles: role of endothelium. *Eur. J. Pharmacol.*, **114**, 9–21
57. Schachter, M. (1980). Kallikreins (kininogenases). A group of serine-proteases with bioregulatory actions. *Pharmacol. Rev.*, **31**, 1–17
58. Goldstein, R. H. and Wall, M. (1984). Activation of protein formation and cell division by bradykinin and des-Arg^9-bradykinin. *J. Biol. Chem.*, **259**, 9263–8
59. Fasolato, C., Pandiella, A., Meldolesi, J. and Pozzan, T. (1988). Generation of inositol phosphates, cytosolic Ca^{2+}, and ionic fluxes in PC12 cells treated with bradykinin. *J. Biol. Chem.*, **263**, 17350–9
60. Cuthbert, A. W. and Margolius, H. S. (1982). Kinins stimulate net chloride secetion by the rat colon. *Br. J. Pharmacol.*, **75**, 587–98
61. Burch, R. M. and Axelrod, J. (1987). Dissociation of bradykinin induced prostaglandin formation from phosphatidyl inositol turnover in Swiss 3T3 fibroblasts: evidence for G protein regulation of phospholipase A_2. *Proc. Natl. Acad. Sci.*, **84**, 6374–8
62. Regoli, D. (1982). Effects of kinins and other peptides in various smooth muscle preparations. *Agents Actions*, **9** (Suppl.), 245–51
63. Tousignant, C., Dion, S., Drapeau, G. and Regoli, D. (1987). Characterization of pre- and postjunctional receptors for neurokinins and kinins in the rat vas deferens. *Neuropeptides*, **9**, 333–43
64. Paegelow, I., Reissman, S., Victinghoff, G., Römer, W. and Arold, H. (1977). Bradykinin action in the rat duodenum through the cyclic AMP system. *Agents Actions*, **7**, 447–51
65. Rhaleb, N.-E., Dion, S., D'Orléans-Juste, P., Drapeau, G., Regoli, D. and Browne, R. E. (1988). Bradykinin antagonism: differentiation between peptide antagonists and antiinflammatory agents. *Eur. J. Pharmacol.*, **151**, 275–9
66. Canklin, B. R., Burch, R. M., Steranka, L. R. and Axelrod, J. (1988). Distinct bradykinin receptors mediate stimulation of prostaglandin synthesis by endothelial cells and fibroblasts. *J. Pharmacol. Exp. Ther.*, **244**, 646–9
67. Staszewska-Wolley, J., Wolley, G. and Regoli, D. (1988). Specific receptors for bradykinin-induced cardiac sympathetic chemoreflexes in the dog. *Eur. J. Pharmacol.*, **156**, 309–14

68. D'Orléans-Juste, P., De Nucci, G. and Vane, J. R. (1989). Kinins act on B_1 and B_2 receptors to release conjointly endothelium-derived relaxing factor and prostacyclin from bovine aortic endothelial cells. *Br. J. Pharmacol.*, **96**, 920–6
69. Tiffany, C. W. and Bursch, R. M. (1989). Bradykinin stimulates tumn necrosis factor and interleukin 1 release from macrophages. *FEBS Lett.* **247**, 189–92
70. Farmer, S. G., Burch, R. M., Meeker, S. N. and Wilkins, D. E. (1989). Evidence for a pulmonary B bradykinin receptor. *Mol. Pharmacol.*, **36**, 1–8
71. Kaplan, A., Kay, A. B. and Austen, K. F. (1972). A prealbunin activator of prekallikrein. III. Appearance of chemstactic activity for human neutrophils by the conversion of human prekallikrein to kallikrein. *J. Exp. Med.*, **135**, 81–97

4
Role of cellular proteinases and their protein inhibitors in inflammation

J. F. WOESSNER, Jr

INTRODUCTION

If immunological events are the trigger for inflammation, then proteinases provide the resultant explosions. The classic signs of inflammation: dolor, rubor, calor, and turgor are all dependent for their production on the action of proteolytic enzymes. There is no possibility of reviewing all of the proteinases involved in inflammation in a single chapter. There are literally scores of enzymes that would have to be considered. In order to reduce the number of proteases to a manageable size the following have been omitted in their entirety: all blood clotting factors, all complement factors (covered in Chapter 2 of this volume), the clot lysing system including plasmin and plasminogen activators, and all proteases that function intracellularly and do not escape to the exterior during inflammation. This latter group includes most membrane-bound proteases and cytoplasmic enzymes such as the calpains.

I propose, then, to consider chiefly those proteinases found within granules of inflammatory cells. The inflammatory cells to be considered, each in a separate section, will be the polymorphonuclear leukocyte, the macrophage/monocyte, the mast cell and the lymphocyte. Fibroblasts, which play an important repair function in inflammation, will not be treated. With respect to proteinase inhibitors, only those which are protein in nature and which are found at the site of inflammation will be considered. These will include the protein inhibitors of the plasma, those of the tissue or tissue secretions, and those produced by the inflammatory cells themselves. An excellent review of such inhibitors may be found in various chapters in the monograph on proteinase inhibitors[1].

Proteinases and proteases

It has been proposed by Barrett and McDonald[2] that the term 'protease' be applied to all hydrolytic enzymes that cleave the peptide bond, regardless of the position of the bond within the peptide. This large group can then be divided into endopeptidases (proteinases) that cleave internally, at least three residues away from either end of large polypeptides, and exopeptidases that cleave at or close to the C- or N-terminal residues. In this review only endopeptidases will be considered. Common usage in the field is to use the terms 'proteinase' and 'protease' interchangeably for the endopeptidases, and that will be the practice here.

The proteinases can be conveniently divided into four classes:[3] the serine, cysteine, aspartic and metalloproteinases. This division is based on the nature of the key catalytic group at the active centre. Thus, in the serine proteinases, a covalent bond is formed between a serine residue at the active site of the enzyme and the peptide to be cleaved. The Enzyme Commission has assigned numbers to each of the well-characterized proteinases based on the specificity of the bonds they cleave[4,5]. These will be indicated in the text for each enzyme, when available. A useful glossary, giving a brief description of each proteinase, is provided by Barrett and McDonald[6].

Proteinase substrates

The proteinases released by inflammatory cells must, by definition, act on substrates in the extracellular space. The major proteins that will be encountered there will be the components of the extracellular matrix, the connective tissue macromolecules. In addition there will be many proteins that have diffused in from the blood, including clotting factors, hormones, and protease inhibitors. Finally, there will be components on the exterior surfaces of cells and even cell receptors for some of the proteinases.

The connective tissue matrix components have not received as much attention as they deserve with respect to their role in inflammation, due in part to the fact that a great number of these components have been characterized only in the past few years. The major component of the matrix is the fibrous protein collagen. Currently, the family of collagens comprises at least 13 members derived from more than 20 distinct genes. Full details of current knowledge of the collagens may be found in the book of Mayne and Burgeson[7]. The interstitial collagens (types I, II and III) form long thin fibrils whose individual molecules have uninterrupted triple helical structures (Figure 4.1). These molecules are most difficult to digest, and require the action of interstitial collagenases[8]. The collagenases typically produce only a single cleavage in the molecule about one-quarter of the way in from the C-terminus. The resultant fragments undergo denaturation at body temperature to form gelatin, which is further digested by gelatinases (Figure 4.1). The basement membrane contains type IV collagen, which is a more complex molecule with non-helical domains that are less resistant to proteolysis. Gelatinases can attack this molecule, as well as type V collagen, a pericellular form[9]. The collagens numbered VI–XIII have not been studied in detail with respect to damage during inflammation, in part because they are present in relatively small amounts. This does not mean that they are unimportant, however. Thus, type IX collagen is found to coat interstitial collagen fibres of type II, and is postulated to regulate fibre size and interactions[10]. When inflammatory cells move to sites of inflammation they typically must degrade basement membranes and interstitial collagens to reach the site of action[11]. This degradation may not be totally controlled, so that excessive damage results, producing swollen tissue, infiltrated with blood and containing chemotactic and immunogenic peptides.

Elastin is a globular protein that is assembled into a fibrous meshwork by covalent crosslinks, the desmosines (Figure 4.1)[12,13]. The hydrophobic nature of elastin and the high density of crosslinks renders this protein also quite difficult to digest, but elastases can hydrolyse it readily. Elastases are not so specific as the collagenases, and are not, as their name might suggest, limited to digesting elastin; rather, they can attack a wide variety of other proteins.

There are many different proteoglycans in the matrix. Current knowledge is summarized in Wight and Mecham[14]. The best-characterized proteoglycan is that of articular cartilage (Figure 4.1). This proteoglycan is a very large molecule of M_r 2 500 000, having a core protein of about M_r 220 000 and about 250 glycosaminoglycan and carbohydrate side-chains. Other proteoglycans include dermatan sulphate and, on the cell surface, heparan sulphate. Most of these are readily susceptible to proteolytic degradation by a wide variety of non-specific proteases. The carbohydrate portions are more resistant, and are usually degraded intracellularly in the lysosomal compartment.

Finally, a great many glycoproteins have been described in recent years; those of the cartilage and bone alone fill a sizeable table[15]. Fibronectin[16] has often been considered in relation to inflammatory changes, and it is likely that many more glycoproteins will be also involved. Fibronectin (Figure 4.1) can form bridges between the fibrous framework of the matrix and the cells due to binding domains with specificity for collagen, heparan sulphate and cell receptors (integrins). Other glycoproteins are involved in attachment of cells to other matrix components and to one another. Disruption of these interactions by proteolysis leads to disorganization of the tissue and release of cells from their site of anchorage within the tissue.

The consequences of the action of proteinases on the connective matrix will be manifold. The basement membrane and vessel wall will be disrupted, resulting in redness, swelling and extravasation of blood products such as clotting factors and kinins. Collagen fibrils will be disrupted, leading to tissue swelling, distortion and loss of mechanical function. Finally, the various degradation products and denatured matrix molecules may act as immunogens and chemotactic agents.

POLYMORPHONUCLEAR LEUKOCYTES

Role of the PMN cells

The neutrophil defends the body against invading pathogens. In response to invasion these cells become activated and pass through the capillary walls

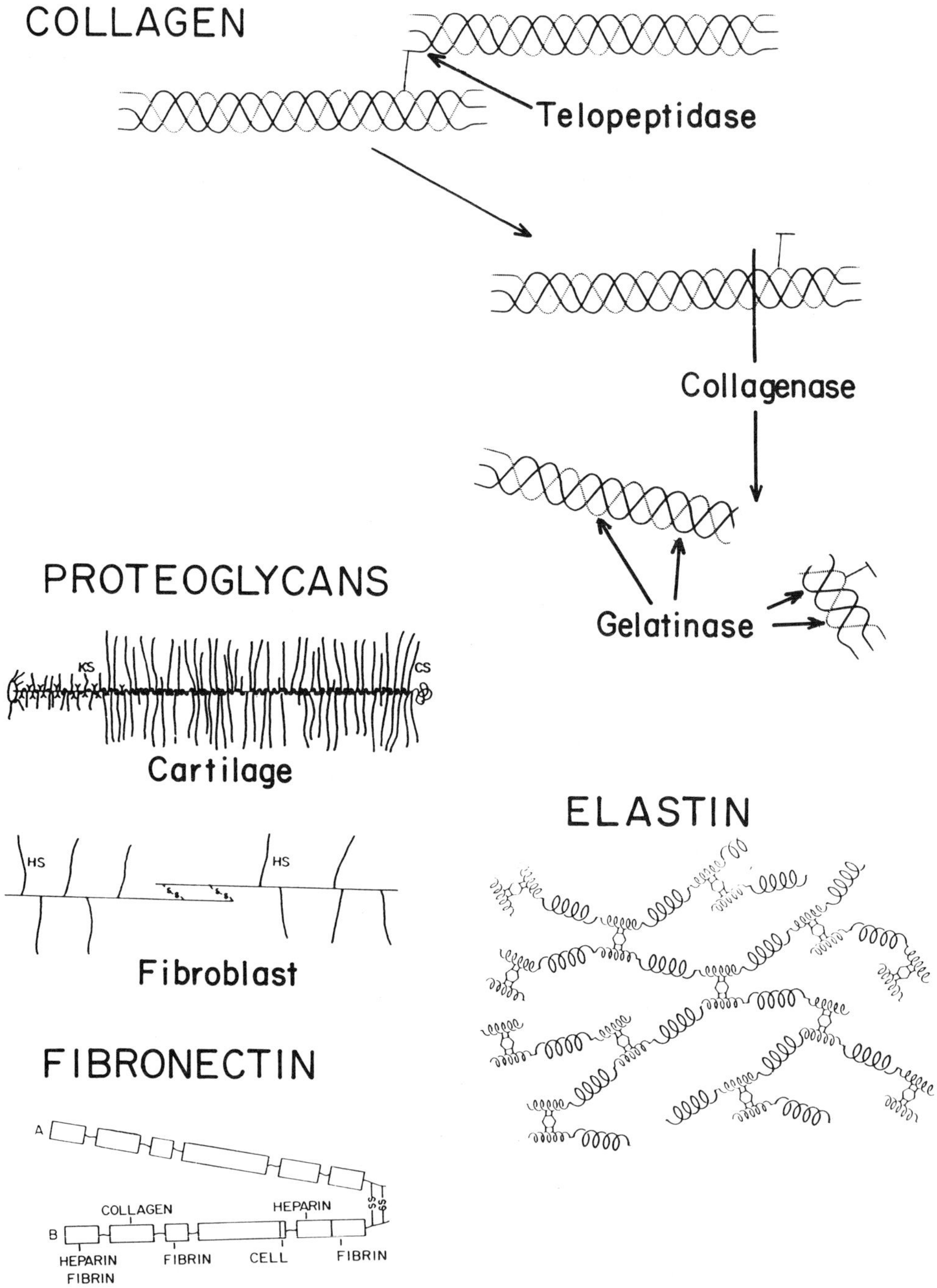
COLLAGEN
Telopeptidase
Collagenase
Gelatinase
PROTEOGLYCANS
KS
CS
Cartilage
HS
HS
Fibroblast
ELASTIN
FIBRONECTIN
A
B
COLLAGEN
HEPARIN
SS
SS
HEPARIN
FIBRIN
FIBRIN
CELL
FIBRIN

and along chemotactic gradients to the foreign material. This material is then phagocytosed and degraded intracellularly by a combination of oxidants and hydrolytic enzymes. The PMN cells are the first to arrive at sites of acute inflammation; indeed, these cells serve as a histological indicator of an inflammatory response[17]. These cells have a powerful battery of proteolytic enzymes able to digest a wide variety of substrates. Since these cells are not very active in protein synthesis, most of their proteinases are synthesized prior to terminal differentiation and stored in cytoplasmic granules[17]. A listing of these enzymes is given in Table 4.1.

The enzyme-containing granules are of several types (azurophil, specific and C-particle) which may be important for the selective release of different activities. The primary granules (azurophilic) are analogous to lysosomes, but contain neutral proteases and myeloperoxidase in addition to acid hydrolases. The secondary granules (specific) are formed at intermediate stages of neutrophil maturation and are more readily exocytosed.[17] These contain the metalloproteinases, which are released to enable the cells to penetrate the capillary walls and the intervening connective tissue matrix on the way to their targets. Some of the most powerful proteases, elastase and cathepsin G, degrade ingested materials, but part of this activity is released, perhaps only incidentally, during the phagocytic events. The various released proteases appear to be important in inflammation. A brief review of the role of human neutrophil proteases in inflammation is found in Rest[18].

Leukocyte elastase

Discussion of neutrophil proteinases will be limited to those of the human, unless otherwise noted. Leukocyte elastase (EC 3.4.21.37) is similar to the

Table 4.1 Polymorphonuclear leukocyte granule proteinases

Granule	*Proteinase*	*Class*
Azurophil	Leukocyte elastase	Serine
	Cathepsin G	Serine
	Proteinase 3	Serine
	Cathepsin B	Cysteine
	Cathepsin D	Aspartic
Specific	Collagenase	Metallo
C-particle	Gelatinase, 72 kD	Metallo
?	Gelatinase, 92 kD	Metallo

Figure 4.1 (*Opposite*) Macromolecules of the connective tissue matrix. *Collagen*: two molecules joined by a covalent crosslink represent the fibrillar structure. Telopeptidase would solubilize the fibril without cutting the helix. Collagenase cuts the helix into two fragments, which become denatured and susceptible to gelatinase attack. *Proteoglycans*: CS, KS and HS refer to chondroitin sulphate, keratan sulphate and heparan sulphate. Y, *N*-linked oligosaccharides; ●, *O*-linked oligosaccharides. *Fibronectin*: binding domains are indicated together with their ligands. The A chain contains corresponding domains. *Elastin*: large helices represent putative beta-coils, small helices represent alpha-helices, hexagons represent desmosine crosslinks.

well-known elastase of the pancreas (EC 3.4.21.36), but it is a different gene product with distinctive properties of its own. The enzyme was first clearly identified by Janoff and Scherer[19]. It is a serine proteinase of M_r 27 000–31 000; as many as five isozyme forms may be found in one preparation due to variable carbohydrate content. The pH optimum for elastin digestion is 8.5, but extensive activity remains at physiological pH. In addition to elastin, a variety of matrix components is cleaved including proteoglycan[20], type I collagen of tendon[21], type III collagen[22], type IV collagen[23], fibronectin[24] and telopeptides of type I collagen[25]. Elastase has been localized to the azurophil granule by density gradient centrifugation[26]. Damiano *et al.*[27] are able to distinguish azurophil granules containing myeloperoxidase from those containing elastase: of 1500 granules/cell, only 400 contain elastase.

Recently, the cDNA sequence and gene structure of human elastase has been described[28]. The initially synthesized protein has 267 amino acid residues of which 27 and 20 are ultimately cleaved from the N- and C-termini, respectively. A further two residues are cleaved from the amino-end in a final activation step that yields a 218-residue active enzyme. The mRNA for elastase is not found in neutrophils or blood monocytes, but only in progenitor cells in the bone marrow[29]. This indicates that elastase must be synthesized and stored before the final step of cell maturation. The X-ray crystal structure of elastase[30] has been resolved at 2.3 Å; it is similar to that of pancreatic elastase.

Elastase appears to play a central role in contributing to inflammatory reactions. In addition to the matrix substrates listed above, it has been noted to degrade fibrinogen[31], complement factors[32], IgG[33], kininogen (to give a bradykinin-like peptide)[34], clotting factors VIII, XII, XIII[35] and IXa and Xa[36], and apolipoprotein A2[37]. Elastase also produces met-enkephalin[38], activates prorenin to renin[39] and destroys clot-promoting activity of high M_r kininogen[40]. The release of elastase from the leukocyte is triggered by many reactions. Cells that phagocytose zymosan particles or immune complexes release up to 25% of their elastase[41]. Antigen–antibody complexes, lipopolysaccharide and concanavalin A all stimulate release of elastase but not of cathepsin[42].

In view of the extensive degradative abilities of elastase, one would expect multiple inhibitors to regulate its activity (see Table 4.2 for a listing of proteinase inhibitors). The PMN cells themselves produce a cytosolic inhibitor of M_r 42 000[43]. This is a member of the serpin (*ser*ine *p*roteinase *in*hibitor) family that binds covalently to the enzyme. The presumed function of this inhibitor is to protect the cell from any enzyme that may escape internally from the granules. Two inhibitors are found in plasma. Alpha$_2$-macroglobulin is an inhibitor of M_r 760 000 that acts by physically and covalently entrapping elastase after it has produced a proteolytic cleavage at a specific peptide bond in the bait region of α_2-macroglobulin[44]. The plasma also contains the inhibitor α_1-proteinase inhibitor (α_1-PI), also commonly known as α_1-antitrypsin (α_1-AT). This is a powerful inhibitor of elastase of M_r 52 000 that is also a member of the serpin family. Both inhibitors are of similar efficacy, but the concentration of α_1-PI makes it quantitatively more important[45]. Close contact of PMN cells with their substrate may physically exclude α_1-PI and α_2-macroglobulin, preventing inhibition[24]. The

PMN cells secrete hypochlorous acid and chloramines that oxidize the methionine at the inhibitory center of α_1-PI, thereby protecting secreted elastase in the vicinity of the cell from inhibition by α_1-PI[46]. However, this protection is not complete, since the circulating levels of elastase–α_1-PI complexes provide a good index of inflammation[47]. Elastase cleaves α_2-plasmin inhibitor, $C\bar{1}$ inhibitor[48], and antithrombin III[49], so these plasma components are not inhibitory. However, the inter-α-trypsin inhibitor can block elastase[50].

The bronchi, salivary glands, etc. contain a leukoproteinase inhibitor of M_r 11 000[51]. α_1-PI will compete against this inhibitor and can even cause dissociation of the elastase–leukoproteinase inhibitor complex[52]. The amino acid sequence of this inhibitor shows two domains of 54 residues each, the C-domain binds elastase and the N-domain binds trypsin and cathepsin G[53]. Again, myeloperoxidase can destroy this inhibitor so that elastase can continue its action in the vicinity of the cell[54]. Yet another way of inactivating elastase is accomplished by macrophages, which bind elastase to surface receptors and internalize it[55].

There is an extensive literature on the role of leukocyte elastase in inflammatory reactions. Its role in emphysema is summarized in Taylor and Mittman[56] and Travis[57]. The absence of α_1-PI in certain individuals (P_iZZ homozygotes) shows the importance of elastase–inhibitor balance in preventing tissue damage. Elastase is also implicated in rheumatoid arthritis[58] and adult respiratory distress syndrome[59].

Table 4.2 Protein inhibitors of proteinases: a listing of inhibitors discussed in this chapter

Source	*Name*	*Class inhibited*
Plasma	α_2-Macroglobulin	All
	α_1-Proteinase inhibitor	Serine
	α_1-Antichymotrypsin	Serine
	Antithrombin III	Serine
Tissues	Leukoproteinase inhibitor	Serine
	TIMP, Tissue inhibitor of metalloproteinases	Metallo
	TIMP-2	Metallo
	Aprotinin, pancreatic trypsin inhibitor	Serine
	Cystatin	Cysteine
Leukocyte	PMN cytosolic inhibitor	Serine
Macrophage	α_1-Proteinase inhibitor	Serine
	α_2-Macroglobulin	All
	TIMP	Metallo
Mast cell	Trypstatin	Serine
	Aprotinin	Serine
T-lymphocyte	Lymphocyte proteinase inhibitor 1	Serine
	α_1-Proteinase inhibitor	Serine
	Cystatin	Cysteine

Cathepsin G

Cathepsin G (EC 3.4.21.20) is a chymotrypsin-like enzyme reported in human PMN granules by Schmidt and Havemann[60] and given its name by Starkey and Barrett[61]. Its M_r is 30 000 and its pH optimum is 7.5. The cDNA sequence of cathepsin G is only 36% identical to that of leukocyte elastase, but is 47% identical to that of rat mast cell protease II, and 56% to mouse cytotoxic T lymphocytic protease[62]. Although no specific function has been assigned to cathepsin G to date, it no doubt acts together with elastase in the killing and digestion of engulfed microbes. However, inactivated enzyme also is bactericidal, apparently due to the extremely basic nature of the protein (pI = 10)[63]. Cathepsin G may be important in the generation and control of inflammation, and in the accompanying remodelling of the connective tissues[62]. Kruse-Jarres and Kinzelmann[64] review its role in inflammation: cathepsin G and elastase appear to work peripherally where blood flow is good, whereas acid cathepsins are limited to the oxygen-poor centre. Many of the factors that cause cells to release elastase also cause the release of cathepsin G.

This inflammatory role is due in part to the ability of cathepsin G to degrade various substrates such as cartilage proteoglycan[65], link protein[66], telopeptides of collagen[67], fibrinogen[68], fibronectin[69], IgG and IgM[33], prothrombin[70] and complement factors 3 and 5[71]. Further contributions to inflammation may be caused by the enzyme's ability to activate latent leukocyte collagenase[72] and to convert angiotensinogen[73] or angiotensin I to angiotensin II[74]. Cathepsin G also has limited action on elastin[75] but does not cause emphysema when instilled in guinea pig lungs[76].

Among the plasma proteinase inhibitors, the most effective are α_2-macroglobulin and α_1-antichymotrypsin (a glycoprotein of M_r 68 000 which binds with 1:1 stoichiometry)[77]. α_1-PI is less effective; in fact, much of the inhibitor is enzymatically modified to a 50 kD inactive form[78]. The tissue leukoproteinase inhibitor is also effective, as mentioned in the previous section. Cathepsin G, like elastase, can be cleared from inflamed tissues by binding tightly to receptors of low specificity on macrophages and being internalized[79].

Leukocyte collagenase (EC 3.4.24.34)

In addition to the serine proteinases of the azurophil granule, the PMN cells also contain a battery of metalloproteinases in the specific granules and C-particles. The first of these to be discovered was leukocyte collagenase[80], a latent enzyme of M_r 70 000 shown to be in specific granules[81]. The latent enzyme can be activated by trypsin or organomercurials[82], and by cathepsin G[72]. In distinction to other collegenases, the leukocyte proenzyme can also be activated by sulphydryl-binding reagents[83], disulphide exchange[84] and hypochlorous acid[11]. This is currently interpreted as pointing to a cysteine residue that binds to the zinc of the active centre; various reactions of this cysteine cause it to be dislodged, thereby exposing the active centre[85]. The leukocyte enzyme is immunologically distinct from tissue collagenases[86]. A

76 000 kD serine 'collagenase' was reported by Ohlsson, but was later found to lack action on intact collagen molecules[87].

Various agents such as phorbol esters and chemotactic peptides cause release of collagenase from the specific granules[88]. The enzyme is elevated in synovial fluid from rheumatoid arthritis patients[89] and in osteoarthritic cartilage[90]. Once released from the cells the enzyme may do extensive damage to the interstitial collagens. Its relative efficacy in degrading collagens of types I, II and III has been reviewed by Hasty *et al.*[91].

Gelatinases (EC 3.4.24.35 and 3.4.24.24)

In addition to collagenase, PMN cells contain two gelatinases of 92 and 72 kD mass[8]. These have been variously described as type IV collagenases (both species) and type V collagenase (92 kD), since they degrade native collagen of these types (basement membrane and pericellular) as well as gelatins of many collagen types. Sopata and Dancewicz noted the latent 72 kD form in 1974[92]; it has no action on casein, elastin, haemoglobin or histone. This enzyme is localized to the C-particles[93]. This gelatinase degrades type IV collagen and basement membrane[94]. The 92-kD gelatinase also digests type V collagen, but has only low activity on casein and albumin[95]. It is not always possible to tell in a given reference which gelatinase is being considered, since the molecular weight determinations are variable due to aggregation and combination with other proteins. SDS-PAGE is required for accurate determination.

It is found that the 92-kD gelatinase occurs as a complex with TIMP, the *t*issue *i*nhibitor of *m*etallo*p*roteinases, and the 72 kD gelatinase, as a complex with TIMP-2. These inhibitor molecules are bound stoichiometrically to the enzymes, but apparently not directly at the active centre which is still in the proenzyme (or concealed) form[95]. When the enzymes are activated they can be further inhibited by adding additional TIMP. Activation by trypsin is generally poor. However, PMN cells generate hypochlorous acid which is a good activator[96]. Thus, the cells can directly regulate the enzyme activity. In the rat, mast cell protease can also activate latent gelatinase[97].

The collagenases and gelatinases are readily inhibited by α_2-macroglobulin[98]. This is surprising in that collagenase has a very circumscribed specificity. Nonetheless, there is a sequence in the bait region of α_2-macroglobulin that is readily susceptible to collagenase cleavage, followed by conformational change and trapping of the enzyme. In addition, most tissues contain TIMP. This is a glycoprotein of M_r 28 500 that is stable to heat and acid, but sensitive to reduction and alkylation[99,100]. It forms a 1:1 complex with the metalloproteinases (or 2:1 in case of 92 kD gelatinase). However, the mechanism of inhibition is not yet clear. In osteoarthritic cartilage the tissue levels of TIMP are not high; elevated metalloproteinase activity may overcome inhibition and produce tissue damage[101].

Weiss and Peppin[11] believe that the metalloproteinases are not important in killing microbes, due to their unusual specificities. Rather, they may be important in the movement of PMN cells to the site of an inflammatory stimulus. The circulating neutrophil must leave the vessel, penetrate through the interstitial matrix and ingest the microbe. The types IV and V collagenases would be useful in penetrating the endothelial cells and basement membrane, whereas the collagenase of interstitial type would be needed to get through the matrix containing types I and III (or type II in cartilage) collagen. It is important that these enzymes be released by separate mechanisms. The response of PMN cells to chemotaxins has been measured *in vitro*. At low concentrations the cells release only gelatinase, but then at higher levels, as would be found when cells near their target, both gelatinase and collagenase are released[88,102]. The azurophil enzymes would not be released during these steps. When the cells arrive at their target, phagocytosis of microbes will release further amounts of metalloproteinases. These have the potential for causing extensive damage to the extracellular matrix, as in fulminating arthritis.

Other proteinases

The PMN azurophil granules contain lysosomal proteases such as cathepsins B (EC 3.4.22.1) and D (EC 3.4.23.5). Cathepsin D has been purified to homogeneity from PMN cells[103]. The digestion of proteoglycan by cathepsin B and D is much poorer than that by cathepsin[104]. The role of acid cathepsins in inflammation was reviewed by the present author[105] in 1979, and there has been little activity in this field since that time.

A third serine enzyme of the leukocyte was recognized by Baggliolini *et al.* in 1978[106] and named proteinase 3. This enzyme was recently purified and was shown to produce emphysema when introduced into the trachea of guinea pigs[107].

MACROPHAGE

Role of the macrophage

By 'macrophage' is meant the mononuclear phagocyte system, with particular reference to the monocytes and macrophages. Unanue and Allen[108] have reviewed the functions of this system. Macrophages are involved in phagocytosis of extracellular proteins and polysaccharides, including those still attached to infectious and foreign agents. They interact with the T lymphocytes as part of the cellular immune response. They are activated by lymphokines, particularly interferon-gamma, to become microbicidal and tumoricidal. In other words, they are involved in the infectious process, immune regulation and inflammation.

Proteolytic activity is implicated in each of these functions (see Table 4.3 for a listing of macrophage proteases). When phagocytosis occurs there is some release (10–25%) of the lysosomal enzymes to the exterior of the cell; certain agents such as zymosan and asbestos cause much greater release[109]. Particles that cause selective release of lysosomal enzymes lead to chronic inflammation[109]. The phagocytosed materials are digested internally, but part is salvaged from degradation and made accessible to T cells by presentation on the macrophage surface. The lysosomal system is presumably important in preparing these denatured and partly digested antigens[108]. When monocytes leave the blood and pass into the tissue to become macrophages, they must penetrate the basement membrane[109], by a process that involves several proteases. When macrophages are stimulated by interferon-gamma from T cells or other factors, they develop cytotoxicity which involves a series of complex reactions involving secretion of cytotoxic proteases[110]. Activation also results in increased secretion of collagenase, acid hydrolases, and plasminogen activator, but decreased release of elastase[110]. Such proteases may also be important in removing tissue debris and in wound repair.

Cytotoxic protease(s)

The macrophage has important microbicidal and tumoricidal functions, which follow its activation by T cells. It is necessary that the macrophage be in physical contact with the target cells to initiate a cytotoxic event. However, once contact is made, soluble factors are released that possess a direct cytotoxic effect[111]. Thus, mouse peritoneal macrophages are activated by bacillus BCG and then release neutral proteases that lyse sarcoma target cells[112,113]. Bovine pancreatic trypsin inhibitor blocks lysis; this indicates that a serine protease is involved. Inflammatory macrophages treated with concanavalin A do not produce lysis, but they do produce lysis when stimulated with lipopolysaccharide[112,113]. Johnson and Pizzo[114] distinguish three proteases secreted by mouse macrophages: plasminogen activator, neutral caseinase and cytolytic protease. If complexes of proteases and α_2-macroglobulin bind to cell receptors, secretion of all three proteases is suppressed. The cytolytic protease(s) are inhibited by soybean trypsin inhibitor[115], elastatinal and chymostatin[116]. These results are consistent with the action of a chymotrypsin-like protease, perhaps of the type described by Rojas-Espinosa *et al.*[117], but no definitive purification appears to have been carried out to date.

Table 4.3 Macrophage proteinases

Proteinase	*Class*
Cytolytic protease(s)	Serine
Plasminogen activator	Serine
Cathepsin B	Cysteine
Cathepsin H	Cysteine
Cathepsin L	Cysteine
Cathepsin D	Aspartic
Collagenase	Metallo
Gelatinase, 72 kD	Metallo
Gelatinase, 92 kD	Metallo
Macrophage elastase	Metallo

Lysosomal protease

The macrophage contains a rich complement of lysosomal proteases of the aspartic and cysteine classes. In the rat the thiol cathepsins B (EC 3.4.22.1), H (EC 3.4.22.16), and L (EC 3.4.22.15) are synthesized and processed to one-chain and two-chain active forms; the cell releases 40% of procathepsins B and L, and 10% of H without processing[118]. The rat macrophage has about 5 times more cathepsin B than L, and its level of L is 5 times that of the neutrophil and 10 times that of the lymphocyte[119]. However, cathepsin D (EC 3.4.23.5) is still more prominent[120]. The transformation of monocytes to macrophages is accompanied by a considerable increase in lysosomal proteases. Thus, in the rat the increase is 25-fold in cathepsin D[121] and 8-fold in cathepsin B[122]. In humans, cathepsin L is not detected in monocytes, but is prominent in alveolar macrophages[123]. The lysosomal system is of particular importance in digesting phagocytosed materials including proteins, polysaccharides and lipids. This system may also be important, due to its acid pH, in denaturing proteins preparatory to presenting them as antigens to the T cells.

In addition to their role in intracellular digestion, the lysosomal proteases will also be released both during processing, as mentioned above, and accompanying phagocytosis[124]. It is often postulated that such released enzymes may damage the extracellular matrix; for example, cathepsins B and L may be implicated in elastin degradation in human emphysema[125,126]. However, Werb *et al.*[127] do not find degradation of elastin and collagen-containing matrices by lysosomal proteases unless the pH is around 5. A simple spillage of the enzymes may not be deleterious to the highly resistant proteins such as collagen and elastin, but there are other matrix components that would be more readily attacked, such as proteoglycans and glycoproteins. However, the macrophage lysosomes may have an important role in matrix degradation in cases where the cell comes in direct contact with the substrate. Thus Roberts and Dean[128] find that macrophages degrade cartilage matrix, but only if in direct contact with the cartilage fragment. Silver *et al.*[129] showed by means of microelectrodes that the pH beneath adherent macrophages, especially beneath cell clumps, may fall as low as 3.7. They postulate a role in collagen degradation for such macrophages, which may release lysosomal cysteine cathepsins into this confined space between the cell and the matrix. Loss of enzyme and acidifying molecules, and entry of inhibitors, would be limited by the relative impermeability of the matrix.

Macrophage metalloproteinases

The macrophage possesses a battery of proteases of the metalloproteinase class, specifically designed to digest the various components of the extracellular matrix. One point where such enzymes may come into play is during the penetration of the basement membrane and the underlying extracellular matrix when the monocyte leaves the blood vessel to take up residence in the tissue. The first member of this class of proteinases to be discovered was interstitial collagenase (EC 3.4.24.7), i.e. collagenase that digests types I, II and III collagens. Collagenase was first shown to be elaborated by guinea pig macrophages stimulated with endotoxin[130]. There is a complex array of signalling factors that regulate the macrophage production of collagenase; these have been reviewed recently by Wahl[131]. Endotoxins and lymphokines initiate a chain of reactions involving prostaglandins, cyclic AMP, putrescine, etc. that leads to collagenase synthesis and secretion. Inhibitors of this sequence include indomethacin, colchicine, retinoic acid, and dexamethasone. Macrophages are prominent in chronic inflammatory lesions such as rheumatoid arthritis and periodontitis; collagenase may play an important role in tissue destruction that accompanies such inflammation. It is frequently concluded that the major role of macrophages in matrix breakdown is to produce cytokines in order to stimulate fibroblasts to release large amounts of collagenase, which then accomplishes most of the digestion. However, Cury *et al.*[132] show that with proper stimulus human alveolar macrophages secrete as much as 20% of the amount of collagenase that fibroblasts produce. Monocytes and U-937 cells also secrete collagenase, although not as much as do macrophages[133]. All three cells also secrete a collagenase inhibitor, TIMP[133].

In 1980, Mainardi *et al.*[134] reported a new type of collagenase, Type V collagenase, from rabbit alveolar macrophages. This enzyme cuts type V collagen into three fragments and also digests gelatins prepared from collagens of type I and V. More recent study shows a similar enzyme in human alveolar macrophages with M_r 92 000. The enzyme crossreacts with an antibody to the 72 kD gelatinase of macrophages; this points to the presence of some common epitopes[135]. Welgus *et al.*[136] showed that human mononuclear cells can produce both 72 kD gelatinase, sometimes referred to as type IV collagenase, and 92 kD gelatinase (type V collagenase), in addition to interstitial collagenase and the proteoglycan-degrading metalloprotease, stromelysin. Lipopolysaccharide stimulates the production of all of these metalloenzymes. U-937 cells and monocytes produce only 92 kD gelatinase and collagenase, whereas alveolar macrophages produce all four enzymes. Various reports of proteoglycan-digesting activity in macrophages have appeared since the early work of Hauser and Vaes[137]; however, there has been insufficient purification to determine the exact nature of these activities. Some reports may have been occasioned by elastase activity (see below); but most likely stromelysin is the responsible enzyme, as suggested by the finding of Welgus *et al.*[136].

Macrophage elastase

Although this enzyme is a metalloproteinase, it is not clear whether it is to be classified with the matrix metalloproteinases discussed in the previous section. It has not been shown to occur in latent form, and it has not yet been identified with any of the matrix metalloproteinases for which the cDNA sequence is known. Macrophage elastase was first described in detail by Banda and Werb[138], who purified the enzyme from mouse macrophages. Three isozymes were noted with M_r 22 000. The enzyme was clearly a metalloproteinase that required both calcium ions (extrinsic) and zinc ions (intrinsic) for activity. No latent form was found, although activity increased 800% during the purification process. The enzyme was not inhibited by TIMP, but was inhibited by serum and by α_2-macroglobulin. Secretion of this enzyme is modulated by IgG receptors on the macrophage surface[139]. Macrophage elastase readily cleaves and inactivates α_1-PI at the Pro^{357}–Met^{358} bond. Cleavage cannot occur if the methionine is first oxidized[140]. The carboxy-terminal peptide released serves as a powerful chemoattractant for neutrophils[141]. This metalloproteinase is found in rat, mouse and human macrophages. Whether the digestion of elastin is a major function remains moot. Its secretion during phagocytosis suggests a broader role. The enzyme also digests IgG, fibronectin, myelin basic protein and other substrates[142].

The metal-dependent elastase makes its appearance in mature macrophages. In human monocytes it is found that 90% of the cell protease is a serine elastase of M_r 30 000 that crossreacts with an antibody to neutrophil elastase[143]. This enzyme is also expressed on the cell surface[144]; but upon transformation to the macrophage there is a shift from the serine elastase to the metalloelastase[145]. The human metalloelastase is inhibited by TIMP and an antibody to TIMP prevents this inhibition[146]. The presence in the macrophage of collagenase, gelatinases, stromelysin and elastase means that this cell is able to digest all major components of the extracellular matrix. This would be of importance when the cell enters the tissue from the vessels and penetrates through the tissue to sites of inflammation or foreign cells.

Proteinase inhibitors of the macrophage

Three distinct types of inhibitor have been reported for macrophages. White *et al.*[147] noted that cultured rat macrophages secreted α_1-PI. This inhibitor has also been found in guinea pig[148] and human[149] macrophages, although it does not appear to make a major contribution to the serum level of this inhibitor. Elastases (of the serine type) stimulate human mononuclear phagocytes to produce α_1-PI; lipopolysaccharide has a similar effect[150]. The role of this inhibitor in regulating any proteinases of the macrophage is not clear.

The human macrophage is reported to produce both α_2-macroglobulin and TIMP, the tissue inhibitor of metalloproteinases[146]. Both inhibitors would be expected to block interstitial collagenase, type IV and type V collagenases, and stromelysin – all products of the macrophage. In addition, both are shown to inhibit the macrophage metalloelastase[146]. TIMP production is quite high in unstimulated monocytes, whereas these cells produce little collagenase[133].

MAST CELL

Role of the mast cell

The mast cell is involved in the allergic immediate hypersensitivity reaction, the inflammatory response and defence against nematodes[151]. In the rat the mast cells can be divided into two types[152]. One is the connective tissue mast cell (CTMC) which is widely distributed in various tissues of the body and can be isolated from the peritoneal fluid. The other is the 'atypical' mucosal mast cell (MMC) found in the lamina propria of the intestinal mucosa. The mast cells are identified by dense membrane-bound secretory granules about 0.1–0.5 μm in diameter. These granules contain heparin in CTMC or chondroitin sulphate E in MMC, which give the granules their basophilic character. Various agents stimulate the release of granule contents. These include antigen bound to specific IgE antibody on the cell surface receptors, anaphylatoxins such as C3a and C5a, endotoxin, etc.[152] In the human, two types of mast cells can also be differentiated, the T type containing tryptase and the TC type containing tryptase and chymase.[153]

Graziano[154] tabulates the mediators that are released from mast cell granules. These can be divided into three groups: preformed mediators that are rapidly released from the granule include histamine, serotonin, superoxide dismutase, tryptase and factors chemotactic for neutrophils and eosinophils. Factors that remain firmly associated with the granule, which is everted and becomes part of the cell membrane, include heparin proteoglycan, peroxidase and the chymases. Finally, there are mediators that are generated after the mast cells become activated. These include prostaglandins, leukotrienes, thromboxanes and platelet-activating factor.

Proteases of the mast cell

The rat mast cell has been the major tissue source for early work on the purification and characterization of chymotrypsin-like proteases. The two types of rat mast cells produce two distinct enzymes: the connective tissue cell CTMC contains RMCP I (EC 3.4.21.39), and the mucosal cell MMC, or atypical mast cell, produces RMCP II. A current review of our knowledge of these two proteases may be found in Woodbury *et al.*[152] and in Table 4.4

Table 4.4 Mast cell serine proteases

Species	*Cell type*	*Protease name*	M_r	*Specificity*	*Sequence reference*
Rat	**CTMC**	**Chymase,RMCP I**	**25 000**	**Arg-X**	**155**
Rat	**MMC**	**GSP, RMCP II**	**24 700**	**Leu-X**	**151, 156**
Rat	MMC	RMPL1	?	Chymotrypsin-like	156
Rat	CTMC	Tryptase	120 000	Arg-X	
Mouse	MMC	MMMCP II	24 900	Leu-X	157
Human	**T, TC**	**Tryptase**	**135 000**	**Arg-X**	
Human	TC	Chymase	28 000	Leu-X	
Dog	**Mastocytoma**	**Tryptase**	**132 000***	**Arg-X**	**158**
Dog	Mastocytoma	DMP	27 800	Trypsin-like	158

* Tetramer comprising four subunits of M_r 27 157 with varying degrees of glycosylation. Enzymes in **bold** are those that have been most extensively characterized. Where the amino acid sequence is known, the reference is given.
Abbreviations (Cell types are given in the text): RMCP, rat mast cell protease; GSP, group specific protease; MMMCP, mouse mucosal mast cell protease; DMP, dog mastocytoma protein; RMPL, rat mast-cell protease-like.

The specificity of the two enzymes is similar, but both are distinct from chymotrypsin and cathepsin G. The amino acid in a protein substrate that contributes the carboxy group to the scissile peptide bond is denominated P_1 and the neighbouring residues to the amino side of P_1 are designated P_2, P_3, etc. The chymases prefer Leu at P_1 and hydrophobic amino acids at $P_2$and P_3, as well. The crystal structure of RCMP II has been elucidated[159] at a resolution of 1.9 Å and shows similarities to chymotrypsin, but with significant differences at the active centre that would be reflected in different specificities. Chymase has also been purified from human skin[160,161]. A further chymotrypsin-like protease has been identified in rat MMC by its partial cDNA sequence[151].

A second type of proteolytic activity, a trypsin-like one, has been found in rat CTMC[162,163]. However, most of our knowledge of tryptase has come from study of the human enzyme. Schwartz *et al.*[164] purified this enzyme from human pulmonary mast cells. They showed that the active enzyme had M_r 140 000 and was made up of four subunits, each with an active centre. Antibody studies show that in the lung 93% of the mast cells are of the T type, which contain only tryptase, and 7% are TC, which contain chymase as well. Skin has about 12% TC[153]. A comparative study of purified skin tryptase and lung tryptase by Tanaka *et al.*[165] indicated that the best substrates are those in which there are two basic groups together, e.g. Lys-Arg-X, where Arg-X is the scissile bond. The tryptases are sensitive to salt; 1 M NaCl raises the K_m for peptide substrates about 100-fold[166]. During studies of the cDNA for dog mastocytoma tryptase, a second trypsin-like DNA was found[158]. The corresponding enzyme has not yet been identified.

Thus, the major proteolytic complement of the granules of various types of mast cells consists of trypsin-like and chymotrypsin-like serine proteases. These can be differentiated not only on the basis of their substrate specificity, but also by the use of selective inhibitors as tabulated in ref. 167. Chymases are completely blocked *in vitro* by chymostatin (a small inhibitor produced by microorganisms) and the protein inhibitors α_1-antichymotrypsin and Bowman–Birk soybean trypsin inhibitor. Tryptase, on the other hand, is insensitive to these three compounds, but is blocked by antipain and leupeptin (additional microbial inhibitors), and by a mast cell protein, trypstatin. Inhibitors such as Kunitz soybean trypsin inhibitor and α_1-antitrypsin give only partial inhibition.

The mast cells appear to produce two protease inhibitors. Rat CTMC produces trypstatin, an inhibitor of tryptase. This inhibitor has 70% identity with inter-α-trypsin inhibitor[168]. The mast cells in bovine lung and liver are a principal source of aprotinin (Trasylol)[169] which, however, has little effect on either type of granule protease.

Biological role of chymase and tryptase

It must be admitted that, although these proteases constitute a major fraction of the mast cell protein, their function is not understood. Their role in allergic inflammation has been reviewed recently by Katunuma[170]. Granule release by mast cells is mediated by IgE-binding to receptors and bridging through antigen. The release of histamine is blocked by chymase inhibitors but not by tryptase inhibitors. These inhibitors act inside the granules. Metalloproteases are also involved in granule release, as shown by this group and by Mundy and Strittmatter[171]. When the granules are released from the cells the chymase tends to remain bound to the everted granule on the cell surface through interaction with heparin proteoglycan, whereas tryptase is released[172]. Chymase action outside the cell is restricted by this barrier to the approach of large protein substrates. There is a relative paucity of inhibitors of the two proteases outside the cell. Both are relatively insensitive to α_1-antitrypsin. Chymase is inhibited by α_1-antichymotrypsin and tryptase is inhibited by trypstatin that is released simultaneously from rat granules.

Purified free chymase can stimulate other mast cells to degranulate[173]; it acts as a trigger to an induction phase but not the secretion phase. Rat chymase can generate a chemotactic factor for neutrophils by its action on IgG[167]. The RMCP II is readily released from granules of the mucosa and enters the gut lumen or blood stream. Human tryptase acts on a number of extracellular proteins. It degrades high molecular weight kininogen[174], cleaves complement factor C3 to the anaphylactic protein C3a[175], and degrades factor XII[176]. It thus has a general anticoagulant effect. In contrast, rat tryptase activates prothrombin to thrombin[177]. The rat granules also release the protein trypstatin which inhibits this action of tryptase on prothrombin. Tryptase would presumably become denatured shortly after leaving the cell, since its association with the stabilizing heparin is concentration-dependent[178]. The production of anaphylatoxin C3a by tryptase stimulates human PMN to secrete lysosomal enzymes, guinea pig macrophages to release thromboxane, guinea pig platelets to release serotonin and rat mast cells to degranulate[179]. However, when C3a binds to rat mast cells it is rapidly degraded by chymase[179].

Dog tryptase cleaves vasoactive intestinal peptide, but not substance P, whereas chymase cleaves both[180]. A role for tryptase in lung bronchospasm and skin neurogenic inflammation is postulated. RMCP I cleaves angiotensin I, substance P, neurotensin, somatostatin, vasoactive intestinal peptide, gastric inhibitory peptide, human pancreatic peptide, human Von Willebrand factor peptide and histone 4; its action appears to be limited to peptides of mass up to about 15 kD as long as the protease remains associated with the granules[181]. Human lung chymase shows angiotensin II converting activity[182].

King *et al.*[183] have made the interesting observation that if worm antigen is administered intravenously to rats infected with the intestinal nematode *Nippostrongylus*, anaphylactic shock ensues, lesions are seen in the gut and RMCP II appears in gut secretions. Corticosteroids can abolish this response, if given prior to antigen, by depleting the MMCs from the gut. CTMCs remain unaffected by these procedures. An observation of considerable importance has recently been made by MacQueen *et al.*[184]. Injection of egg albumin antigen into rats causes mucosal mast cells to secrete RMCP II. The injection is combined with an audiovisual stimulus so that a Pavlovian response develops in which protease is released without any albumin injection.

This is a potential means whereby the central nervous system can be an effector of mast cell function in allergic states!

Effects of mast cell protease on the extracellular matrix

Rat chymase can digest both soluble and matrix fibronectins[185]. It also cleaves type VIII collagen of endothelial origin[186]. According to Seppä[187] chymase has no action on elastin, but does cleave fibrin clots. It plays a role in inflammatory vasopermeability. RMCP II is reported to digest type IV collagen[188]. Tryptase has no action on proteoglycan core protein or on type I collagen[189].

There are various reports on the activation of matrix metalloproteinases by mast cell enzymes. Birkedal-Hansen *et al.*[190] noted that dog mast cell granules could activate human procollagenase and could also prevent serum inhibition of active collagenase. Human skin chymase can activate skin procollagenase[191]. Sopata *et al.*[192] found that rat chymase can activate human PMN gelatinase. However, there is conflicting evidence with respect to human tryptase: Johnson and Cawston[189] could not produce any activation of procollagenase with human tryptase, whereas Gruber *et al.*[193] claimed to observe such activation.

LYMPHOCYTE

Cytotoxic T lymphocytes (CTL) and natural killer cells (NK)

CTLs bind to cells bearing foreign antigens and cause such cells to lyse. Various lines of evidence point to a role of cytoplasmic granules in such lysis[194,195]. After antigens bind to cells there is transmembrane signalling. CTL granules then fuse to the CTL cytoplasmic membrane and transfer their contents into the pocket formed between it and the target cell. This process involves calcium and energy. The target cell is exposed to a high concentration of granular proteins. Perforin is present and is believed to behave like the C9 component of complement to produce transmembrane channels. The target cell develops membrane lesions and undergoes lysis.

Serine granzymes of the mouse CTL

The granules of CTL and NK cells contain as many as six distinct serine esterases/proteinases (Table 4.5). Ester substrates provide a convenient assay for proteinases; however, not every esterase is capable of digesting protein substrates. Pasternack and Eisen[196] showed the presence of a serine esterase in T cells that was low in B cells and non-cytotoxic T cells. Activity was blocked by diisopropyl fluorophosphate (DFP) but not by tosyl-lysyl-chloromethyl ketone (TLCK, a trypsin inhibitor). In 1986 the first cDNA clones for serine esterases were sequenced[197–199], and by 1988 all six sequences had been completed. mRNA transcripts of such genes were found

Table 4.5 Equivalencies of CTL serine proteinases

Mouse enzymes	*Related names*	*Amino acid sequence*	*Human enzymes*	*cDNA sequence*
Granzyme A	HF, CTLA-3, TSP-1	197*	HuHF, HuTSP	200, 201
Granzyme B	CCP1, CTLA-1	198, 199	HLP	211
Granzyme C	CCP2	198, 203		
Granzyme D		194, 207		
Granzyme E	CCP3, MCSP-2	204, 207		
Granzyme F	CCP4, MCSP-3	204, 207		
Granzyme G	Glycosylated form of B			
Granzyme H	Glycosylated form of B			
—	MCSP-1	204		

* Sequence, based on cDNA, given in the reference with this number.
Abbreviations: CCP, cytotoxic cell proteinase; CTLA, cytotoxic T-cell lymphocyte A; HF, Hanukah factor; HLP, human lymphocyte proteinase; MCSP, mouse cytotoxic serine proteinase; TSP, T-cell serine proteinase.

in CTL, nude mouse spleen, and 2 or 8 T-helper clones, but not in normal spleen or in tumours of B or T cells[198]. Concurrent with work on cloning the genes for these putative enzymes, work was in progress on isolating corresponding proteins from CTL. Simon *et al.*[205] isolated a serine protease of M_r 60000 from CTL that was not found in resting T cells. Upon reduction one monomeric subunit of M_r 30000 was obtained, indicating that this enzyme (TSP-1) is a dimer. Hydrolytic activity was demonstrated on D-Pro-Phe-Arg-nitroanalide. Masson and Tschopp[206] review their work in describing the protein granzymes A–F; G and H proved to be glycosylated forms of B. The enzymes are closely related in immunological properties. Antibodies against granzyme B crossreact with A, and those against D recognize C, E and F. Partial sequence analyses have permitted the identification of the isolated proteins with the cDNA clones. Immunoelectron microscopic studies have demonstrated that granzymes D, E and F are localized to the same cytoplasmic granules of CTL that contain perforin[207]. The other granzymes are similarly localized.

The sequences of HF (granzyme A) and CCP1 (granzyme B) have been used to construct putative three-dimensional models of these enzymes based on X-ray crystallographic structures of trypsin and rat mast cell proteinase-II[208]. It is concluded that HF should display trypsin-like specificity, while CCP1, although closely related to the chymotrypsins, should bind Glu or Asp at the active centre. No enzymatic activity has yet been demonstrated for this second enzyme.

Serine granzymes of the human CTL and NK

The number of such enzymes in the human appears to be smaller than in the mouse; only two have been characterized in detail. Hatcher *et al.*[209] were apparently the first to isolate an enzyme of this class from human peripheral blood lymphocytes. The enzyme, isolated by soybean trypsin inhibitor affinity chromatography, had M_r 30 000. It was inhibited by α_1-AT and α_2-macroglobulin, but not by aprotinin or tosyl-phenylalanyl chloromethylketone (TPCK, a chymotrypsin inhibitor). It proved to be highly cytotoxic to human bladder carcinoma cells. Fruth *et al.*[210] obtained a purified preparation of HuTSP of M_r 50 000 that dissociated to a monomeric subunit of 25–30 kD upon reduction. This enzyme cleaves Tosyl-Gly-Pro-Arg-p-nitroanilide. It is induced by lectin and released from effector cells upon ligand binding to CD3–T-cell receptor complex. Krähenbühl *et al.*[211] purified two enzymes from human $CD8^+$ CTL. N-terminal amino acid sequences showed that the larger enzyme, a homodimer, is the Hanukah factor corresponding to mouse granzyme A, and that the smaller, monomeric enzyme corresponds to HLP or granzyme B. The sequences of HF and HLP have been deduced from cDNA as referenced in Table 4.1.

Although Krähenbühl *et al.*[211] did not detect further granzymes, it is likely that the list must be lengthened. Hameed *et al.*[212] distinguish three serine esterases in NK cells. Granzymes 1 and 2 correspond to mouse A and B. However, there is a monomeric granzyme 3 that acts on the same substrate as granzyme 1, i.e. it is trypsin-like. Poe *et al.*[213] have purified a dimeric tryptase, similar to HF. However, it differs in its N-terminal sequence. A large table of natural and synthetic inhibitors and synthetic substrates is presented for this enzyme. Finally, Hudig *et al.*[214] demonstrated a protease of chymotrypsin-like specificity in NK cells.

Natural inhibitors of CTL proteinases

The granzymes appear to be of two general types: tryptase or trypsin-like and chymase or chymotrypsin-like. General inhibition of both should be produced by α_1-AT. The trypsin-like enzymes should be inhibited by aprotinin and antithrombin III[215,216] and the chymotrypsin-like enzymes, by α_1-antichymotrypsin; but there have not been extensive systematic studies of the various granzymes and these inhibitors. The synthetic inhibitors TLCK, useful for the trypsin-like proteinases and TPCK, for the chymotrypsin type, have not been found to be particularly effective in blocking the granzymes.

Ganea *et al.*[217] show that the human T cell line C91/PL produces a proteinase inhibitor (LPI 1) that blocks trypsin and kallikrein, but not thrombin, plasmin, chymotrypsin or pancreatic elastase. It is comparable to the rabbit inhibitor. This cell line is a T4 line that has been transformed with HTLV 1 virus; other T4 cells do not produce the inhibitor. An immunoregulatory role is assigned to this inhibitor, but it is not known if it inhibits any of the lymphocytic enzymes. The human lymphocyte is able to synthesize α_1-AT[218].

Role of serine proteinases in cell lysis

It must first be noted that, while all the granzymes are esterases, not all possess proteolytic activity. Thus, in the mouse only granzyme A has been shown to digest proteins and extracellular matrix[219]. Granzyme D also has esterase activity at lysine and arginine bonds. These two enzymes react strongly with diisopropyl fluorophosphate (DFP), whereas B and C react weakly, and E and F not at all. This, of course, does not exclude their being serine enzymes: tonin, from rat submaxillary glands, is a good example of a serine protease that reacts extremely slowly with DFP[220]. The absence of general peptide cleavage could be due to the possibility that these enzymes have extreme specificity and are designed to digest only certain (unknown) protein substrates. Chymotrypsin-like specificity of peptide cleavage has been noted for mouse, rat and human enzymes[221,222], but no correspondence with known granzymes has been established.

What is the role of the granzymes in the cytotoxic action of CTL? In fact, this remains a mystery. Certainly the granzymes are found almost exclusively in the CTL[196]. The enzymes are not detected in cell assays until after the post-bonding events; this indicates that the granules have been released[223]. Treatment of CTL with α_1-PI has no effect on binding, but does inhibit the subsequent lysis[223]. HuTSP is released from cell upon ligand binding to the CD3–T-cell receptor complex[210]. Arakawa *et al.*[224] use the guanidinobenzoate compound Camostat mesilate to block lysis of target cells. The chymotrypsin inhibitor CBZ-Phe-Pro-Arg-chloromethylketone has been shown[222] to block cytolysis by the rat CTL, as do inhibitors of trypsin. Thus, serine proteases are essential to cytolysis. But how do they participate?

Brogan and Targan[225] suggest three possible roles for serine enzymes in human NK: trigger, amplification cascade and cytolytic complex. TPCK does not affect cell proliferation or binding to target cells but does inhibit cytolysis. If one dissociates the NK cell from the target after initiation of event, lysis continues, and this lysis is blocked by *p*-chloromercuribenzoate, pointing to thiol protease involvement. With respect to an amplification cascade it must be noted that there is no objective evidence for one of these enzymes activating another with an amplifying effect. With respect to cytolysis, it must be noted that there is only a single instance in which cytotoxicity has been demonstrated. Hatcher *et al.*[209] showed that a 30 000 D proteinase purified from human T cells had high cytotoxic activity. Cytolysis is generally explained on the basis of the release of perforin from the granule[226]. The blocking of cytolysis by protease inhibitors does not prove a direct role in membrane or cell breakdown, since the role could be at steps 1 or 2.

What about the concept that the granzymes act as triggers? This idea receives support from the work of Utsunomiya and Nakanishi[227], who showed by fluorescent techniques that early changes within 1 s of cell binding include increased membrane fluidity and influx of calcium ions. These early steps are blocked by inhibitors of trypsin- and chymotrypsin-like proteases. It is postulated that a cell-surface protease is responsible, not a granzyme. If CTL are treated with reversible inhibitors then washed, no effects are noted; but if irreversible inhibitors are used, cytolysis is blocked[224]. This would support the trigger hypothesis, since granzymes would not be exposed at this stage. One candidate cell-surface enzyme has been described earlier by Tokes[228].

Other possible roles for granzymes have been suggested. They may serve to stimulate B cell proliferation[205]. They degrade extracellular matrix by digesting heparan sulphate proteoglycan and thus allow cells to pass through the blood vessel walls[229]. They can also degrade fibronectin[230]. Finally, they may enter the target cell after membrane breakdown and lead to the release of nuclear DNA, as illustrated by the experiments of Munger *et al.*[231]. The preparation of large amounts of proteases in the near future should help to clarify the role of these enzymes.

Other lymphocyte proteinases

There appear to be several cell surface proteinases on lymphocytes. A serine enzyme is reported by Bata *et al.*[232]. Depleting the lymphocyte population of T cells leaves a population enriched in this enzyme. The T cell surface enzyme of Tokes[228] is not stimulated by mitogen. Thymocytes contain the metalloproteinase 24.11 (EC 3.4.24.11) on their surface; possibly this acts to inactivate interleukin 1[233]. An insulin-degrading enzyme is found on the surface of cultured human lymphocytes, but has not been further characterized[234].

With respect to secreted metalloproteinases, the mouse T lymphocyte has been reported[235] to produce a proteoglycan-degrading metalloproteinase (perhaps stromelysin). It is released in latent form and is not stimulated by antigen or mitogen. The high level of T lymphocytes in the rheumatoid synovium suggests a possible role for this enzyme. Collagenase is also found in the human lymphocyte at levels about one-third of those found in PMN cells[236]. Simpson *et al.*[237] separated B and T cells, and found that the former produced high collagenase activity.

Lysosomal cathepsins are also found in lymphocytes. Cathepsin D in human lymphocytes[238] is not stimulated by phytohaemagglutinin[239]. Rat lymphocytes appear to contain a unique heavy form of cathepsin D of M_r 95 000[240]. The thiol cathepsins B, H and L are found in human peripheral blood lymphocytes[241] and decrease in specific activity after PHA stimulation. Kominami *et al.*[242] find lymphocyte B and H similar to neutrophil content and much lower than macrophage in the rat. The lymphocytes contain a cystatin similar in amount to the amount of cathepsins. Cathepsin L in the rat lymphocyte is only 10% of the amount found in resident macrophages[119].

Acknowledgement

This review was prepared with support from grants from the National Institutes of Health, US Public Health Service, HD-06773 and AM-16940.

References

1. Barrett, A. J. and Salvesen, G. (eds) (1986). *Proteinase Inhibitors*. Research Monographs in Cell and Tissue Physiology, Vol. 12. (Amsterdam: Elsevier)
2. Barrett, A. J. and McDonald, J. K. (1986). Nomenclature: protease, proteinase and peptidase. *Biochem. J.*, **237**, 935
3. Hartley, B. S. (1970). Proteolytic enzymes. *Ann. Rev. Biochem.*, **29**, 45–72

4. Nomenclature Committee – International Union of Biochemistry (1984). *Enzyme Nomenclature* (New York: Academic Press)
5. Nomenclature Committee – International Union of Biochemistry (1989). Enzyme Nomenclature. Supplement 2: Corrections and Additions. *Eur. J. Biochem.*, **179**, 489–533
6. Barrett, A. J. and McDonald, J. K. (1980). *Mammalian Proteases: A Glossary and Bibliography*, Vol. 1: *Endopeptidases* (London: Academic Press)
7. Mayne, R. and Burgeson, R. E. (eds) (1987). *Structure and Function of Collagen Types* (New York: Academic Press)
8. Jeffrey, J. J. (1986). The biological regulation of collagenase activity. In Mecham R. P. (ed.), *Regulation of Matrix Accumulation*, pp. 53–98 (New York: Academic Press)
9. Tschesche, H., Fedrowitz, J., Honert, U., Michaelis, J. and Macartney, H. W. (1986). Matrix degrading proteinases from human granulocytes: type I, II, III collagenase, gelatinase and type IV, V collagenase. A survey of recent findings and inhibition by γ-anticollagenase. *Folia Histochem. Cytobiol.*, **24**, 125–31
10. van der Rest, M. and Mayne, R. (1987). Type IX collagen. In Mayne, R. and Burgeson, R. E. (eds), *Structure and Function of Collagen Types*, pp. 195–221 (New York: Academic Press)
11. Weiss, S. J. and Peppin, G. J. (1985). Collagenolytic metalloenzymes of the human neutrophil. Characteristics, regulation and potential function *in vivo*. *Biochem. Pharmacol.*, **35**, 3189–98
12. Davidson, J. M. (1987). Elastin. Structure and biology. In Uitto, J. and Perejda, A. J. (eds), *Connective Tissue Disease. Molecular Pathology of the Extracellular Matrix*, pp. 29–54 (New York: Marcel Dekker)
13. Gosline, J. M. and Rosenbloom, J. (1984). Elastin. In Piez, K. A. and Reddi, A. H. (eds), *Extracellular Matrix Biochemistry*, pp. 191–227 (New York: Elsevier)
14. Wight, T. N. and Mecham, R. P. (eds) (1987). *Biology of the Proteoglycans* (New York: Academic Press)
15. Heinegård, D. and Oldberg, Å. (1989). Structure and biology of cartilage and bone matrix noncollagenous macromolecules. *FASEB J.*, **3**, 2042–51
16. Mosher, D. R. (ed.) (1988). *Fibronectin* (New York: Academic Press)
17. Wright, D. G. (1988). Human neutrophil degranulation. *Methods Enzymol.*, **162**, 538–51
18. Rest, R. F. (1988). Human neutrophil and mast cell proteases implicated in inflammation. *Methods Enzymol.*, **163**, 309–27
19. Janoff, A. and Scherer, J. (1968). Mediators of inflammation in leukocyte lysosomes. IX. Elastinolytic activity in granules of human polymorphonuclear leukocytes. *J. Exp. Med.*, **128**, 1137–55
20. Janoff, A. and Blondin, J. (1970). Depletion of cartilage matrix by a neutral protease fraction of human leukocyte lysosomes. *Proc. Soc. Exp. Biol. Med.*, **135**, 302–6
21. Janoff, A. (1970). Mediators of tissue damage in leukocyte lysosomes. X. Further studies on human granulocyte elastase. *Lab. Invest.*, **22**, 228–36
22. Gadek, J. E., Fells, G. A., Wright, D. G. and Crystal, R. G. (1980). Human neutrophil elastase functions as a type III collagen 'collagenase'. *Biochem. Biophys. Res. Commun.*, **95**, 1815–22
23. Mainardi, C. L., Dixit, S. M. and Kang, A. H. (1980). Degradation of type IV (basement membrane) collagen by a proteinase isolated from human polymorphonuclear leukocyte granules. *J. Biol. Chem.*, **255**, 5435–41
24. Campbell, E. J., Senior, R. M., McDonald, J. A., Cox, D. L., Greco, J. M. and Landis, J. A. (1982). Proteolysis by neutrophils. Relative importance of cell–substrate contact and oxidative inactivation of proteinase inhibitors *in vitro*. *J. Clin. Invest.*, **70**, 845–52
25. Scott, P. G. and Pearson, H. (1983). Cleavage of the C-terminal cross-linking region of type I collagen by tissue proteinases. *Biochem. Soc. Trans.*, **11**, 746–7
26. Dewald, B., Rindler-Ludwig, R., Bretz, U. and Baggiolini, M. (1975). Subcellular localization and heterogeneity of neutral proteases in neutrophilic polymorphonuclear leukocytes. *J. Exp. Med.*, **141**, 709–23
27. Damiano, V. V., Kucich, U., Murer, E., Laudenslager, N. and Weinbaum, G. (1988). Ultrastructural quantitation of peroxidase- and elastase-containing granules in human neutrophils. *Am. J. Pathol.*, **131**, 235–45
28. Takahashi, H., Nukiwa, T., Kunihiko, N., Yoshimura, K., Quick, C. D., States, D. J., Holmes, M. D., Whang-Peng, J., Knutsen, T. and Crystal, R. G. (1988). Structure of the

human neutrophil elastase gene. *J. Biol. Chem.*, **263**, 14739–47
29. Takahasi, H., Nukiwa, T., Basset, P. and Crystal, R. G. (1988). Myelomonocytic cell lineage expression of the neutrophil elastase gene. *J. Biol. Chem.*, **263**, 2543–7
30. Wei, A.-Z., W. Mayr, I. and Bode, W. (1988). The refined 2.3 Å crystal structure of human leukocyte elastase in a complex with a valine chloromethyl ketone inhibitor. *FEBS Lett.*, **234**, 367–73
31. Nagamatsu, A. and Soeda, S. (1981). Effects of human granulocyte elastase on fibrinolysis. *Chem. Pharm. Bull. Tokyo*, **29**, 1121–9
32. Johnson, U., Ohlsson, K. and Olsson, I. (1976). Effects of granulocyte neutral proteases on complement components. *Scand. J. Immunol.*, **5**, 421–6
33. Baici, A., Knöpfel, M., Fehr, K., Skvaril, F. and Böni, A. (1980). Kinetics of different susceptibilities of the four human immunoglobulin G subclasses to proteolysis by human lysosomal elastase. *Scand. J. Immunol.*, **12**, 41–50
34. Movat, H. Z., Habal, F. M. and MacMorine, D. R. L. (1976). Generation of a vasoactive peptide by a netural protease of human neutrophil leukocytes. *Agents Actions*, **6**, 183–90
35. Schmidt, W., Egbring, R. and Havemann, K. (1975). Effect of elastase-like and chymotrypsin-like neutral proteases from human granulocytes on isolated clotting factors. *Thromb. Res.*, **6**, 315–26
36. Karpati, J., Varadi, K. and Elodi, S. (1982). Effect of granulocyte proteases on human coagulation factors IX and X. The protective effect of calcium. *Hoppe-Seyler's Z. Physiol. Chem.*, **363**, 521–6
37. Byrne, R. E., Polacek, D., Gordon, J. I. and Scanu, A. M. (1984). The enzyme that cleaves apolipoprotein A-II upon *in vitro* incubation of human plasma high-density lipoprotein-3 with blood polymorphonuclear cells is an elastase. *J. Biol. Chem.*, **259**, 4537–43
38. Watorek, W. and Travis, J. (1987). The action of neutrophil elastase on intact and oxidized (Met)-enkephalin-Arg^6-Gly^7-Leu^8 peptide. *Biochem. Biophys. Res. Commun.*, **147**, 416–21
39. Takada, Y., Maruta, H., Wagner, B., Fa, X. G., James, H. L. and Erdös, E. G. (1987). Activation of human prorenin by neutrophil elastase. *J. Clin. Endocrinol. Metab.*, **65**, 1225–30
40. Kleniewski, J. and Donaldson, V. (1988). Granulocyte elastase cleaves human high molecular weight kininogen and destroys its clot-promoting activity. *J. Exp. Med.*, **167**, 1895–907
41. Ohlsson, K. and Olsson, I. (1977). The extracellular release of granulocyte collagenase and elastase during phagocytosis and inflammatory processes. *Scand. J. Haematol.*, **19**, 145–52
42. Schmidt, W. (1978). Differential release of elastase and chymotrypsin from polymorphonuclear leukocytes. In Havemann, K. and Janoff, A. (eds), *Neutral Proteases of Human Polymorphonuclear Leukocytes*, pp. 77–81 (Munich: Urban & Schwarzenberg)
43. Remold-O'Donnell, E., Nixon, J. C. and Rose, R. M. (1989). Elastase inhibitor. Characterization of the human elastase inhibitor molecule associated with monocytes, macrophages, and neutrophils. *J. Exp. Med.*, **169**, 1071–86
44. Virca, G. D., Salvesen, G. S. and Travis, J. (1983). Human neutrophil elastase and cathepsin G cleavage sites in the bait region of α_2-macroglobulin. Proposed structural limits of the bait region. *Hoppe-Seyler's Z. Physiol. Chem.*, **364**, 1297–302
45. Ohlsson, K. and Olsson, I. (1974). Neutral proteases of human granulocytes. III. Interaction between granulocyte elastase and plasma protease inhibitors. *Scand. J. Clin. Lab. Invest.*, **34**, 349–56
46. Weiss, S. J., Curnutte, J. T. and Regiani, S. (1986). Neutrophil-mediated solubilization of the subendothelial matrix: oxidative and nonoxidative mechanisms of proteolysis used by normal and chronic granulomatous disease phagocytes. *J. Immunol.*, **136**, 636–41
47. Hochstrasser, K., Schuster, R., Reichert, R. and Heimberger, N. (1972). Detection and quantitative determination of complexes between leukocyte proteases and α_1-antitrypsin in body secretions and body fluids. *Hoppe-Seyler's Z. Physiol. Chem.*, **353**, 1120–5
48. Brower, M. S. and Harpel, P. C. (1982). Proteolytic cleavage and inactivation of α2-plasmin inhibitor and $C\bar{1}$ inactivator by human polymorphonuclear leukocyte elastase. *J. Biol. Chem.*, **257**, 9849–54
49. Jordan, R. E., Kilpatrick, J. and Nelson, R. M. (1987). Heparin promotes the inactivation of antithrombin by neutrophil elastase. *Science*, **237**, 777–9
50. Albrecht, G. J., Hochstrasser, K. and Salier, J.-P. (1983). Elastase inhibition by the inter-α-trypsin inhibitor and derived inhibitors of man and cattle. *Hoppe-Seyler's Z. Physiol. Chem.*, **364**, 1703–8

51. Hochstrasser, K. and Schorn, K. (1976). Characterization of proteinase-inhibitor complexes in the purulent secretions of mucous membranes as complexes between leukocytic elastase and proteinase inhibitors. *Protides Biol. Fluids*, **23**, 231–4
52. Gauthier, F., Fryksmark, U., Ohlsson, K. and Bieth, J. G. (1982). Kinetics of the inhibition of leukocyte elastase by the bronchial inhibitor. *Biochim. Biophys. Acta.*, **700**, 178–83
53. Thompson, R. C. and Ohlsson, K. (1986). Isolation, properties, and complete amino acid sequence of human secretory leukocyte protease inhibitor, a potent inhibitor of leukocyte elastase. *Proc. Natl. Acad. Sci. USA*, **83**, 6692–6
54. Kramps, J. A., Van Twisk, C., Klasen, E. C. and Dijkman, J. H. (1988). Interactions among stimulated human polymorphnuclear leukocytes, released elastase and bronchial antileukoprotease. *Clin. Sci.*, **75**, 53–62
55. Campbell, E. J., White, R. R., Senior, R. M., Rodriguez, R. J. and Kuhn, C. (1979). Receptor-mediated binding and internalization of leukocyte elastase by alveolar macrophages *in vitro*. *J. Clin. Invest.*, **64**, 824–33
56. Taylor, J. C. and Mittman, C. (eds) (1987). *Pulmonary Emphysema and Proteolysis: 1986* (New York: Academic Press)
57. Travis, J. (1988). Structure, function, and control of neutrophil proteinases. *Am. J. Med.*, **84** (Suppl. 6A), 37–42
58. Velvart, M. and Fehr, K. (1987). Degradation *in vivo* of articular cartilage in rheumatoid arthritis and juvenile chronic arthritis by cathepsin-G and elastase from polymorphonuclear leukocytes. *Rheumatol. Int.*, **7**, 195–202
59. Bonney, R. J. and Smith, R. J. (1986). Evidence for the role of neutral proteases in chronic inflammatory diseases in humans. In Otterness, I., Lewis, A. and Capetola, R. (eds), *Advances in Inflammation Research*, Vol. 11, pp. 127–133 (New York: Raven Press)
60. Schmidt, W. and Havemann, K. (1974). Isolation of elastase-like and chymotrypsin-like neutral proteases from human granulocytes. *Hoppe-Seyler's Z. Physiol. Chem.*, **355**, 1077–82
61. Starkey, P. M. and Barrett, A. J. (1976). Human cathepsin G. Catalytic and immunological properties. *Biochem. J.*, **155**, 273–8
62. Salvesen, G., Farley, D., Shuman, J., Przybyla, A., Reilley, C. and Travis, J. (1987). Molecular cloning of human cathepsin G: structural similarity to mast cell and cytotoxic T lymphocyte proteinases. *Biochemistry*, **26**, 2289–93
63. Odeberg, H. and Olsson, I. (1976). Microbicidal mechanisms of human granulocytes: synergistic effects of granulocyte elastase and myeloperoxidase or chymotrypsin-like cationic protein. *Infect. Immun.*, **14**, 1276–83
64. Kruse-Jarres, J. D. and Kinzelmann, T. (1986). Pathobiochemistry and clinical role of granulocytes and their lysosomal neutral proteinases in inflammatory processes. *Aerztl. Lab.*, **32**, 185–96
65. Malemud, C. J. and Janoff, A. (1975). Identification of neutral proteases in human neutrophil granules that degrade articular cartilage proteoglycan. *Arthritis Rheum.*, **18**, 361–8
66. Keiser, H., Greenwald, R. A., Feinstein, G. and Janoff, A. (1976). Degradation of cartilage proteoglycan by human leukocyte granule neutral proteases — a model of joint injury. II. Degradation of isolated bovine nasal cartilage proteoglycan. *J. Clin. Invest.*, **57**, 625–32
67. Starkey, P. M., Barrett, A. J. and Burleigh, M. C. (1977). The degradation of articular collagen by neutrophil proteinases. *Biochim. Biophys. Acta*, **483**, 386–97
68. Gramse, M., Bingenheimer, C. and Havemann, K. (1980). Degradation of human fibrinogen by chymotrypsin-like neutral protease from human granulocytes. *Thromb. Res.*, **19**, 201–9
69. Vartio, T., Seppä, H. and Vaheri, A. (1981). Susceptibility of soluble and matrix fibronectins to degradation by tissue proteinases, mast cell chymase, and cathepsin G. *J. Biol. Chem.*, **256**, 471–7
70. Turkington, P. T., Blumsom, N. L. and Elmore, D. T. (1986). The degradation of bovine and human prothrombin by human polymorphonuclear leukocyte cathepsin G. *Thromb. Res.*, **44**, 339–46
71. Venge, P. (1978). Polymorphonuclear proteases and their effects on complement components and neutrophil function. In Havemann, K. and Janoff, A. (eds), *Neutral Proteases of Human Polymorphonuclear Leukocytes*, pp. 264–82 (Munich: Urban & Schwarzenberg)
72. Stančiková, M. and Trnavský, K. (1979). Activation of latent collagenase from polymorphonuclear leukocytes by cathepsin G. *Collect. Czech. Chem. Commun.*, **44**, 3177–82
73. Wintroub, B. U., Klickstein, L. B., Dzau, V. J., and Watt, K. W. K. (1984).

Granulocyte–angiotensin system. Identification of angiotensinogen as the plasma protein substrate of leukocyte cathepsin G. *Biochemistry*, **23**, 227–32

74. Klickstein, L. B., Kaempfer, C. E. and Wintroub, B. U. (1982). The granulocyte angiotensin system. Angiotensin I-converting activity of cathepsin G. *J. Biol. Chem.*, **257**, 15042–6
75. Reilly, C. F. and Travis, J. (1980). The degradation of human lung elastin by neutrophil proteinases. *Biochim. Biophys. Acta.*, **621**, 147–57
76. Lucey, E. C., Stone, P. J., Breuer, R., Christensen, T. G., Calore, J. D., Catanese, A., Franzblau, C. and Snider, G. L. (1985). Effect of combined human neutrophil cathepsin-G and elastase on induction of secretory cell metaplasia and emphysema in hamsters, with *in vitro* observations on elastolysis by these enzymes. *Am. Rev. Respir. Dis.*, **132**, 362–6
77. Travis, J., Bowen, J. and Baugh, R. (1978). Human α-1-antichymotrypsin: interaction with chymotrypsin-like proteinases. *Biochemistry*, **17**, 5651–6
78. Ohlsson, K. and Åkesson, U. (1976). α1-Antichymotrypsin interaction with cationic proteins from granulocytes. *Clin. Chim. Acta*, **73**, 285–92
79. Campbell, E. J. (1982). Human leukocyte elastase, cathepsin G and lactoferrin: family of neutrophil granule glycoproteins that bind to an alveolar macrophage receptor. *Proc. Natl. Acad. Sci. USA*, **79**, 6941–5
80. Lazarus, G. S., Brown, R. S., Daniels, J. R. and Fullmer, H. M. (1968). Human granulocyte collagenase. *Science*, **159**, 1483–5
81. Robertson, P. B., Ryel, R. B., Taylor, R. F., Shyu, K. W. and Fullmer, H. M. (1972). Collagenase localization in polymorphonuclear leukocyte granules in the rabbit. *Science*, **177**, 64–5
82. Murphy, G., Bretz, U., Baggiolini, M. and Reynolds, J. J. (1980). The latent collagenase and gelatinase of human polymorphonuclear neutrophil leukocytes. *Biochem. J.*, **192**, 517–25
83. Uitto, V.-J., Turto, H., Huttenen, A., Lindy, S. and Uitto, J. (1980). Activation of human leukocyte collagenase by compounds reacting with sulfhydryl groups. *Biochim. Biophys. Acta*, **613**, 168–77
84. Macartney, H. W. and Tschesche, H. (1982). Latent and active human polymorphonuclear collagenases. Isolation, purification and characterization. *Eur. J. Biochem.*, **130**, 71–8
85. Springman, E., Angleton, E., Birkedal-Hansen, H. and Van Wart, H. E. (1990). Multiple modes of activation of latent human fibroblast collagenase: evidence for the role of a Cys_{73}-active site zinc complex in latency and a 'cysteine switch' mechanism for activation. *Proc. Natl. Acad. Sci. USA*, **87**, 364–8
86. Hasty, K. A., Hibbs, M. S., Kang, A. H. and Mainardi, C. L. (1984). Heterogeneity among human collagenases demonstrated by monoclonal antibody that selectively recognizes and inhibits human neutrophil collagenase. *J. Exp. Med.*, **159**, 1455–63
87. Ohlsson, K. (1980). Polymorphonuclear leukocyte collagenase. In Woolley, D. E. and Evanson, J. M. (eds), *Collagenase in Normal and Pathological Connective Tissues*, pp. 209–222 (Chichester: Wiley)
88. Hibbs, M. A., Hasty, K. A., Kang, A. H. and Mainardi, C. L. (1984). Secretion of collagenolytic enzymes by human polymorphonuclear leukocytes. *Collagen Rel. Res.*, **4**, 467–78
89. Harris, E. D. Jr., DiBona, D. R. and Krane, S. M. (1969). Collagenases in human synovial fluid. *J. Clin. Invest.*, **48**, 2104–13
90. Pelletier, J.-P., Martel-Pelletier, J., Howell, D. S., Ghandur-Mnaymneh, L., Enis, J. E. and Woessner, J. F., Jr (1983). Collagenase and collagenolytic activity in human osteoarthritic cartilage. *Arthritis Rheum.*, **26**, 63–8
91. Hasty, K. A., Jeffrey, J. J., Hibbs, M. S. and Welgus, H. G. (1987). The collagen substrate specificity of human neutrophil collagenase. *J. Biol. Chem.*, **262**, 10048–52
92. Sopata, I. and Dancewicz, A. (1974). A neutral protease from human leukocytes involved in collagen degradation. *Przegl. Lek.*, **31**, 435–9
93. Uitto, V.-J., Schwartz, D. and Veis, A. (1980). Degradation of basement-membrane collagen by neutral proteases from human leukocytes. *Eur. J. Biochem.*, **105**, 409–17
94. Hibbs, M. S., Hasty, K. A., Seyer, J. M., Kang, A. H. and Mainardi, C. L. (1985). Biochemical and immunological characterization of the secreted forms of human neutrophil gelatinase. *J. Biol. Chem.*, **260**, 2493 –2500
95. Wilhelm, S. M., Collier, I. E., Marmer, B. L., Eisen, A. Z., Grant, G. A. and Goldberg, G. I. (1989). SV40 transformed human lung fibroblasts secrete a 92-kDa type IV collagenase which is identical to that secreted by normal human macrophages. *J. Biol. Chem.*, **264**, 17213–21

96. Peppin, G. J. and Weiss, S. J. (1986). Activation of the endogenous metalloproteinase, gelatinase, by triggered human neutrophils. *Proc. Natl. Acad. Sci. USA*, **83**, 4322–26
97. Sopata, I., Wojteka-Lukasik, E. and Maslinski, S. (1986). Activation of latent human granulocyte gelatinase by rat mast cell protease. *Folia Histochem. Cytobiol.*, **24**, 133–7
98. Sottrup-Jensen, L. and Birkedal-Hansen, H. (1989). Human fibroblast collagenase-α-macroglobulin interactions. Localization of cleavage sites in the bait regions of five mammalian α-macroglobulins. *J. Biol. Chem.*, **264**, 393–401
99. Cawston, T. E., Galloway, W. A., Mercer, E., Murphy, G. and Reynolds, J. J. (1981). Purification of rabbit bone inhibitor of collagenase. *Biochem. J.*, **195**, 159–65
100. Dean, D. D. and Woessner, J. F., Jr (1983). Extracts of human articular cartilage contain an inhibitor of tissue metalloproteinases. *Biochem. J.*, **218**, 277–80
101. Dean, D. D., Martel-Pelletier, J., Pelletier, J.-P., Howell, D. S. and Woessner, J. F., Jr (1989). Evidence for metalloproteinase and metalloproteinase inhibitor imbalance in human osteoarthritic cartilage. *J. Clin. Invest.*, **84**, 678–85
102. Dewald, B., Bretz, U. and Baggiolini, M. (1982). Release of gelatinase from a novel secretory compartment of human neutrophils. *J. Clin. Invest.*, **70**, 518–25
103. Ishikawa, I. and Cimasoni, G. (1977). Isolation of cathepsin D from human leukocytes. *Biochim. Biophys. Acta*, **480**, 228–40
104. Roughley, P. J. (1977). The degradation of cartilage proteoglycans by tissue proteinases. Proteoglycan heterogeneity and the pathway of proteolytic degradation. *Biochem. J.*, **167**, 639–46
105. Woessner, J. F., Jr (1979). Acid cathepsins. In: Houck, R. J. (ed.) *Handbook of Inflammation*, Vol. 1: *Chemical Messengers of the Inflammatory Process*, pp. 261–84 (Amsterdam: Elsevier)
106. Baggiolini, M., Bretz, U., Dewald, B. and Feigenson, M. E. (1978). The polymorphonuclear leukocyte. *Agents Actions*, **3**, 3–11
107. Kao, R. C., Wehner, N. G., Skubitz, K. M., Gray, B. H. and Hoidal, J. R. (1988). Proteinase 3. A distinct human polymorphonuclear leukocyte proteinase that produces emphysema in hamsters. *J. Clin. Invest.*, **82**, 1963–73
108. Unanue, E. R. and Allen, P. M. (1987). The basis for the immunoregulatory role of macrophages and other accessory cells. *Science*, **236**, 551–7
109. Roska, A. K. and Lipsky, P. E. (1989). Monocytes and macrophages. In Kelley, W. N., Harris, E. D., Jr, Ruddy, S. and Sledge, C. B. (eds) *Textbook of Rheumatology*, 3rd edn, pp. 346–66 (Philadelphia: W. B. Saunders)
110. Johnston, R. B., Jr (1988). Current concepts: immunology. Monocytes and macrophages. *N. Engl. J. Med.*, **318**, 747–52
111. De Weger, R. A., Runhaar, B. A. and Den Otter, W. (1986). Cytotoxicity by macrophages and monocytes. *Methods Enzymol.*, **132**, 458–66
112. Adams, D. O. (1980). Effector mechanisms of cytolytically activated macrophages. I. Secretion of neutral proteases and effect of protease inhibitors. *J. Immunol.*, **124**, 286–92
113. Adams, D. O., Kao, K.-J., Farb, R. and Pizzo, S. V. (1980). Effector mechanisms of cytolytically activated macrophages. II. Secretion of a cytolytic factor by activated macrophages and its relationship to secreted neutral proteases. *J. Immunol.*, **124**, 293–300
114. Johnson, W. J., Pizzo, S. V., Imber, M. J. and Adams, D. O. (1982). Receptors for maleylated proteins regulate secretion of neutral proteases by murine macrophages. *Science*, **218**, 574–6
115. Reidarson, T. H., Granger, G. A. and Klostergaard, J. (1982). Inducible macrophage cytotoxins. II. Tumor lysis mechanism involving target cell-binding proteases. *J. Natl. Cancer Inst.*, **69**, 889–94
116. Okawa, Y., Ozeki, Y., Suzuki, K., Sakai, K., Suzuki, S. and Suzuki, M. (1987). Correlation between tumor cell cytotoxicity and serine protease activity of peritoneal macrophages from mice treated with bakers' yeast mannans. *Chem. Pharm. Bull.*, **35**, 1138–43
117. Rojas-Espinosa, O., Arce-Paradez, P., Dannenberg, A. M., Jr and Kamenetz, R. L. (1975). Macrophage esterase: identification, purification and properties of a chymotrypsin-like esterase from lung that hydrolyses and transfers nonpolar amino acid esters. *Biochim. Biophys. Acta*, **403**, 161–79
118. Kominami, E., Tsukahara, T., Hara, K. and Katunuma, N. (1988). Biosynthesis and processing of lysosomal cysteine proteinases in rat macrophages. *FEBS Lett.*, **231**, 225–8
119. Bando, Y., Kominami, E. and Katunuma, N. (1986). Purification and tissue distribution of rat cathepsin L. *J. Biochem.*, **100**, 35–42

120. Kato, T., Kojima, K. and Murachi, T. (1972). Proteases of macrophages in rat peritoneal exudate, with special reference to the effects of actinomycete protease inhibitors. *Biochim. Biophys. Acta*, **289**, 187–94
121. Orlowski, M., Orlowski, R., Chang, J. C., Wilk, E. and Lesser, M. (1984). A sensitive procedure for determination of cathepsin D: activity in alveolar and peritoneal macrophages. *Mol. Cell. Biochem.*, **64**, 155–62
122. Lesser, M., Chang, J. C., Orlowski, J., Kilburn, K. H. and Orlowski, M. (1983). Cathepsin B and prolyl endopeptidase activity in rat peritoneal and alveolar macrophages. *J. Lab. Clin. Med.*, **101**, 327–34
123. Reilly, J. J., Jr, Mason, R. W., Chen, P., Joseph, L. J., Sukhatme, V. P., Yee, R. and Chapman, H. A., Jr (1989). Synthesis and processing of cathepsin L, and elastase, by human alveolar macrophages. *Biochem. J.*, **257**, 493–8
124. Cohn, Z. A. and Wiener, E. (1963). The particulate hydrolases of macrophages. II. Biochemical and morphological response to particulate ingestion. *J. Exp. Med.*, **118**, 1009–20
125. Chapman, H. A. and Stone, O. L. (1984). Co-operation between plasmin and elastase in elastin degradation by intact murine macrophages. *Biochem. J.*, **222**, 721–8
126. Mason, R. W. (1988). The role of cysteine proteinases in elastin degradation. In Glauert, A. M. (ed.), *Control of Tissue Damage. Res. Monogr. Cell Tissue Physiol.*, **15**, pp. 259–67 (Amsterdam: Elsevier)
127. Werb, Z., Banda, M. J. and Jones, P. A. (1980). Degradation of connective tissue matrices by macrophages. I. Proteolysis of elastin, glycoproteins and collagen by proteinases isolated from macrophages. *J. Exp. Med.*, **152**, 1340–57
128. Roberts, C. R. and Dean, R. T. (1986). Degradation of cartilage by macrophages in culture: evidence for the involvement of an enzyme which is associated with the cell surface. *Connect. Tissue Res.*, **14**, 199–212
129. Silver, I. A., Murrills, R. J. and Etherington, D. J. (1988). Microelectrode studies on the acid microenvironment beneath adherent macrophages and osteoclasts. *Exp. Cell. Res.*, **175**, 266–76
130. Wahl, L. M., Wahl, S. M., Mergenhagen, S. E. and Martin, G. R. (1974). Collagenase production by endotoxin activated macrophages. *Proc. Natl. Acad. Sci. USA*, **71**, 3598–601
131. Wahl, L. M. and Mergenhagen, S. E. (1988). Regulation of monocyte/macrophage collagenase. *J. Oral Pathol.*, **17**, 452–5
132. Cury, J. D., Campbell, E. J., Lazarus, C. J., Albin, R. J. and Welgus, H. G. (1988). Selective up-regulation of human alveolar macrophage collagenase production by lipopolysaccharide and comparison to collagenase production by fibroblasts. *J. Immunol.*, **141**, 4306–12
133. Campbell, E. J., Cury, J. D., Lazarus, C. J. and Welgus, H. G. (1987). Monocyte procollagenase and tissue inhibitor of metalloproteinases: identification, characterization and regulation of secretion. *J. Biol. Chem.*, **262**, 15862–8
134. Mainardi, C. L., Seyer, J. M. and Kang, A. H. (1980). Type-specific collagenolysis: a type V collagen-degrading enzyme from macrophages. *Biochem. Biophys. Res. Commun.*, **97**, 1108–15
135. Hibbs, M. S., Hoidal, J. R. and Kang, A. H. (1987). Expression of a metalloproteinase that degrades native type V collagen and denatured collagens by cultured human alveolar macrophages. *J. Clin. Invest.*, **80**, 1644–50
136. Welgus, H. G., Campbell, E. J., Cury, J. D., Eisen, A. Z., Senior, R. M., Wilhelm, S. M. and Goldberg, G. I. (1988). Neutral metalloproteinases produced by human mononuclear phagocytes. *J. Cell Biol.*, **107** (6, part III), 376A
137. Hauser, P. and Vaes, G. (1978). Degradation of cartilage proteoglycans by a neutral proteinase secreted by rabbit bone-marrow macrophages in culture. *Biochem. J.*, **172**, 275–84
138. Banda, M. J. and Werb, Z. (1981). Mouse macrophage elastase. Purification and characterization as a metalloproteinase. *Biochem. J.*, **193**, 589–605
139. Takemura, R. and Werb, Z. (1984). Regulation of elastase and plasminogen activator secretion in resident and inflammatory macrophages by receptors for the Fc domain of immunoglobulin G. *J. Exp. Med.*, **159**, 152–66
140. Banda, M. J., Clark, E. J., Sinha, S. and Travis, J. (1987). Interaction of mouse macrophage elastase with native and oxidized human α_1-proteinase inhibitor. *J. Clin. Invest.*, **79**, 1314–7
141. Banda, M. J., Rice, A. G., Griffin, G. L. and Senior, R. M. (1988). α_1-Proteinase inhibitor is a neutrophil chemoattractant after proteolytic inactivation by macrophage elastase. *J. Biol. Chem.*, **263**, 4481–4

142. Werb, Z., Banda, M. J., McKerrow, J. H. and Sandhaus, R. A. (1982). Elastases and elastin degradation. *J. Invest. Dermatol.*, **79** (Suppl. 1), 154s–159s
143. Senior, R. M., Campbell, E. J., Landis, J. A., Cox, F. R., Kuhn, C. and Koren, H. S. (1982). Elastase of U-937 monocyte-like cells: comparisons with elastases derived from human monocytes and neutrophils and murine macrophage-like cells. *J. Clin. Invest.*, **69**, 384–93
144. Fuks, A., Zucker-Franklin, D. and Franklin, E. C. (1983). Identification of elastases associated with purified plasma membranes isolated from human monocytes and lymphocytes. *Biochim. Biophys. Acta*, **755**, 195–203
145. Sandhaus, R. A., McCarthy, K. M., Musson, R. A. and Henson, P. M. (1983). Elastolytic proteinases of the human macrophage. *Chest*, **83** (5, Suppl.), 60s–62s
146. Albin, R. J., Senior, R. M., Welgus, H. G., Connolly, N. L. and Campbell, E. J. (1987). Human alveolar macrophages secrete an inhibitor of metalloproteinase elastase. *Am. Rev. Respir. Dis.*, **135**, 1281–5
147. White, R., Lee, D., Habicht, G. S. and Janoff, A. (1981). Secretion of α_1-proteinase inhibitor by cultured rat alveolar macrophages. *Am. Rev. Resp. Dis.*, **123**, 447–9
148. Remold-O'Donnell, E. and Lewandrowski, K. (1983). Two proteinase inhibitors associated with peritoneal macrophages. *J. Biol. Chem.*, **258**, 3251–7
149. Krivit, W., Miller, J., Nowicki, M. and Freier, E. (1988). Contribution of monocyte-macrophage system to serum α_1-antitrypsin. *J. Lab. Clin. Med.*, **112**, 437–42
150. Perlmutter, D. H., Travis, J. and Punsal, P. I. (1988). Elastase regulates the synthesis of its inhibitor, α_1-proteinase inhibitor, and exaggerates the defect in homozygous PiZZ α_1PI deficiency. *J. Clin. Invest.*, **81**, 1774–80
151. Benfey, P. N., Yin, F. H. and Leder, P. (1987). Cloning of the mast cell protease RMCP II. Evidence for cell specific expression and a multigene family. *J. Biol. Chem.*, **262**, 5377–84
152. Woodbury, R. G., Le Trong, H. and Neurath, H. (1987). Structure and function of mast cell proteases. *Acta Histochem. Cytochem.*, **20**, 261–9
153. Irani, A. A., Schechter, N. M., Craig, S. S., DeBlois, G. and Schwartz, L. B. (1986). Two types of human mast cells that have distinct neutral protease compositions. *Proc. Natl. Acad. Sci. USA*, **83**, 4464–8
154. Graziano, F. M. (1988). Mast cells and mast cell products. *Methods Enzymol.*, **162**, 501–22
155. Le Trong, H., Parmalee, D. C., Walsh, K. A., Neurath, H. and Woodbury, R. G. (1987). Amino acid sequence of rat mast cell protease I (chymase). *Biochemistry*, **26**, 6988–94
156. Woodbury, R. G., Katunuma, N., Kobayashi, K., Titani, K. and Neurath, H. (1978). Covalent structure of a group-specific protease from rat small intestine. *Biochemistry*, **17**, 811–19
157. Le Trong, H., Newlands, G. F. J., Miller, H. R. P., Charbonneau, H., Neurath, H. and Woodbury, R. G. (1989). Amino acid sequence of a mouse mucosal mast cell protease. *Biochemistry*, **28**, 391–5
158. Vanderslice, P., Craik, C. S., Nadel, J. A. and Caughey, G. H. (1989). Molecular cloning of dog mast cell tryptase and a related protease: structural evidence of a unique mode of serine protease activation. *Biochemistry*, **28**, 4148–55
159. Remington, S. J., Woodbury, R. G., Reynolds, R. A., Matthews, B. W. and Neurath, H. (1988). The structure of the rat mast cell protease II at 1.9 Å resolution. *Biochemistry*, **27**, 8097–104
160. Schechter, N. M., Fräki, J. E., Geesin, J. C. and Lazarus, G. S. (1983). Human skin chymotryptic proteinase. Isolation and relation to cathepsin G and rat mast cell proteinase I. *J. Biol. Chem.*, **258**, 2973–8
161. Johnson, L. A., Moon, K. E. and Eisenberg, M. (1986). Purification to homogeneity of the human skin chymotryptic proteinase 'chymase'. *Anal. Biochem.*, **155**, 358–64
162. Kido, H., Fukusen, N. and Katunuma, N. (1985). Chymotrypsin- and trypsin-type serine proteases in rat mast cells: properties and functions. *Arch. Biochem. Biophys.*, **239**, 436–43
163. Muramatu, M., Itoh, T., Takei, M. and Endo, K. (1988). Tryptase in rat mast cells: properties and inhibition by various inhibitors in comparison with chymase. *Biol. Chem. Hoppe-Seyler*, **369**, 617–26
164. Schwartz, L. B., Lewis, R. A. and Austen, K. F. (1981). Tryptase from human pulmonary mast cells. Purification and characterization. *J. Biol. Chem.*, **256**, 11939–43
165. Tanaka, T., McRae, B. J., Cho, K., Cook, R., Fraki, J. E., Johnson, D. A. and Powers, J. C. (1983). Mammalian tissue trypsin-like enzymes. Comparative reactivities of human skin tryptase, human lung tryptase, and bovine trypsin with peptide 4-nitroanilide and thioester

substrates. *J. Biol. Chem.*, **258**, 13552–7

166. Cromlish, J. A., Seidah, N. G., Marcinkiewicz, M., Hamelin, J., Johnson, D. A. and Chretien, M. (1987). Human pituitary tryptase: molecular forms, NH_2-terminal sequence, immunocytochemical localization and specificity with prohormone and fluoregenic substrates. *J. Biol. Chem.*, **262**, 1363–73
167. Katunuma, N., Fukusen, N. and Kido, H. (1986). Biological functions of serine proteases in the granules of rat mast cells. *Adv. Enzyme Regul.*, **25**, 241–55
168. Kido, H., Yokogoshi, Y. and Katunuma, N. (1988). Kunitz-type protease inhibitor found in rat mast cells. Purification, properties and amino acid sequences. *J. Biol. Chem.*, **263**, 18104–7
169. Fritz, H., Kruck, J., Rüsse, I. and Liebich, H. G. (1979). Immunofluorescence studies indicate that the basic trypsin-kallikrein-inhibitor of bovine organs (Trasylol) originates from mast cells. *Hoppe-Seyler's Z. Physiol. Chem.*, **360**, 437–44
170. Katunuma, N. and Kido, H. (1988). Biologic functions of serine proteases in mast cells in allergic inflammation. *J. Cell. Biochem.*, **38**, 291–302
171. Mundy, D. I. and Strittmatter, W. J. (1985). Requirement for metalloendoprotease in exocytosis: evidence in mast cells and adrenal chromaffin cells. *Cell*, **40**, 645–56
172. Kido, H., Fukusen, N. and Katunuma, N. (1985). Antibody and inhibitor of chymase inhibit histamine release in immunoglobulin E-activated mast cells. *Biochem. Int.*, **10**, 863–72
173. Schick, B. and Austen, K. F. (1985). Pharmacological modulation of activation-secretion of rat serosal mast cells by chymase, an endogenous secretory granule protease. *Immunology*, **56**, 513–22
174. Maier, M., Spragg, J. and Schwartz, L. B. (1983). Inactivation of human high molecular weight kininogen by human mast cell tryptase. *J. Immunol.*, **130**, 2352–6
175. Schwartz, L. B., Kawahara, M. S., Hugli, T. E., Vik, D., Fearon, D. T. and Austen, K. F. (1983). Generation of C3a anaphylatoxin from human C3 by human mast cell tryptase. *J. Immunol.*, **130**, 1891–5
176. Majima, M., Tani, Y. and Katori, M. (1987). Loss of the activity of human coagulation factor XII by a chymotrypsin-like protease activated in rat mast cells during degranulation with compound 48/80. *Thromb. Res.*, **46**, 855–68
177. Kido, H., Fukusen, N., Katunuma, N., Morita, T. and Iwanaga, S. (1985). Tryptase from rat mast cells converts bovine prothrombin to thrombin. *Biochem. Biophys. Res. Commun.*, **132**, 613–19
178. Alter, S. C., Metcalfe, D. D., Bradford, T. R. and Schwartz, L. B. (1987). Regulation of human mast cell tryptase. Effects of enzyme concentration, ionic strength and the structure and negative charge density of polysaccharides. *Biochem. J.*, **248**, 821–8
179. Gervasoni, J. E., Jr, Conrad, D. H., Hugli, T. E., Schwartz, L. B. and Ruddy, S. (1986). Degradation of human anaphylatoxin C3a by rat peritoneal mast cells: a role for the secretory granule enzyme chymase and heparin proteoglycan. *J. Immunol.*, **136**, 285–92
180. Caughey, G. H., Leidig, F., Viro, N. F. and Nadel, J. A. (1988). Substance P and vasoactive intestinal peptide degradation by mast cell tryptase and chymase. *J. Pharmacol. Exp. Ther.*, **244**, 133–7
181. Le Trong, H., Neurath, H. and Woodbury, R. G. (1987). Substrate specificity of the chymotrypsin-like protease in secretory granules isolated from rat mast cells. *Proc. Natl. Acad. Sci. USA*, **84**, 364–7
182. Wintroub, B. U., Kaempfer, C. E., Schechter, N. M. and Proud, D. (1986). A human lung mast cell chymotrypsin-like enzyme – identification and partial characterisation. *J. Clin. Invest.*, **77**, 196–201
183. King, S. J., Miller, H. R. P., Newlands, G. F. J. and Woodbury, R. G. (1985). Depletion of mucosal mast cell protease by corticosteroids: effect on intestinal anaphylaxis in the rat. *Proc. Natl. Acad. Sci. USA*, **82**, 1214–8
184. MacQueen, G., Marshall, J., Perdue, M., Siegel, S. and Bienenstock, J. (1989). Pavlovian condition of rat mucosal mast cells to secrete rat mast cell protease II. *Science*, **243**, 83–5
185. Vartio, T., Seppä, H. and Vaheri, A. (1981). Susceptibility of soluble and matrix fibronectins to degradation by tissue proteinases, mast cell chymase, and cathepsin G. *J. Biol. Chem.*, **256**, 471–7
186. Sage, H., Balian, G., Vogel, A. M. and Bornstein, P. (1984). Type VIII collagen. Synthesis by normal and malignant cells in culture. *Lab. Invest.*, **50**, 219–31
187. Seppä, H. (1979). The role of chymotrypsin-like protease of rat mast cells in inflammatory

vasopermeability and fibrinolysis. *Inflammation*, **4**, 1–8

188. Sage, H., Woodbury, R. G. and Bornstein, P. (1979). Structural studies on human type IV collagen. *J. Biol. Chem.*, **254**, 9893–900
189. Johnson, D. A. and Cawston, T. E. (1985). Human lung mast cell tryptase fails to activate procollagenase or degrade proteoglycan. *Biochem. Biophys. Res. Commun.*, **132**, 453–9
190. Birkedal-Hansen, H., Cobb, C. M., Taylor, R. E. and Fullmer, H. M. (1975). Activation of fibroblast procollagenase by mast cell proteases. *Biochim. Biophys. Acta*, **438**, 273–86
191. Eisenberg, M., Johnson, L. and Moon, K. E. (1984). Serine proteinase activation of latent human skin collagenase. *Biochem. Biophys. Res. Commun.*, **125**, 279–85
192. Sopata, I., Wojteka-Lukasik, E. and Maslinski, S. (1986). Activation of latent human granulocyte gelatinase by rat mast cell protease. *Folia Histochem. Cytobiol.*, **24**, 133–7
193. Gruber, B. L., Schwartz, L. B., Ramamurthy, N. S., Irani, M. and Marchese, M. J. (1988). Activation of latent rheumatoid synovial collagenase by human mast cell tryptase. *J. Immunol.*, **140**, 3936–42
194. Bleackley, R. C., Duggan, B., Ehrman, N. and Lobe, C. G. (1988). Isolation of two cDNA sequences which encode cytotoxic cell proteases. *FEBS Lett.*, **234**, 153–9
195. Gershenfeld, H. K., Hershberger, R. J., Mueller, C. and Weissman, I. L. (1988). A T cell- and natural killer cell-specific, trypsin-like serine protease. Implications of a protease cascade. *Ann. N.Y. Acad. Sci.*, **532**, 367–79
196. Pasternack, M. S. and Eisen, H. N. (1985). A novel serine esterase expressed by cytotoxic T lymphocytes. *Nature (London)*, **314**, 743–5
197. Gershenfeld, H. K. and Weissman, I. L. (1986). Cloning of a cDNA for a T cell-specific serine protease from a cytotoxic T lymphocyte. *Science*, **232**, 854–8
198. Lobe, C. G., Finlay, B. B., Paranchych, W., Paetkau, V. H. and Bleackley, R. C. (1986). Novel serine proteases encoded by two cytotoxic T lymphocyte-specific genes. *Science*, **232**, 858–62
199. Brunet, J., Dosetto, F., Denizot, F., Mattei, M.-G., Clark, W. R., Haqqi, T. M., Ferrier, P., Nabholz, M., Schmitt-Verhulst, A. M., Luciani, M.-F. and Goldstein, P. (1986). The inducible cytotoxic T-lymphocyte-associated gene transcript CTLA-1 sequence and gene localization to mouse chromosome 14. *Nature*, **322**, 268–71
200. Gershenfeld, H. K., Hershberger, R. J., Shows, T. B. and Weissman, I. L. (1988). Cloning and chromosomal assignment of a human cDNA encoding a T cell- and natural killer cell-specific trypsin-like serine protease. *Proc. Natl. Acad. Sci. USA*, **85**, 1184–8
201. Trapani, J. A., Klein, J. L., White, P. C. and Dupont, B. (1988). Molecular cloning of an inducible serine esterase gene from human cytotoxic lymphocytes. *Proc. Natl. Acad. Sci. USA*, **85**, 6924–8
202. Schmid, J. and Weissmann, C. (1987). Induction of mRNa for a serine protease and a beta-thromboglobulin-like protein in mitogen-stimulated human leukocytes. *J. Immunol.*, **139**, 250–6
203. Jenne, D., Rey, C., Masson, D., Stanley, K., Plaetinck, G. and Tschopp, J. (1988). cDNA cloning of granzyme C, a granule associated serine protease of cytolytic T lymphocytes. *J. Immunol.*, **140**, 318–23
204. Kwon, B. S., Kestler, D., Lee, E., Wakulchik, M. and Young, J. D. (1988). Isolation and sequence analysis of serine protease cDNAs from mouse cytolytic lymphocytes-T. *J. Exp. Med.*, **168**, 1839–54
205. Simon, M. M., Hoschützky, H., Fruth, U., Simon, H. G. and Kramer, M. D. (1986). Purification and characterization of a T-cell-specific serine proteinase (TSP-1) from cloned cytolytic T-lymphocytes. *EMBO J.*, **5**, 3267–74
206. Masson, D. and Tschopp, J. (1987). A family of serine esterases in lytic granules of cytolytic T lymphocytes. *Cell*, **49**, 679–85
207. Jenne, D., Rey, C., Haefliger, J. A., Qiao, B. Y., Groscurth, P. and Tschopp, J. (1988). Identification and sequencing of cDNA clones encoding the granule-associated serine proteases granzymes D, E, and F of cytolytic T lymphocytes. *Proc. Natl. Acad. Sci. USA*, **84**, 4814–8
208. Murphy, M. E. P., Moult, J., Bleackley, R. C., Gershenfeld, H., Weissman, I. L. and James, M. N. G. (1988). Comparative molecular model building of 2 serine proteinases from cytotoxic lymphocytes T. *Proteins*, **4**, 190–204
209. Hatcher, V. B., Oberman, M. S., Lazarus, G. S. and Grayzel, A. I. (1978). A cytotoxic

proteinase isolated from human lymphocytes. *J. Immunol.*, **120**, 665–70

210. Fruth, U., Sinigaglia, F., Schlesier, M., Kilgus, J., Kramer, M. D. and Simon, M. M. (1987). A novel serine proteinase (HuTSP) isolated from a cloned human $CD8^+$ cytolytic T cell line is expressed and secreted by activated $CD4^+$ and $CD8^+$ lymphocytes. *Eur. J. Immunol.*, **17**, 1625–33
211. Krähenbühl, O., Rey, C., Jenne, D., Lanzavecchia, A., Groscurth, P., Carrel, S. and Tschopp, J. (1988). Characterization of granzymes A and B isolated from granules of cloned human cytotoxic T lymphocytes. *J. Immunol.*, **141**, 3471–7
212. Hameed, A., Lowrey, D. M., Lichtenheld, M. and Podack, E. R. (1988). Characterization of three serine esterases isolated from human IL-2 activated killer cells. *J. Immunol.*, **141**, 3142–7
213. Poe, M., Bennett, C. D., Biddison, W. E., Blake, J. T., Norton, G. P., Rodkey, J. A., Sigal, N. H., Turner, R. V., Wu, J. K. and Zweerink, H. J. (1988). Human cytotoxic lymphocyte tryptase. Its purification from granules and the characterization of inhibitor and substrate specificity. *J. Biol. Chem.*, **263**, 13215–22
214. Hudig, D., Redelman, D. and Minning, L. L. (1984). The requirement for proteinase activity for human lymphocyte-mediated natural cytotoxicity (NK): evidence that the proteinase is serine dependent and has aromatic amino acid specificity of cleavage. *J. Immunol.*, **133**, 2647–54
215. Masson, D. and Tschopp, J. (1988). Inhibition of lymphocyte protease granzyme A by antithrombin III. *Mol. Immunol.*, **25**, 1283–90
216. Ganea, D., Cearlock, D., Minowada, J. and Dray, S. (1987). A serine proteinase inhibitor produced by an HTLV 1 virus-transformed human T lymphocyte line. *J. Immunol.*, **138**, 1208–14
217. Ganea, D., Teodorescu, M. and Dray, S. (1986). A low molecular weight proteinase inhibitor produced by T lymphocytes. *Immunology*, **57**, 85–92
218. Ikuta, T., Okubo, H., Kudo, J., Ishibashi, H. and Inoue, T. (1982). $Alpha_1$-antitrypsin synthesis by human lymphocytes. *Biochem. Biophys. Res. Commun.*, **104**, 1509–16
219. Jenne, D. E. and Tschopp, J. (1988). Granzymes, a family of serine proteases released from granules of cytolytic T lymphocytes upon T cell receptor stimulation. *Immunol. Rev.*, **103**, 53–72
220. Thibault, G. and Genest, J. (1981). Tonin, an esteroprotease from rat submaxillary glands. *Biochim. Biophys. Acta*, **660**, 23–9
221. Ashe, B. M., Biddison, W. E., Blake, J. T., Norton, G., Poe, M., Sigal, N. H. and Zweerink, H. J. (1988). A comparison of trypsin-like protease activities in extracts of human and murine cytolytic T-cells. *Ann. N.Y. Acad. Sci.*, **532**, 439–41
222. Zunino, S. J., Allison, N. J., Kam, C. M., Powers, J. C. and Hudig, D. (1988). Localization, implications for function and gene expression of chymotrypsin-like proteinases of cytotoxic RNK-16 lymphocytes. *Biochim. Biophys. Acta*, **967**, 331–40
223. Hudig, D., Minning, L. and Redelman, D. (1985). A serine proteinease as a trigger for human natural killer lymphocyte-mediated cytolysis. In Henkart, P. and Martz, E. (eds), *Mechanisms of Cell-Mediated Toxicity, II. Adv. Exp. Med. Biol.*, Vol. 184, pp. 271–80 (New York: Plenum Press)
224. Arakawa, K., Nakajima, H., Yoshida, T., Yasumuta, T., Aikawa, I., Ohmori, Y. and Oka, T. (1989). Inhibitory effect of reversible serine protease inhibitors on the activity of cytotoxic lymphocytes-T. *Transplant. Proc.*, **21**, 1152–3
225. Brogan, M. and Targan, S. (1986). Evidence for involvement of serine proteases in the late stages of the natural killer cell lytic reaction. *Cell Immunol.*, **103**, 426–33
226. Podack, E. R. and Königsberg, P. J. (1984). Cytolytic T cell granules. Isolation, structural, biochemical and functional characterization. *J. Exp. Med.*, **160**, 695–710
227. Utsunomiya, N. and Nakanishi, M. (1986). A serine protease triggers the initial step of transmembrane signalling in cytotoxic T cells. *J. Biol. Chem.*, **261**, 16514–17
228. Tokes, Z. A. (1981). Cell surface-associated protease activity in lymphocyte interactions. In Steinberg, C. M. and Lefkovits, I. (eds), *Immune Systems*, Vol. 2, pp. 239–48 (Basel: Karger)
229. Simon, M. M., Simon, H. G., Fruth, U., Epplen, J., Müller-Hermelink, H. K. and Kramer, M. D. (1987). Cloned cytolytic T-effector cells and their malignant variants produce an extracellular matrix degrading trypsin-like serine proteinase. *Immunology*, **60**, 219–30
230. Simon, M. M., Prester, M., Nerz, G., Kramer, M. D. and Fruth, U. (1988). Release of biologically active fragments from human plasma-fibronectin by murine T-cell-specific proteinase-1 (TSP-1). *Biol. Chem. Hoppe-Seyler*, **369** (Suppl.), 107–12

231. Munger, W. E., Berrebi, G. A. and Henkart, P. A. (1988). Possible involvement of CTL granule proteases in target cell DNA breakdown. *Immunol. Rev.*, **103**, 99–100
232. Bata, J., Martin, J. P. and Revillard, J. P. (1981). Cell surface protease activity of human lymphocytes; its inhibition by α_1-antitrypsin. *Experientia*, **37**, 518–19
233. Pierart, M. E., Najdovski, T., Appleboom, T. E. and Deschodt-Lanckman, M. M. (1988). Effect of human endopeptidase 24.11 (enkephalinase) in IL-1 induced thymocyte proliferation activity. *J. Immunol.*, **140**, 3808–11
234. Yaso, S., Yokono, K., Hari, J., Yonezawa, K., Shii, K. and Baba, S. (1987). Possible role of cell surface insulin degrading enzyme in cultured human lymphocytes. *Diabetologia*, **30**, 27–32
235. Kammer, G. M., Sapolsky, A. I. and Malemud, C. J. (1985). Secretion of an articular cartilage proteoglycan-degrading enzyme activity by murine lymphocytes-T *in vitro*. *J. Clin. Invest.*, **76**, 395–402
236. Oronsky, A. L. and Perper, R. J. (1975). Connective tissue-degrading enzymes of human leukocytes. *Ann. N.Y. Acad. Sci.*, **256**, 233–53
237. Simpson, J. W., Mackler, B. F., O'Neill, P. A., Mailman, M. L., Adams, S. and Harris, J. (1978). Collagenase production by human peripheral-blood mononuclear cells. *J. Dent. Res.*, **57**, 264
238. Govindarajan, K. R., Offner, H., Clausen, J., Fog, T. and Hyllested, K. (1974). The lymphocytic cathepsin B-1 and D activities in multiple sclerosis. *J. Neurol.*, **23**, 81–7
239. Grayzel, A. I., Hatcher, V. B. and Lazarus, G. S. (1976). Protease activity of normal and PHA (phytohemagglutinin) stimulated human lymphocytes. *Cell. Immunol.*, **18**, 210–19
240. Yago, N. and Bowers, W. E. (1975). Unique cathepsin D-type proteases in rat thoracic duct lymphocytes and in rat lymphoid tissues. *J. Biol. Chem.*, **250**, 4749–54
241. Langner, J., Kirschke, H. and Neumann, V. (1983). Cysteine proteinases in peripheral blood lymphocytes (PBL). *Wiss. Z. Martin-Luther-Univ. Halle-Wittenberg. Math.-Naturwiss. Reihe*, **32**, 23–25
242. Kominami, E., Stukahara, T., Bando, Y. and Katunuma, N. (1985). Distribution of cathepsin B and H in rat tissues and peripheral blood cells. *J. Biochem.*, **98**, 87–94

5
Eicosanoids (prostaglandins and leukotrienes)

E. R. PETTIPHER, G. A. HIGGS and J. A. SALMON

INTRODUCTION

The importance of locally produced prostaglandins (PGs) in the inflammatory response has been well recognized since the observation by Vane and colleagues that aspirin and other non-steroidal anti-inflammatory drugs (NSAIDs) inhibit PG synthesis[1-3]. More recently, it has been suggested that other products of arachidonic acid metabolism, such as leukotrienes, are also mediators of allergic and inflammatory reactions. Inhibitors of leukotriene synthesis and antagonists of their action have recently been developed and are presently undergoing clinical evaluation; the exact role and importance of these mediators in human disease will be clarified only when the outcome of these clinical studies is known. In this review we will describe the pharmacological effects of selective lipoxygenase inhibitors in tests conducted in animals, and will discuss the possible relevance to humans.

Although the prostaglandins have pro-inflammatory effects, it is also clear that prostaglandins (particularly PGE_2 and prostacyclin, PGI_2) can down-regulate the inflammatory response, probably by suppression of the activity of a range of leukocytes including neutrophils, lymphocytes and macrophages. For example, there is some evidence that PGE_2 and PGI_2 inhibit the generation from macrophages of cytokines such as interleukin 1 (IL 1) and tumour necrosis factor α (TNF-α), cytokines which may play a central role in chronic inflammation[4]. Therefore, in this review we will also discuss the importance of interactions of eicosanoids with cytokines and the cells involved in chronic inflammation.

PATHWAYS OF EICOSANOID BIOSYNTHESIS

The important pathways of eicosanoid synthesis are shown in Figure 5.1. The unsaturated fatty acid, arachidonic acid, is the precursor for the synthesis

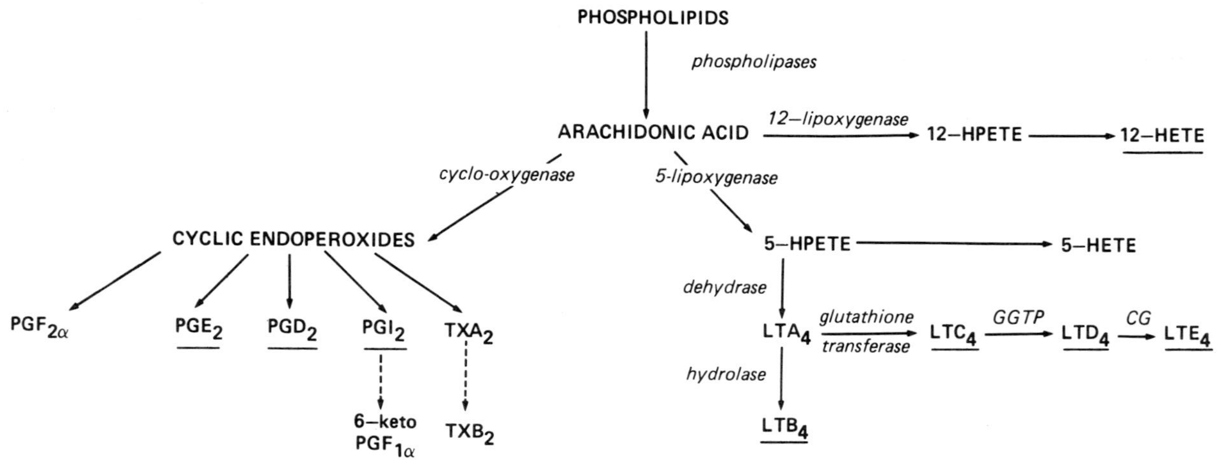

Figure 5.1 Pathways of arachidonic acid metabolism. The enzymes responsible for metabolic transformations are shown in italics (GGTP, gamma-glutamyl transpeptidase; CG, cysteinyl-glycinase). The dashed lines represent non-enzymatic transformations and the mediators underlined represent those with biological activity relevant to inflammation.

of the major classes of both prostaglandins and leukotrienes. The level of free arachidonic acid in cells is very low, but it is stored in an esterified form in membrane phospholipids. The arachidonyl moiety is located almost exclusively at the 2-acyl position of the phospholipids and consequently the action of phospholipase A_2 causes the liberation of arachidonic acid. Lipocortin I and II, which are proteins synthesized by macrophages and possibly other cell types in response to glucocorticoids, inhibit phospholipase A_2 (see Flower[5]). The inhibition of phospholipase A_2 activity by these polypeptides is due to substrate sequestration rather than to a direct enzyme–inhibitor interaction[6]. Recombinant lipocortin I (or calpactin II) inhibits eicosanoid synthesis in guinea-pig lung[7] but not in murine macrophages[8], which suggests that phospholipase A_2 may be responsible for the mobilization of arachidonic acid in some cell types but not in others. Arachidonic acid can also be liberated from phospholipids in some systems by the sequential action of phospholipase C and a diacylglycerol lipase[9]. Whatever the mechanism that initiates eicosanoid synthesis, it can occur extremely rapidly: for example, in platelets 75–80% of liberated arachidonic acid is converted to eicosanoids with 10 s of stimulation[9].

Arachidonic acid is often found esterified in the 2 position of the ether-linked phosphatide which is also the substrate for the formation of platelet-activating factor (PAF)[10]. Consequently, cleavage by phospholipase will lead to the liberation of arachidonic acid and lyso-PAF, the precursor substrates for eicosanoid and PAF synthesis respectively. The pathways of PAF synthesis are discussed in more detail in Chapter 9.

Free arachidonic acid can be converted to a variety of metabolites ('eicosanoids'). Two major groups (cyclooxygenase and lipoxygenase products) can be formed, and these are classified according to the enzyme reaction which initiates their synthesis. The biosynthetic pathways leading to the formation of cyclooxygenase and lipoxygenase products are complex (see Figure 5.1) and are described only briefly here; readers are referred to more detailed reviews for further information[11–13]. The cyclooxygenase enzyme complex is present in the 'microsomal' fraction of most mammalian cells and converts arachidonic acid to the cyclic endoperoxides, PGG_2 and PGH_2. Prostaglandin G_2 and H_2 can degrade non-enzymatically to the primary prostaglandins PGD_2, PGE_2 and $PGF_{2\alpha}$. However, there are distinct isomerases which catalyse the conversion of endoperoxides to PGD_2 and PGE_2. Also, the reduction of the endoperoxides to $PGF_{2\alpha}$ may be catalysed by aldoketoreductases[14]. Some cell types (e.g. mast cells) produce PGD_2, but not PGE_2, which suggests that the relative distribution of these isomerases is important in determining which prostaglandin is formed.

In endothelial cells, prostacyclin (PGI_2) is enzymatically produced from the endoperoxides by the action of the enzyme prostacyclin synthase. Prostacyclin is unstable under physiological conditions and is rapidly hydrolysed to 6-keto-$PGF_{1\alpha}$.

Thromboxane A_2 (TXA_2) is produced from the endoperoxides in platelets, PMNs, macrophages and some other cell types, by an enzyme termed thromboxane synthase. Thromboxane A_2 is also very unstable and decomposes rapidly to TXB_2.

There are several enzymes which can catalyse the formation of positional isomers of hydroperoxy analogues of arachidonic acid (or hydroperoxyeicosatetraenoic acids; HPETEs). The most extensively studied reaction is the conversion of arachidonic acid to 15-HPETE by soybean lipoxygenase[15]. The first reports of a mammalian lipoxygenase was of the enzyme present in blood platelets which catalysed the formation of 12-HPETE[16,17]. However, the most important enzyme in this class is probably the 5-lipoxygenase because it controls the initial step in the biosynthesis of the leukotrienes.

The 5-lipoxygenase is not so widely distributed as the cyclooxygenase, it appears to be restricted mainly to neutrophils, eosinophils, monocyte/macrophages and mast cells. The enzyme introduces a molecule of oxygen at the 5-position of arachidonic acid to produce 5-HPETE. This hydroperoxy acid can then be reduced enzymatically to 5-hydroxyeicosatetraenoic acid (5-HETE) or dehydrated to leukotriene A_4 (LTA_4). The latter can be converted to the peptido-leukotrienes, LTC_4, LTD_4 and LTE_4. Leukotriene A_4 can also be enzymatically hydrolysed to the potent chemotactic lipid, LTB_4.

Although the metabolites described above are considered to be the most biologically important, arachidonic acid can be metabolized to many other derivatives. The lipoxins, which are formed via the 15- and 5-lipoxygenase pathways, are reported to have potent biological activities[18], but it has not yet been confirmed that they are formed *in vivo* and consequently their relevance to pathophysiological processes is uncertain. A 12-HETE was detected in the involved skin of patients with psoriasis[19] but an investigation of the stereochemistry of the hydroxy acid revealed that it was the R-enantiomer[20] whereas 12-lipoxygenase action yields 12(S)-HETE. Therefore, a different enzyme system is probably involved in the biosynthesis of the product observed in psoriasis. Since 12(R)-HETE has more marked inflammatory properties than the S-enantiomer[21] the identification of the enzyme responsible for the formation of 12(R)-HETE is important. Other investigators have detected 12(R)-HETE in incubations of arachidonic acid with kidney homogenates, and evidence was presented indicating that the reaction was catalysed by a cytochrome P-450 hydroxylase[22]. Cytochrome P-450 enzymes have also been implicated in the synthesis of epoxide derivatives of arachidonic acid[23].

The above discussion has focused on arachidonic acid, but some other unsaturated fatty acids may also be substrates for the cyclooxgenase and lipoxygenase enzymes. Although it is not as good a substrate as arachidonic acid, dihomogammalinoleic acid is converted by the cyclooxygenase to monoenoic prostaglandins. In contrast, eicosapentaenoic acid (EPA) is a poor substrate for the cyclooxygenase but can be metabolized efficiently by the 5-lipoxygenase to produce the pentaenoic leukotrienes[24,25]. The efficiency of the formation of the peptido-leukotrienes from EPA is similar to that for synthesis from arachidonic acid, but conversion of EPA to LTB_5 is relatively inefficient[24,25]. The use of EPA in the treatment of inflammatory disorders will be considered later.

CELLULAR SOURCES OF EICOSANOIDS IN INFLAMMATION

Cyclooxygenase products

Elevated levels of cyclooxygenase products including PGE_2, $PGF_{2\alpha}$, PGD_2, 6-keto-$PGF_{1\alpha}$ and TXB_2 have been found in experimental models of inflammation and in human diseases. Prostaglandins E_2 and TXB_2 have been detected in carrageenan-induced inflammatory exudate in rats[26], and PGE_2 has been detected in the inflamed joints of rabbits with antigen-induced arthritis[27,28]. The inflamed synovial lining from arthritic rabbits produces PGE_2, TXB_2 and 6-keto-$PGF_{1\alpha}$ *ex vivo*[27,28]. Synovial effusions from both rheumatoid and osteoarthritic patients contain high concentrations of PGE_2 but lower levels of $PGF_{2\alpha}$, TXB_2 and 6-keto-$PGF_{1\alpha}$ (see Higgs[29]). Synovial tissues from rheumatoid patients produce elevated levels of PGE_2, 6-keto-$PGF_{1\alpha}$ and TXB_2[30]. In most inflammatory lesions PGE_2 appears to be the most abundant cyclooxygenase product but in systemic mastocytosis very high levels of PGD_2 and/or its metabolites have been detected in plasma and urine[31].

Although it is clear that cyclooxygenase products are abundant in inflamed tissues and exudate, it is not always clear which cell type(s) is responsible for the production of a particular eicosanoid. The capacity of various cell types to produce cyclooxygenase products is shown in Table 5.1, but this information does not always indicate the contribution of each cell type *in vivo*. For example, in inflammatory reactions is the thromboxane detected in inflammatory exudate produced by platelets or neutrophils? Does PGE_2 originate from infiltrating leukocytes or from resident connective tissue cells? Attempts have been made to determine the source of cyclooxygenase products in inflammatory responses by depleting various types of cell in animal models of inflammation. In rats which were made thrombocytopenic with antiplatelet serum the TXB_2 generated in clotted blood was markedly inhibited, but the levels of cyclooxygenase products, including TXB_2, in the inflammatory exudate were not reduced compared to control[32]. In contrast, when rats were rendered neutropenic by prior treatment with methotrexate, or when leukocyte migration was prevented by the administration of colchicine, the level of TXB_2 in the exudate was reduced by $>95\%$ compared to control. These results strongly suggest that neutrophils, rather than platelets, are the source of TXB_2 in this model of irritant-induced inflammation. Neutrophil depletion also prevented the rise in the levels of PGE_2 by some 60–70%. This is

Table 5.1 Cellular sources of cyclooxygenase products

Cell type	*Major cyclooxygenase product*
Platelet	TXA_2
Neutrophil	TXA_2
Endothelial cell	$PGI_2 > PGE_2$
Mast cell	PGD_2
Fibroblast	PGE_2
Chondrocyte	$PGE_2 > PGI_2$
Monocyte/macrophage	TXA_2, PGE_2, PGI_2

surprising since PMN produce little PGE_2 compared to resident fibroblasts. However, this result could indicate that PMNs are indirectly responsible for PGE_2 synthesis by producing factors such as lysosomal phospholipase A_2 which initiate eicosanoid synthesis in the resident tissue. Similar results have been obtained in immune arthritis in the rabbit; neutropenia inhibited the rise in PGE_2 levels in the synovial fluid after antigen challenge[33]. Also, in a rabbit model of myocardial infarction neutropenia significantly suppressed the generation of PGE_2 and 6-keto-$PGF_{1\alpha}$ by infarcted tissue *ex vivo*[34]. However, it should be noted that under some experimental conditions the rise in PGE_2 is independent of PMN migration[26].

In summary, it is suggested that migrating PMN, rather than platelets, are responsible for TXA_2 synthesis in inflammation, and PGE_2 is produced by the resident tissue in response to the presence of activated PMN.

Lipoxygenase products

The cell types that can produce leukotrienes are more limited in number than those that can produce cyclooxygenase products. Neutrophils produce large amounts of LTB_4 and this chemotactic lipid is present in neutrophil-rich exudates in experimental models[26,28] and in human diseases such as arthritis[35] and psoriasis[36]. Human alveolar macrophages also produce LTB_4 (but little LTC_4), and this is probably responsible for their PMN chemotactic activity[37,38]. In contrast, peripheral human monocytes produce similar amounts of LTB_4 and LTC_4 in response to stimulation with the calcium ionophore A23187, or the bacterial tripeptide, F-Met-Leu-Phe[39,40]. Human eosinophils produce LTC_4 but little LTB_4[41,42]. Leukotriene C_4 is also the predominant lipoxygenase product of purified human mast cells[43]. However, when human lung fragments or unpurified dispersed cells are stimulated, LTD_4 and LTE_4 are also detected[44], which suggests that LTC_4 released from the mast cell is metabolized to LTD_4 and LTE_4 by the other cells present[45]. As mentioned previously, 12(R)-hydroxyeicosatetraenoic acid is now recognized as a major chemotactic lipid present in psoriatic scale[20].

ROLE OF EICOSANOIDS IN ACUTE INFLAMMATORY RESPONSES

Vasodilatation

Prostaglandin E_2 and PGI_2 cause dilatation of the microcirculation; effects are observed at doses of 0.1–10 ng. When injected into human skin, both PGE_2 and PGI_2 induce erythema[46,47]. Prostaglandin D_2 also induces erythema in human skin, although it is less potent than PGE_2[48]. Blood flow changes induced by PGs in rabbit skin have been measured directly using ^{133}xenon clearance; it was found that PGE_2 and PGI_2 were potent vasodilators whereas $PGF_{2\alpha}$ and PGD_2 were effective only at high doses[49]. The relative contribution of different PGs to hyperaemia may depend on the species, the tissues involved and on the nature of the inflammatory/allergic response. The effects of PGE_2 and/or PGI_2 probably predominate in most instances. However, in conditions where mast cell degranulation is central to the pathology, PGD_2 may play an important role because PGD_2 is the main cyclooxygenase product produced by mast cells. In general aspirin-like drugs reduce erythema in a variety of inflammatory responses in experimental animals and in humans; this beneficial effect can be explained by the ability of this class of therapeutic agents to inhibit the synthesis of cyclooxygenase products, thereby confirming the role of prostaglandins in mediating erythematous responses in inflammation.

The role of lipoxygenase products in the control of vascular tone is less clear. This, in part, is due to the fact that marked species and tissue differences have been reported. Leukotrienes C_4 and D_4 are potent vasoconstrictors in some *in vivo* preparations such as guinea pig skin[50] and in the exposed cheek pouch of the hamster[51]. In human skin, LTC_4, LTD_4 and LTE_4 induce rapid onset wheal-and-flare responses[52,53] with evidence of increased blood flow rather than vasoconstriction[54]. The pallor associated with the wheal response is believed to be indirect due to constriction of the vasculature caused by the increased volume of extravascular fluid, rather than by direct vasoconstriction[55]. Leukotriene D_4 also increases blood flow in human nasal mucosa, which may contribute to the symptoms of rhinitis[56].

Vascular permeability and leukocyte emigration

Prostaglandins are only weak inducers of vascular permeability *in vivo*. Early studies indicated that PGEs injected at doses greater than 0.1 μg could induce oedema in rat skin, and this effect was mediated by the release of histamine and 5-HT[57]. Later studies in the guinea-pig and rabbit indicated that PGEs had little effect on vascular permeability directly, but could dramatically enhance the effects of histmaine or bradykinin by increasing blood flow[58–60]. In human skin, PGE_2 can enhance oedema caused by other mediators, such as bradykinin, without having any overt effects itself[61]. Prostaglandin E_2 also enhances oedema in response to chemotactic factors such as C5a or LTB_4 which increase vascular permeability by a PMN-dependent mechanism[62].

Prostaglandins are generally weak inducers of leukocyte accumulation. However, as in the case of oedema formation, local injections of PGE_2 or PGI_2 can enhance leukocyte accumulation induced by chemotactic factors, presumably by increasing the supply of blood to the inflamed site[63,64]. This may be particularly important for tissues with low basal blood flow, but in other circumstances the contribution of endogenous PGs to leukocyte emigration is less clear, since doses of NSAIDs which prevent the generation of PGE_2 do not inhibit leukocyte accumulation[65,66]. Furthermore, in response to the irritant, carrageenan, indomethacin enhanced leukocyte accumulation[65]. Since infiltrating leukocytes may contribute to the pathogenesis of chronic inflammation by releasing toxic oxygen radicals and lysosomal enzymes, the observation that NSAIDs may increase cell influx suggests that these drugs could exacerbate some symptoms of chronic inflammation: the clinical implications of this possibility are considered later.

The peptido-leukotrienes can induce vascular permeability directly. Leukotrienes C_4 and D_4 induce plasma leakage from postcapillary venules in the hasmster cheek pouch at low doses; LTC_4 is slightly more potent than LTD_4[51]. These LTs are at least 1000 times more potent than histamine in eliciting this response, but LTE_4 is equipotent with histamine in inducing vessel 'leakiness' in guinea pig skin[67]. However, the peptido-leukotrienes do not cause neutrophil chemotaxis or adhesion. In contrast, LTB_4 potently stimulates neutrophil motility and adhesion to endothelial cells *in vitro*[68,69]. Although LTB_4 causes chemokinesis and chemotaxis by a direct action on PMN, the stimulation of adhesion by LTB_4 may be mediated by an action on the endothelial cell[70]. This is similar to the effects of the cytokine, IL-1[71], but, interestingly, differs from other chemotactic factors such as FMLP or C5a, which effect neutrophil adhesion to the endothelium by stimulating the neutrophil[72]. Leukotriene B_4 also causes neutrophil adhesion to the endothelium of postcapillary venules of the hamster cheek pouch[51] and causes neutrophil infiltration when injected into the rabbit eye[73] and rabbit skin[63,74].

Since the leukotrienes appear to be important mediators of inflammatory and allergic reactions, much effort has been directed towards developing selective inhibitors of their generation. A series of acetohydroxamic acids inhibit 5-lipoxygenase *in vitro* and *ex vivo*[75], and these have been used as experimental tools to explore the role of leukotrienes in mediating inflammatory processes. The acetohydroxamic acids BWA4C and BWA797C did not suppress leukocyte-dependent oedema in response to carrageenan in the rat at doses which blocked LTB_4 generation[76]: this suggests that LTB_4 may not be an important mediator of the oedematous response. However, at high doses these acetohydroxamic acids did suppress leukocyte accumulation in a sponge-implant model. Similarly, selective inhibition of leukotriene generation did not suppress the oedema associated with a delayed-type hypersensitivity response in the mouse[77]. Furthermore, eicosanoids do not seem to be involved in the inflammatory responses stimulated by the cytokine, IL 1: inhibition of leukotriene generation did not affect leukocyte accumulation in response to IL 1 in the rabbit[78] or the mouse[79]. Selective lipoxygenase inhibitors need to be tested in a range of animal models, and ultimately in humans, before firm conclusions about the role of leukotrienes in inflammation can be made. For example, leukotrienes may be important mediators of pulmonary oedema in asthma since the peptido-leukotriene antagonist, FPL 55712, inhibited plasma leakage in guinea pig lungs after antigen challenge[80].

Pain and hyperalgesia

Prostaglandins do not cause overt pain, but can sensitize pain receptors to the effects of other mediators such as histamine or bradykinin[81]. The PGs can also sensitize pain receptors to mechanical stimuli so that a normally non-painful stimulus becomes painful; for example the rubbing of clothes on sunburnt skin. The hyperalgesic effect of PGE_2 is cumulative and long-lasting whereas prostacyclin, which is a more potent hyperalgesic agent, has a short-lasting action[82,83]. Direct evidence supporting a role for PGs in mediating the pain of the joint was obtained from experiments performed in dogs[84]. Infusions of bradykinin into the dog knee produced a reflex nociceptive response which manifested itself as a rise in blood pressure: the response became more intense with time or when PGE_1 or PGE_2 was co-infused. Aspirin or indomethacin reduced the time-dependent increase in nociceptive activity but not that produced by the injection of exogenous prostaglandins. These experiments suggest that endogenous prostaglandins are responsible for hyperalgesia, and this can be reduced by aspirin-like drugs.

Leukotriene B_4, but not LTD_4, can induce hyperalgesia by a PMN-dependent mechanism[85]. However, inhibition of LTB_4 production by selective lipoxygenase inhibitors did not inhibit pain responses induced by the irritant, carrageenan, whereas cyclooxygenase inhibitors greatly reduced the response[76].

In summary, the anti-inflammatory and analgesic actions of NSAIDs can be accounted for by inhibition of PG synthesis, but it is not clear whether inhibition of LT generation will lead to an improvement in anti-inflammatory thereapy.

ROLE OF EICOSANOIDS IN CHRONIC INFLAMMATION: INTERACTIONS WITH CYTOKINES

Anti-inflammatory/immunosuppressive action of prostaglandins

Prostaglandins of the E series and PGI_2, when given systemically, can suppress acute and chronic inflammatory reactions. Early experiments indicated that high systemic doses of PGE_1 or PGE_2 could suppress adjuvant arthritis in rats[86,87]. Although it could be interpreted that these effects were due to a non-specific reduction in blood pressure, recent evidence indicates that leukocyte-dependent oedema in the rabbit can be suppressed by 15-methyl PGE_1 (a synthetic analogue of PGE_1) or PGI_2 at doses which are not hypotensive[88]. The latter data are consistent with the finding that PGEs and PGI_2 suppress neutrophil responses to a range of stimuli *in vitro*[89]. However, much lower doses of PGE_2 are required to inhibit the proliferation of lymphocytes[90] and the production of lymphokines[91] than required to suppress neutrophil function. Therefore, inhibition of lymphocyte function by PGEs *in vivo* may be a more likely explanation for the effect of these prostanoids on adjuvant arthritis. Also, the finding that PGE treatment suppressed cartilage degradation[92], as well as joint swelling, suggests that the prostanoids exert an effect in addition to suppressing neutrophil function, because cartilage damage in arthritis is probably not due to infiltrating neutrophils[33]. It is clear that PGEs and PGI_2 reduce neutrophil-dependent inflammatory responses *in vivo* such as the tissue injury that occurs in models of myocardial infarction[93]. Prostaglandin E_2 also suppresses other autoimmune diseases such as murine nephritis, and this correlates with inhibition of T cell function rather than inhibition of immune complex formation[94].

Prostaglandins E_1 and E_2 and PGI_2 also decrease macrophage activation. In particular, there are many reports that PGE_2 reduces the production of IL 1[95,96] which is a potent inducer of arthritic changes in the joint[78]. However, recent evidence suggests that PGEs may not affect IL 1 production directly, but that they interfere with the ability of responder thymocytes to detect IL 1 produced by macrophages[97]. On the other hand, PGE_2 may inhibit the secretion of mature IL 1 protein rather than inhibit the production of IL 1 in some systems[98]. The effect of PGE_2 on the production of TNF-α from macrophages appears to be more clear-cut; it inhibits the production of mature TNF-α protein activity[99] and down-regulates the level of TNF-α mRNA[100] in macrophages. Tumour necrosis factor α is a less potent inflammatory agent than IL 1, although it can dramatically enhance leukocyte infiltration in response to IL 1 after intra-articular injection[101].

Treatment of arthritic rabbits with indomethacin leads to an enhancement of lymphocyte infiltration in the synovial tissue and accelerated cartilage damage[102] (see Figures 5.2 and 5.3). Clearly, the findings that PGs can suppress lymphocyte and macrophage function may have serious implications for patients treated with NSAIDs, such as those with chronic arthritis.

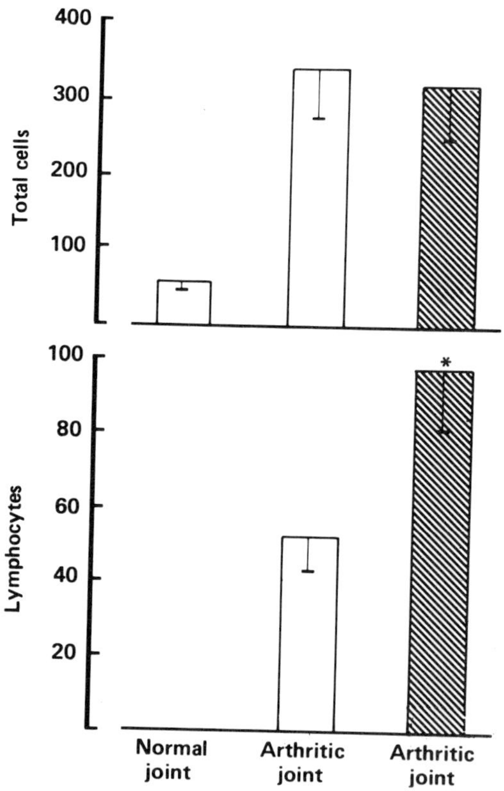

Figure 5.2 The effect of indomethacin on the cellular content of synovial tissues from rabbits with antigen-induced arthritis. The numbers of total cells (upper panel) and lymphocytes (lower panel) counted in 10 bands of synovial membrane (250 μm wide) taken from arthritic joints of untreated (open columns) and indomethacin-treated (hatched columns) rabbits 14 days after the induction of arthritis. Each column represents the mean ± SEM of data from the six to 19 animals (*$p < 0.05$ compared to control).

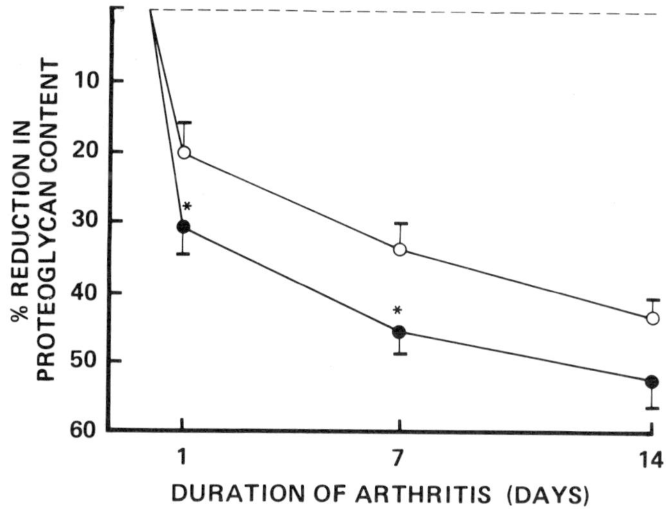

Figure 5.3 The effect of indomethacin on degradation of cartilage in rabbits with antigen-induced arthritis. Proteoglycan depletion from the articular cartilage from arthritic joints of untreated (○) and indomethacin-treated (●) rabbits. Each point is the mean ± SEM of data from five to 18 animals (*$p < 0.05$ compared to control).

Leukotrienes as immunomodulators

The first indication that lipoxygenase products may participate in immune responses came from experiments using non-selective cyclooxygenase/lipoxygenase inhibitors, such as BW 755C, *in vitro*. These compounds inhibited thymocyte replication in response to IL 1[103] and suppressed the production of IL 1-like activity from macrophages[104]. However, it is not yet known whether selective inhibitors of the 5-lipoxygenase also suppress the activity of these immunocompetent cells.

Other studies examined the effects of exogenous leukotrienes on macrophage and lymphocyte function. Addition of LTB_4 to cultures of human monocytes enhanced IL 1 production in response to a range of stimuli including lipopolysaccharide and zymosan[105]. Leukotriene D_4 was less effective at eliciting this response. Leukotriene B_4 can also augment TNF-α production[106].

At low concentrations, LTB_4 induces suppressor cell activity in human lymphocyte cultures[107,108]. Separation of T cells into subtypes revealed that LTB_4 inhibited the proliferation of helper cells (CD4 positive cells) but stimulated the proliferation of suppressor cells (CD8 positive cells)[109]. Furthermore, LTB_4 induced the expression of the CD8 antigen on a proportion of CD4-positive lymphocytes[110]. It is not clear whether the ability of non-selective lipoxygenase inhibitors to inhibit thymocyte replication can be explained by interference with any of the above LT-dependent activities. Clearly, there is a need to investigate the effect of specific lipoxygenase inhibitors on the responses of different lymphocyte subsets in order to establish whether LTs do indeed play a significant role in modulating lymphocyte function.

The effects of selective lipoxygenase inhibitors on cell-mediated immune responses *in vivo* have not yet been evaluated fully. The selective lipoxygenase inhibitor, L-551,896, when given alone or in combination with indomethacin, did not modify oxazalone-induced delayed hypersensitivity in the mouse, despite inhibiting the production of LTB_4[77]. Dietary manipulation of LTB_4 production by feeding fish oil (rich in EPA) has been attempted in models of autoimmune diseases. Prickett *et al.*[111] found that the incidence, but not the severity, of collagen-induced arthritis in rats was increased by EPA-feeding. This was attributed to the reduced production of PGE_2 which has immunosuppressant activity. However, collagen-induced arthritis in mice was suppressed by EPA when given prophylactically or therapeutically[112,113]. Similarly, EPA suppresses murine lupus[114]. Some symptomatic benefit has been observed in rheumatoid patients fed fish oil[115-117]. Although EPA-feeding does reduce the generation of LTB_4 from neutrophils and monocytes[118] it is not clear if this is the mechanism underlying the observed clinical effects of fish oil. A fish oil diet has also been shown to give moderate improvement in psoriatic patients, and the degree of improvement correlated with the level of incorporation of EPA and docosahexaenoic acid into the epidermis[119]. A fish oil diet given to healthy volunteers also reduced the generation of IL 1 and TNF-α from mononuclear cells *ex vivo*[120].

SUMMARY

Locally produced PGs, particularly PGE_2 and PGI_2, participate in acute inflammatory responses by increasing the flow of blood to the site of injury and by sensitizing pain receptors to chemical and mechanical stimuli. Indeed, the anti-inflammatory activity of NSAIDs correlates with their ability to inhibit PG synthesis. However, there is some evidence that PGs may serve to downregulate the chronic inflammatory response by inhibiting lymphocyte activation and possibly by inhibiting the production of cytokines, such as IL 1 and TNF-α, from macrophages. This view is supported by the observation that NSAIDs may exacerbate some aspects of chronic inflammatory diseases. Therefore, there is a need for improved anti-inflammatory therapy. Recently developed lipoxygenase inhibitors could represent a new class of anti-inflammatory drug. However, selective lipoxygenase inhibitors do not appear to be very effective in the models of acute inflammation in which they have so far been tested. The compounds have not yet been thoroughly tested in models of chronic inflammation; nor have they been subjected to clinical evaluation. It is possible that, when given in combination with conventional NSAIDs, they could offer improved anti-inflammatory activity compared to NSAIDs alone. It is also possible that selective lipoxygenase inhibitors may prevent the exacerbation of tissue damage seen with NSAID therapy. Therefore, the outcome of the clinical trials being conducted presently with several 5-lipoxygenase inhibitors and LT antagonists is awaited with interest. Dietary manipulation, for example by the increased intake of EPA, may also offer a modest symptomatic improvement for patients suffering from inflammatory disorders, but further placebo-controlled, double-blind clinical trials are required to confirm the earlier interesting observations.

References

1. Vane, J. R. (1971). Inhibition of prostaglandin synthesis as a mechanism of action for the aspirin-like drugs. *Nature*, **231**, 232–5
2. Smith, J. B. and Willis, A. L. (1971). Aspirin selectively inhibits prostaglandin synthesis in human platelets. *Nature*, **231**, 235–7
3. Ferreira, S. H., Moncada, S. and Vane, J. R. (1971). Indomethacin and aspirin abolish prostaglandin release from the spleen. *Nature*, **231**, 237–9
4. Henderson, B., Pettipher, E. R. and Higgs, G. A. (1987). Mediators of rheumatoid arthritis. *Br. Med. Bull.*, **43**, 415–28
5. Flower, R. J. (1988). Lipocortin and the mechanism of action of the glucocorticoids. *Br. J. Pharmacol.*, **94**, 987–1015
6. Davidson, F. F., Dennis, E. A., Powell, M. and Glenney, J. R. (1987). Inhibition of phospholipase A_2 by 'lipocortins' and calpactins. *J. Biol. Chem.*, **262**, 1698–1705
7. Cirino, G., Flower, R. J., Browning, J. L., Sinclair, L. K. and Pepinsky, R. B. (1987). Recombinant human lipocortin 1 inhibits thromboxane release from guinea-pig isolated perfused lung. *Nature*, **328**, 270–2
8. Northup, J. K., Valentine-Braun, K. A., Johnson, L. K., Severson, D. L. and Hollenberg, M. D. (1988). Evaluation of the anti-inflammatory and phospholipase-inhibitory activity of calpactin II/lipocortin I. *J. Clin. Invest.*, **82**, 1347–52
9. Irvine, R. F. (1982). How is the level of free arachidonic acid controlled in mammalian cells? *Biochem. J.*, **204**, 3–16
10. Albert, D. H. and Snyder, F. (1984). Release of arachidonic acid from 1-alkyl-2-acyl-sn-glycero-3-phosphocholine, a precursor of platelet-activating factor, in rat alveolar macrophages. *Biochim. Biophys. Acta*, **796**, 92–101
11. Samuelsson, B., Goldyne, M., Granstrom, E., Hamberg, M., Hammarstrom, S. and Malmsten, C. (1978). Prostaglandins and thromboxanes. *Ann. Rev. Biochem.*, **47**, 997–1029
12. Samuelsson, B. (1983). Leukotrienes: mediators of immediate hypersensitivity reactions and inflammation. *Science*, **220**, 568–75
13. Hammarstrom, S. (1983). Leukotrienes. *Ann. Rev. Biochem.*, **52**, 355–7
14. Hayashi, H., Fujii, Y., Watanabe, K., Urade, Y. and Hayaishi, O. (1989). Enzymatic conversion of prostaglandin H_2 to prostaglandin $F_{2\alpha}$ by aldehyde reductase from human liver: comparison to the prostaglandin F synthetase from bovine lung. *J. Biol. Chem.*, **264**, 1036–40
15. Hamberg, M. and Samuelsson, B. (1967). On the specificity of the oxygenation of unsaturated fatty acids catalyzed by soybean lipoxidase. *J. Biol. Chem.*, **242**, 5329–35
16. Hamberg, M. and Samuelsson, B. (1974). Prostaglandin endoperoxides. Novel transformations of arachidonic acid in human platelets. *Proc. Natl. Acad. Sci. USA*, **71**, 3400–4
17. Nugteren, D. H. (1975). Arachidonate lipoxygenase in blood platelets. *Biochim. Biophys. Acta*, **380**, 299–307
18. Serhan, C. N., Hamberg, M., Ramstedt, U. and Samuelsson, B. (1986). Lipoxins: stereochemistry, biosynthesis and biological activities. *Adv. Prostaglandin, Thromboxane Leukotriene Res.*, **16**, 83–97
19. Hammarstrom, S., Hamberg, M., Samuelsson, B., Duell, E. A., Stawiski, M. and Voorhees, J. J. (1975). Increased concentrations of non-esterified arachidonic acid, 12 L-hydroxy, 5,8,10,14-eicosatetraenoic acid, prostaglandin E_2 and prostaglandin $F_{2\alpha}$ in epidermis of psoriasis. *Proc. Natl. Acad. Sci. USA*, **72**, 5130–4
20. Woollard, P. M. (1986). Stereochemical difference between 12-hydroxy-5,8,10,14-eicosatetraenoic acid in platelets and psoriatic lesions. *Biochem. Biophys. Res. Commun.*, **136**, 169–76
21. Cunningham, F. M. and Woollard, P. M. (1987). 12(R)-hydroxy-5,8,10,14-eicosatetraenoic acid is a chemoattractant for human polymorphonuclear leukocytes in vitro. *Prostaglandins*, **34**, 71–8

22. McGiff, J. C. and Carroll, M. A. (1987). Cytochrome P-450-related arachidonic acid metabolites. *Am. Rev. Respir. Dis.*, **136**, 488–91
23. Chacos, N., Falck, J. R., Wixtrom, C. and Capdevila, J. (1982). Novel epoxides formed during the liver cytochrome P-450 oxidation of arachidonic acid. *Biochem. Biophys. Res. Commun.*, **104**, 916–21
24. Prescott, S. M. (1984). The effect of eicosapentaenoic acid on leukotriene B production by human neutrophils. *J. Biol. Chem.*, **259**, 7615
25. Terano, T., Salmon, J. A. and Moncada, S. (1984). Biosynthesis and biological activity of leukotriene B_5. *Prostaglandins*, **27**, 217–32
26. Simmons, P. M., Salmon, J. A. and Moncada, S. (1983). The release of leukotriene B_4 during experimental inflammation. *Biochem. Pharmacol.*, **32**, 1353–59
27. Blackham, A., Farmer, J. B., Radziwonik, H. and Westwick, J. (1974). The role of prostaglandins in rabbit monoarticular arthritis. *Br. J. Pharmacol.*, **51**, 35–44
28. Henderson, B. and Higgs, G. A. (1987). Synthesis of arachidonate oxidation products by synovial joint tissues during the development of chronic erosive arthritis. *Arthritis Rheum.*, **30**, 1149–56
29. Higgs, G. A., Moncada, S. and Vane, J. R. (1984). Eicosanoids in inflammation. *Ann. Clin. Res.*, **16**, 287–99
30. Salmon, J. A., Higgs, G. A., Vane, J. R., Bitensky, L., Chayen, J., Henderson, B. and Cashman, B. (1983). Synthesis of arachidonate cyclo-oxygenase products by rheumatoid and non-rheumatoid synovial lining in nonproliferative organ culture. *Ann. Rheum. Dis.*, **42**, 36–9
31. Roberts, L. J., Sweetman, B. J., Lewis, R. A., Austen, K. F. and Oates, J. A. (1980). Increased production of prostaglandin D_2 in patients with systemic mastocytosis. *N. Engl. J. Med.*, **303**, 1400–4
32. Higgs, G. A., Moncada, S., Salmon, J. A. and Seager, K. (1983). The source of thromboxane and prostaglandins in experimental inflammation. *Br. J. Pharmacol.*, **79**, 863–8
33. Pettipher, E. R., Henderson, B., Moncada, S. and Higgs, G. A. (1988). Leucocyte infiltration and cartilage proteoglycan loss in immune arthritis in the rabbit. *Br. J. Pharmacol.*, **95**, 169–76
34. Freed, M. S., Needleman, P., Dunkel, C. G., Saffitz, J. E. and Evers, A. S. (1989). Role of invading leukocytes in enhanced atrial eicosanoid production following rabbit left ventricular myocardial infarction. *J. Clin. Invest.*, **83**, 205–12
35. Rae, S. A., Davidson, E. M. and Smith, M. J. H. (1982). Leukotriene B_4, an inflammatory mediator in gout. *Lancet*, **2**, 1122–4
36. Brain, S. D., Camp, R. D. R., Dowd, P. M., Black, A. K., Woollard, P. M., Mallett, A. I. and Greaves, M. W. (1982). Psoriasis and leukotriene B_4. *Lancet*, **2**, 762–3
37. Fels, A. O. S., Pawlowski, N. A., Cramer, E. B., King, T. K. C., Cohn, Z. A. and Smith, W. A. (1982). Human alveolar macrophages produce leukotriene B_4. *Proc. Natl. Acad. Sci. USA*, **79**, 7866–70
38. Martin, T. R., Raugi, G., Merritt, T. L. and Henderson, W. R. (1987). Relative contribution of leukotriene B_4 to the neutrophil chemotactic activity produced by the resident human alveolar macrophage. *J. Clin. Invest.*, **80**, 1114–24
39. Goldyne, M. E., Burrish, G. F., Poubelle, P. and Borgeat, P. (1984). Arachidonic acid metabolism among human mononuclear leukocytes: lipoxygenase related pathways. *J. Biol. Chem.*, **259**, 8815–19
40. Williams, J. D., Robin, J.-L., Lewis, R. A., Lee, T. H. and Austen, K. F. (1986). Generation of leukotrienes by human monocytes pretreated with cytochalasin B and stimulated with formyl-methionyl-leucyl-phenylalanine. *J. Immunol.*, **136**, 642–8
41. Weller, P. F., Lee, C. W., Foster, D. W., Corey, E. J., Austen, K. F. and Lewis, R. A. (1983). Generation and metabolism of 5-lipoxygenase pathway leukotrienes by human eosinophils: predominant production of leukotriene C_4. *Proc. Natl. Acad. Sci. USA*, **80**, 7626–30
42. Shaw, R. J., Cromwell, O. and Kay, A. B. (1984). Preferential generation of leukotriene C_4 by human eosinophils. *Clin. Exp. Immunol.*, **56**, 716–22
43. Peters, S. P., MacGlashan, D. W., Schulman, E. S., Schleimer, R. P., Hayes, E. C., Rokash, J., Adkinson, N. F. and Lichtenstein, L. M. (1984). Arachidonic acid metabolism in purified human lung mast cells. *J. Immunol.*, **132**, 1972–9
44. Lewis, R. A., Austen, K. F., Drazen, J. M., Clark, D. A. and Corey, E. J. (1980). Slow reacting substance of anaphylaxis: identification of leukotrienes C and D from human and

rat sources. *Proc. Natl. Acad. Sci. USA*, **77**, 3710–14
45. Sirois, P., Brousseau, Y., Chagnon, M., Gentile, J., Gladu, M., Salari, H., Borgeat, P. (1985). Metabolism of leukotrienes by adult and fetal human lungs. *Exp. Lung Res.*, **9**, 17–30
46. Solomon, L. M., Juhlin, L. and Kirschenbaum, M. B. (1968). Prostaglandins on cutaneous vasculature. *J. Invest. Dermatol.*, **51**, 280–2
47. Higgs, G. A., Cardinal, D. C., Moncada, S. and Vane, J. R. (1979). Microvascular effects of prostacyclin (PGI_2) in the hamster cheek pouch. *Microvasc. Res.*, **18**, 245–54
48. Flower, R. J., Harvey, E. A. and Kingston, W. P. (1976). Inflammatory effects of Prostaglandin D_2 in rat and human skin. *Br. J. Pharmacol.*, **56**, 229–33
49. Williams, T. J. (1979). Prostaglandin E_2, prostaglandin I_2 and the vascular changes of inflammation. *Br. J. Pharmacol.*, **65**, 517–24
50. Peck, M. J., Piper, P. J. and Williams, T. J. (1981). The effect of leukotrienes C_4 and D_4 on the microvasculature of guinea-pig skin. *Prostaglandins*, **21**, 315–21
51. Dahlen, S. E., Bjork, J., Hedqvist, P., Arfors, K. E., Hammarstrom, S., Lindgren, J. A. and Samuelsson, B. (1981). Leukotrienes promote plasma leakage and leukocyte adhesion in postcapillary venules: In vivo effects with relevance to the acute inflammatory response. *Proc. Natl. Acad. Sci.*, **78**, 3887–91
52. Soter, N. A., Lewis, R. A., Corey, E. J. and Austen, K. F. (1983). Local effects of synthetic leukotrienes (LTC_4, LTD_4, LTE_4 and LTB_4) in human skin. *J. Invest. Dermatol.*, **80**, 115–19
53. Camp, R. D. R., Coutts, A. A., Greaves, M. W., Kay, A. B. and Walport, M. J. (1983). Responses of human skin to intradermal injection of leukotrienes C_4, D_4 and B_4. *Br. J. Pharmacol.*, **80**, 497–502
54. Bisgaard, H., Kristensen, J., Sondergaard, J. (1982). The effect of leukotrine C_4 and D_4 on cutaneous blood flow in humans. *Prostaglandins*, **23**, 797–801
55. Camp, R. D. R. and Greaves, M. W. (1987). Inflammatory mediators in the skin. *Br. Med. Bull.*, **43**, 401–14
56. Bisgaard, H., Olsson, P. and Bende, M. (1984). Leukotriene D_4 increases nasal blood flow in humans. *Prostaglandins*, **29**, 611–19
57. Crunkhorn, P. and Willis, A. L. (1971). Cutaneous reactions to intradermal prostaglandins. *Br. J. Pharmacol.*, **41**, 49–56
58. Williams, T. J. and Morley, J. (1973). Prostaglandins as potentiators of increased vascular permeability in inflammation. *Nature*, **246**, 215–17
59. Johnston, M. G., Hay, J. B. and Movat, H. Z. (1976). The modulation of enhanced vascular permeability by prostaglandins through alterations in blood flow (hyperemia). *Agents Actions*, **6**, 705–11
60. Williams, T. J. and Peck, M. J. (1977). Role of prostaglandin-mediated vasodilatation in inflammation. *Nature*, **270**, 530–2
61. Basran, G. S., Morley, J., Paul, W. and Turner-Warwick, M. (1982). Evidence in man of synergistic interaction between mediators of acute inflammation and asthma. *Lancet*, **1**, 935–7
62. Wedmore, C. V. and Williams, T. J. (1981). Control of vascular permeability by polymorphonuclear leukocytes in inflammation. *Nature*, **289**, 646–50
63. Movat, H. Z., Rettl, C., Burrowes, C. E. and Johnston, M. G. (1984). The in vivo effect of leukotriene B_4 on polymorphonuclear leukocytes and the microcirculation: comparison with activated complement (C5a des arg) and enhancement by prostaglandin E_2. *Am. J. Pathol.*, **115**, 233–44
64. Rampart, M. and Williams, T. J. (1987). The effect of PGI_2 on polymorphonuclear leukocyte (PMNL) accumulation in rabbit skin. *Br. J. Pharmacol.*, **90**, 56P
65. Higgs, G. A., Eakins, K. E., Mugridge, K. G., Moncada, S. and Vane, J. R. (1980). The effects of non-steroid anti-inflammatory drugs on leukocyte migration in carrageenan-induced inflammation. *Eur. J. Pharmacol.*, **66**, 81–6
66. Salmon, J. A., Simmons, P. M. and Moncada, S. (1983). The effects of BW 755C and other anti-inflammatory drugs on eicosanoid concentrations and leukocyte accumulation in experimentally-induced acute inflammation. *J. Pharm. Pharmacol.*, **35**, 808–13
67. Joris, I., Majno, G., Corey, E. J. and Lewis, R. A. (1987). The mechanism of vascular leakage induced by leukotriene E_4. *Am. J. Pathol.*, **126**, 19–24
68. Ford-Hutchinson, A. W., Bray, M. A., Doig, M. V., Shipley, M. E. and Smith, M. J. H. (1980). Leukotriene B, a potent chemokinetic and aggregating substance released from polymorphonuclear leukocytes. *Nature*, **286**, 264–5

69. Gimbrone, M. A., Brock, A. F. and Schafer, A. I. (1984). Leukotriene B_4 stimulates polymorphonuclear leukocyte adhesion to cultured vascular endothelial cells. *J. Clin. Invest.*, **74**, 1551–5
70. Hoover, R. L., Karnovsky, M. J., Austen, K. F., Corey, E. J. and Lewis, R. A. (1984). Leukotriene B_4 action on endothelium mediates augmented neutrophil/endothelial adhesion. *Proc. Natl. Acad. Sci. USA*, **81**, 2191–3
71. Bevilacqua, M. P., Pober, J. S., Wheeler, M. E., Cotran, R. S. and Gimbrone, M. A. (1985). Interleukin 1 acts on cultured human vascular endothelial cells to increase the adhesion of polymorphonuclear leukocytes, monocytes and related cell lines. *J. Clin. Invest.*, **76**, 2003–11
72. Tonnessen, M. G., Smedly, L. A. and Henson, P. M. (1984). Neutrophil-endothelial cell interactions: modulation of neutrophil adhesiveness induced by complement fragments C5a and C5a des arg and formyl-methionyl-leucyl-phenylalanine in vitro. *J. Clin. Invest.*, **74**, 1581–92
73. Bhattacherjee, P., Hammond, B., Salmon, J. A., Stepney, R. and Eakins, K. E. (1981). Chemotactic response to some arachidonate lipoxygenase products in the rabbit eye. *Eur. J. Pharmacol.*, **73**, 21–8
74. Higgs, G. A., Salmon, J. A. and Spayne, J. A. (1981). The inflammatory effects of hydroperoxy and hydroxy acid products of arachidonate lipoxygenase in rabbit skin. *Br. J. Pharmacol.*, **74**, 429–33
75. Tateson, J. E., Randall, R. W., Reynolds, C. H., Jackson, W. P., Bhattacherjee, P., Salmon, J. A. and Garland, L. G. (1988). Selective inhibition of arachidonate 5-lipoxygenase by novel acetohydroxamic acids: biochemical assessment in vitro and ex vivo. *Br. J. Pharmacol.*, **94**, 528–39
76. Higgs, G. A., Follenfant, R. L. and Garland, L. G. (1988). Selective inhibition of arachidonate 5-lipoxygenase by novel acetohydroxamic acids:effects on acute inflammatory responses. *Br. J. Pharmacol.*, **94**, 547–51
77. Meurer, R., Opas, E. E. and Humes, J. L. (1988). Effects of cycloxygenase and lipoxygenase inhibitors on inflammation associated with oxazolone-induced delayed hypersensitivity. *Biochem. Pharmacol.*, **37**, 3511–14
78. Pettipher, E. R., Higgs, G. A. and Henderson, B. (1986). Interleukin 1 induces leukocyte infiltration and cartilage proteoglycan degradation in the synovial joint. *Proc. Natl. Acad. Sci. USA*, **83**, 8749–53
79. Sayers, T. J., Wiltrout, T. A., Bull, C. A., Denn, A. C., Pilaro, A. M. and Lokesh, B. (1988). Effect of cytokines on polymorphonuclear neutrophil infiltration in the mouse: prostaglandin- and leukotriene-independent induction of infiltration by IL-1 and tumour necrosis factor. *J. Immunol.*, **141**, 1670–7
80. Evans, T. W., Rogers, D. F., Aursudky, B., Chung, K. F. and Barnes, P. J. (1988). Inflammatory mediators involved in antigen-induced airway microvascular leakage in guinea pigs. *Am. Rev. Respir. Dis.*, **138**, 395–9
81. Ferreira, S. H. (1972). Prostaglandins, aspirin-like drugs and analgesia. *Nature*, **240**, 200–3
82. Ferreira, S. H., Nakamura, M. and Abreu-Castro, M. S. (1978). The hyperalgesic effects of prostacyclin and PGE_2. *Prostaglandins*, **16**, 31–7
83. Higgs, E. A., Moncada, S. and Vane, J. R. (1978). Inflammatory effects of prostacyclin (PGI_2) and 6-oxo-$PGF_{1\alpha}$ in the rat paw. *Prostaglandins*, **16**, 153–62
84. Moncada, S., Ferreira, S. H. and Vane, J. R. (1975). Inhibition of prostaglandin biosynthesis as the mechanism of analgesia of aspirin-like drugs in the dog knee joint. *Eur. J. Pharmacol.*, **31**, 250–60
85. Levine, J. D., Lau, W., Kiviat, G. and Goetzl, E. J. (1984). Leukotriene B_4 produces hyperalgesia that is dependent on polymorphonuclear leukocytes. *Science*, **225**, 743–5
86. Aspinall, R. L. and Cammarata, P. S. (1969). Effect of prostaglandin E_2 on adjuvant arthritis. *Nature*, **224**, 1320–1
87. Zurier, R. B. and Quagliata, F. (1971). Effect of prostaglandin E_1 on adjuvant arthritis. *Nature*, **234**, 304–5
88. Rampart, M. and Williams, T. J. (1986). Polymorphonuclear leukocyte-dependent plasma leakage in the rabbit skin is enhanced or inhibited by prostacyclin, depending on the route of administration. *Am. J. Pathol.*, **124**, 66–73
89. Fantone, J. C., Marasco, W. A., Elgas, L. J. and Ward, P. A. (1984). Stimulus specificity of prostaglandin inhibition of rabbit polymorphnuclear leukocyte lysosomal enzyme release

and superoxide anion production. *Am. J. Pathol.*, **115**, 9–16

90. Goodwin, J. S., Bankhurst, A. D. and Messner, R. P. (1977). Suppression of human T-cell mitogenesis by prostaglandin: existence of a prostaglandin-producing suppressor cell. *J. Exp. Med.*, **146**, 1719–34
91. Gordon, D., Bray, M. and Morley, J. (1976). Control of lymphokine secretion of prostaglandins. *Nature*, **262**, 401–2
92. Zurier, R. B. and Ballas, M. (1973). Prostaglandin E_1 (PGE_1) suppression of adjuvant arthritis: histopathology. *Arthritis Rheum.*, **16**, 251–8
93. Simpson, P. J., Mickelson, J., Fantone, J. C., Gallagher, K. P. and Lucchesi, B. R. (1988). Reduction of experimental canine myocardial infarct size with prostaglandin E_1: inhibition of neutrophil migration and activation. *J. Pharmacol. Exp. Ther.*, **244**, 619–24
94. Kelly, C. J., Zurier, R. B., Krakauer, K. A., Blanchard, N. and Neilson, E. G. (1987). Prostaglandin E_1 inhibits effector T cell induction and tissue damage in experimental murine interstitial nephritis. *J. Clin. Invest.*, **79**, 782–9
95. Kunkel, S. L., Chensue, S. W. and Phan, S. H. (1986). Prostaglandins as endogenous mediators of interleukin 1 production. *J. Immunol.*, **136**, 186–92
96. Brandwein, S. R. (1986). Regulation of interleukin 1 production by mouse peritoneal macrophages: effects of arachidonic acid metabolites, cyclic nucleotides and interferons. *J. Biol. Chem.*, **261**, 8624–32
97. Otterness, I. G., Bliven, M. L., Eskra, J. D., Reinke, M. and Hanson, D. C. (1988). The pharmacologic regulation of interleukin-1 production: the role of prostaglandins. *Cell Immunol.*, **114**, 385–97
98. Knudsen, P. J., Dinarello, C. A. and Strom, T. B. (1986). Prostaglandins post-transcriptionally inhibit monocyte expression of interleukin 1 activity by increasing intracellular cyclic adenosine monophosphate. *J. Immunol.*, **137**, 3189–94
99. Kunkel, S. L., Wiggins, R. C., Chensue, S. W. and Larrick, J. (1986). Regulation of macrophage tumour necrosis factor production by prostaglandin E_2. *Biochem. Biophys. Res. Commun.*, **137**, 404–10
100. Kunkel, S. W., Spengler, M., May, M. A., Spengler, R., Larrick, J. and Remick, D. (1987). Prostglandin E_2 regulates macrophage-derived tumour necrosis factor gene expression. *J. Biol. Chem.*, **263**, 5380–4
101. Henderson, B. and Pettipher, E. R. (1989). Arthritogenic actions of recombinant IL-1 and tumour necrosis factor α in the rabbit: evidence for synergistic interactions between cytokines in vivo. *Clin. Exp. Immunol.*, **75**, 306–10
102. Pettipher, E. R., Henderson, B., Edwards, J. C. W. and Higgs, G. A. (1989). Effect of indomethacin on swelling, lymphocyte influx, and cartilage proteoglycan depletion in experimental arthritis. *Ann. Rheum. Dis.*, **48**, 623–7
103. Dinarello, C. A., Marnoy, S. O. and Rosenwasser, L. J. (1983). Role of arachidonate metabolism in the immunoregulatory function of human leukocytic pyrogen/lymphocyte-activating factor/interleukin 1. *J. Immunol.*, **130**, 890–5
104. Dinarello, C. A., Bishai, I., Rosenwasser, L. J. and Coceano, F. (1984). The influence of lipoxygenase inhibitors on the in vitro production of human leukocytic pyrogen and lymphocyte-activating factor (interleukin 1). *Int. J. Immunopharmacol.*, **6**, 43–8
105. Rola-Pleszczynski, M. and Lemaire, I. (1985). Leukotrienes augment interleukin 1 production by human monocytes. *J. Immunol.*, **135**, 3958–61
106. Gagnon, L., Fillion, L. G., Dubois, C. and Rola-Pleszczynski, M. (1989). Leukotrienes and macrophage activation: augmented cytotoxic activity and enhanced interleukin 1, tumour necrosis factor and hydrogen peroxide production. *Agents Actions*, **26**, 141–7
107. Rola-Pleszczynski, M., Borgeat, P. and Sirois, P. (1982). Leukotriene B_4 induces human suppressor lymphocytes. *Biochem. Biophys. Res. Commun.*, **108**, 1531–7
108. Payan, D. G. and Goetzl, E. J. (1983). Specific suppression of human lymphocyte function by leukotriene B_4. *J. Immunol.*, **131**, 551–3
109. Payan, D. G., Missivian-Bastian, A. and Goetzl, E. J. (1984). Human T-lymphocyte subset specificity of the regulatory effects of leukotriene B_4. *Proc. Natl. Acad. Sci. USA*, **81**, 3501–3
110. Rola-Pleszczynski, M. (1985). Differential effects of Leukotriene B_4 on $T4^+$ and $T8^+$ lymphocyte phenotype and immunoregulatory functions. *J. Immunol.*, **135**, 1357–60
111. Prickett, J. D., Trentham, D. E. and Robinson, D. R. (1984). Dietary fish oil augments the induction of arthritis in rats immunised with type II collagen. *J. Immunol.*, **132**, 725–9

112. Leslie, C. A., Gonnerman, W. A., Ullman, M. D., Hayes, K. C., Franzblau, C. and Cathcart, E. S. (1985). Dietary fish oil modulates macrophage fatty acids and decreases arthritis susceptibility in mice. *J. Exp. Med.*, **163**, 1336–49
113. Leslie, C. A., Conte, J. M., Hayes, K. C. and Cathcart, E. S. (1988). A fish oil diet reduces the severity of collagen induced arthritis after onset of disease. *Clin. Exp. Immunol.*, **73**, 328–32
114. Robinson, D. R., Prickett, J. D., Makoul, R. T., Steinberg, A. D. and Colvin, R. B. (1986). Dietary fish oil reduces progression of established renal disease in (NZB × NZW) F_1 mice and delays renal disease in BXSB and MRL/1 strains. *Arthritis Rheum.*, **29**, 539–46
115. Kremer, J. M., Bigauoette, J., Michalek, A. V., Timchalk, M. A., Lininger, L., Rynes, R. I., Huyck, C., Zieminski, J. and Bartholomew, L. E. (1985). Effects of manipulation of dietary fatty acids on clinical manifestations of rheumatoid arthritis. *Lancet*, **1**, 184–7
116. Sperling, R. I., Weinblatt, M., Robin, J. L., Coblyn, J., Fraser, P., Lewis, R. A. and Austen, K. F. (1986). Effects of dietary fish oil on in vitro leukocyte function, leukotriene generation and activity of disease in rheumatoid arthritis. *Arthritis Rheum.*, **29**, S18
117. Belch, J. J., Ansell, D., Madhok, R., O'Dowd, A. and Sturrock, R. D. (1988). Effects of altering dietary essential fatty acids on requirements on non-steroidal anti-inflammatory drugs in patients with rheumatoid arthritis: a double blind placebo controlled study. *Ann. Rheum. Dis.*, **47**, 96–104
118. Lee, T. H., Hoover, R. L., Williams, J. D., Sperling, R. I., Ravelese, J., Spur, B. W., Robinson, D. R., Corey, E. J., Lewis, R. A. and Austen, K. F. (1985). Effect of dietary enrichment with eicosapentaenoic acid and docosahexanoic acids on in vitro neutrophil and monocyte leukotriene generation and neutrophil function. *N. Engl. J. Med.*, **312**, 1217–21
119. Ziboh, V. A., Cohen, K. A., Ellis, C. N., Miller, C., Hamilton, T. A., Kragbelle, K., Hydrick, C. R. and Voorhees, J. J. (1986). Effect of dietary supplementation of fish oil on neutrophil and epidermal fatty acids: modulation of clinical course of psoriatic subjects. *Arch Dermatol.*, **122**, 1277–82
120. Endres, S., Ghorbani, R., Kelley, V. E., Georgilis, K., Lonnemann, G., Van der Meer, J. W. M., Cannon, J. D., Rogers, T. S., Klempner, M. S., Weber, P. C., Schaefer, E. J., Wolff, S. M. and Dinarello, C. A. (1989). The effect of dietary supplementation with n-3 polyunsaturated fatty acids on the synthesis of interleukin-1 and tumor necrosis factor by mononuclear cells. *N. Engl. J. Med.*, **320**, 265–71

6
The role of toxic oxygen species in inflammation with special reference to DNA damage

P. G. WINYARD, D. PERRETT, G. HARRIS and D. R. BLAKE

Paradoxically, oxygen is both necessary for aerobic life and a toxic hazard at higher than atmospheric concentrations. In mammalian systems the controlled reduction of oxygen is essential for the production of energy. The quantum chemistry of oxygen (see below) provides for this molecule to undergo univalent reduction more readily than divalent reduction. Mammalian cells control this process by virtue of an array of enzymes – the mitochrondrial respiratory chain – which supplies electrons to O_2 singly. This system is imperfect and up to 5% of the electrons 'leak' out, forming toxic $O_2^{\cdot -}$ radicals. Furthermore, other enzymes have the specific function of releasing toxic oxygen species under certain conditions. For example the bactericidal capacity of neutrophils is, in part, dependent on the generation of toxic oxygen species by a membrane NADPH oxidase. Thus, in some circumstances, the production of oxygen free radicals may be desirable. However, protective mechanisms normally deal effectively with toxic oxygen species when they escape their intended sphere of action. These 'antioxidant defences' consist of both enzymes and low-molecular-weight compounds which may either 'scavenge' oxygen radicals or 'repair' oxidative damage to biomolecules. Recent evidence suggests that many inflammatory disorders may be linked to an increase in the production of oxygen radicals and/or deficiencies of antioxidant defence systems.

Chronic inflammatory diseases may be characterized by populations of cells with altered regulation and function. This might be explained by several different free-radical-mediated processes. First, oxygen radicals might be selectively toxic to certain susceptible cell types and/or certain subpopulations within a given cell type. This could involve alterations in the energy charge state of the cell, and here oxidative DNA damage is likely to play a critical role[1,2]. Secondly, cell disorder might occur without cytotoxicity or cell killing by alteration of important cell surface structures (e.g. receptors) by oxidants[3]. (However, it seems unlikely that doses of oxygen radicals sufficient to cause loss of cell surface receptor function would not be toxic.) Finally, oxidative DNA damage to target cells might give rise to mutations, the so-called 'somatic mutation theory' put forward by F. M. Burnet (reviewed in ref. 4). The possible roles of these processes will be considered below.

THE CHEMISTRY OF OXYGEN RADICALS

A free radical may be defined as an atom or molecule with one or more unpaired electrons, capable of an independent existence. They may be positively charged, negatively charged or neutral. Examples include the ground state diatomic oxygen molecule, the hydrogen atom and most transition metals. The unpaired electron(s) that characterizes an oxygen free radical, which may be denoted by a superscripted dot (e.g. $^{\cdot}OH$ denotes the hydroxyl radical), confers on the molecule a high level of instability and thus a high chemical reactivity.

While oxygen is clearly essential for aerobic life, it is toxic when supplied at concentrations greater than those in the atmosphere. Its toxicity relates to its almost unique electronic configuration. Molecular oxygen possesses two unpaired electrons each located in a π^* antibonding orbital. The two unpaired electrons have a parallel spin (the same spin quantum number). This we depict as (↑) (↑). Consider the case where oxygen oxidizes another atom or molecule by accepting a pair of electrons from it. A pair of incoming electrons with the more usual configuration (↑) (↓) would fit into both vacant spaces only if one electron inverted its spin (↓) (↓). This imposes a 'spin restriction' on oxygen's ability to take up electrons simultaneously, and hence it has a tendency to accept electrons singly (↑) (↑↓), generating a free radical species – $O_2^{\cdot -}$ (the superoxide anion radical). Superoxide is capable of undergoing further one electron reductions to produce other oxygen free radicals and these reactions are given in equations (1) to (4).

$$O_2 + e + H^+ \rightarrow HO_2^{\cdot} \leftrightarrow O_2^{\cdot -} + H^+ \qquad (1)$$

perhydroxyl radical in equilibrium with superoxide radical ($pK_a = 4.8$)

$$HO_2^{\cdot} + e + H^+ \rightarrow H_2O_2 \qquad (2)$$

hydrogen peroxide

$$H_2O_2 + e + H^+ \rightarrow {}^{\cdot}OH + H_2O \qquad (3)$$

hydroxyl radical

$$^{\cdot}OH + e + H^+ \rightarrow H_2O \qquad (4)$$

water

Clearly, hydrogen peroxide is not a free radical as it has no unpaired electrons. However, it is an oxidant with a good diffusion ability and is classified as a reactive oxygen species (ROS), a collective term that also encompasses oxygen free radicals. Since ROS are short-lived they are difficult to detect directly in biological systems and usually the *characteristic products* of oxygen radical reactions with biomolecules are detected. For example, the technique of electron spin resonance (ESR) may be used, which is an unequivocal means of detecting the unpaired electrons of radical species. ESR can be applied to the study of radical generation (e.g. $O_2^{\cdot-}$ or $^{\cdot}OH$) in biological samples, using a non-radical substance (e.g. nitrone or nitroso compound) to perform 'spin trapping' experiments. In this system an oxygen radical reacts with a non-radical substance, with the transfer of a single electron and the formation of a further radical – in this case a more stable and easily detectable species. This principle illustrates the propensity of oxygen radicals to produce radical chain reactions.

FREE RADICAL THEORIES OF OXYGEN TOXICITY

The superoxide theory of oxygen toxicity

In 1954, Daniel Gilbert and Rebecca Gerschman formulated the theory that most of the toxic effects of oxygen were attributable to the formation of oxygen radicals. The discovery in aerobic cells of superoxide dismutase (SOD), an enzyme which specifically scavenges $O_2^{\cdot-}$, led Irwin Fridovich to refine this idea into the 'superoxide theory of oxygen toxicity' (reviewed in ref. 5). In aqueous media at neutral pH, the main reaction of $O_2^{\cdot-}$ is a relatively slow spontaneous dismutation to H_2O_2 and O_2:

$$O_2^{\cdot-} + O_2^{\cdot-} + 2H^+ \rightarrow H_2O_2 + O_2 \qquad (5)$$

SOD increases the rate of this reaction almost as far as the diffusion-controlled limit. It was found that SOD activity was a requirement for life in the presence of oxygen; the involvement of superoxide in causing damage to many different biomolecules was inferred by virtue of the ability of SOD to inhibit the damaging reaction. However, subsequent studies suggest that most of the damaging effects of superoxide in aqueous media are not mediated *directly* by this species, but rather by another oxidant derived from $O_2^{\cdot-}$.

The Haber–Weiss reaction

Superoxide will react with H_2O_2 (formed by the dismutation of $O_2^{\cdot-}$) to give highly reactive $^{\cdot}OH$, which will oxidize virtually all biomolecules.

$$O_2^{\cdot-} + H_2O_2 \rightarrow O_2 + OH^- + {}^{\cdot}OH \qquad (6)$$

This reaction, known as the Haber–Weiss reaction, has a rate constant of virtually zero in aqueous solution[6]. However, a modification of the Haber–Weiss reaction, in which a transition metal (e.g. iron or copper) acts as a redox catalyst, allows the reaction to proceed at a much faster rate. This is known as the 'iron catalysed Haber–Weiss reaction'. Thus, superoxide reduces any iron complexes present to the Fe^{2+} valency state:

$$O_2^{\cdot -} + Fe^{3+} \rightarrow Fe^{2+} + O_2 \quad (7)$$

Iron(II) ions and H_2O_2 react to generate $^{\cdot}OH$ by the Fenton reaction:

$$H_2O_2 + Fe^{2+} \rightarrow {}^{\cdot}OH + OH^- + Fe^{3+} \quad (8)$$

The sum of reactions (5), (7) and (8) is reaction (6).

The high reactivity of $^{\cdot}OH$ means that it has a very short lifetime and a diffusion radius of only 2.3 nm. Thus $^{\cdot}OH$ produced in a Haber–Weiss reaction catalysed by iron or copper bound to protein or DNA, will react close to its site of formation. This is a 'site-specific' mechanism of $^{\cdot}OH$ attack[7].

MECHANISMS OF OXYGEN RADICAL PRODUCTION IN INFLAMMATION

There is no doubt that oxygen radicals are formed in inflammatory diseases such as rheumatoid arthritis (RA). A wide variety of oxidized biomolecules, known to be specific products of free radical reactions, have been detected in extracellular fluids from patients with inflammatory conditions (*see below*). Whether such damage is a primary aetiological event or contributes to the development/persistence of chronic inflammation still remains to be established. However, the discussion below indicates our reasons for believing that radical damage *could* be involved in aetiology and act as mediators and modulators of inflammatory reactions.

It has now become clear that, in mammalian systems, oxygen can be reduced to ROS by a wide variety of both enzymic and non-enzymic pathways, as a result of normal metabolic processes. It is also thought that in a variety of diseases, including many which involve acute or chronic inflammation, one pathogenetic factor might be a disruption of the normal metabolic balance between production and removal of oxygen radicals, leading to cell damage. Some of the pathways by which oxidants may be produced are listed below.

Activation of NADPH oxidase and myeloperoxidase systems

Polymorphonuclear leukocytes (PMNs) are sequestered at sites of inflammation and are stimulated by immune complexes or bacteria to undergo a 'respiratory burst', so called because it involves a sharp increase in the consumption of oxygen by these cells. This phenomenon is responsible for the killing of microbial pathogens.

The mechanism involves the generation of oxidant species by two separate enzyme systems[8]. First, a plasma membrane-bound NADPH oxidase system containing cytochrome b_{-245}. This enzyme catalyses the univalent reduction of molecular oxygen to generate $O_2^{\cdot -}$. Secondly, myeloperoxidase, a haemoprotein located within the azurophilic granules, which catalyses the production of the oxidant hypochlorous acid:

$$Cl^- + H_2O_2 \rightarrow ClO^- + H_2O \tag{9}$$

In the inherited syndrome of chronic granulomatous disease (CGD), cytochrome b_{-245} is absent and consequently the respiratory burst cannot take place[9]. Persistent, but selective, bacterial infections are seen in these patients. NADPH oxidase is useful as part of a controlled acute inflammatory response to bacterial invasion, but excessive activity of this enzyme might lead to tissue destruction. In addition to PMNs, other inflammatory cell types, e.g. lymphocytes and macrophages, possess a membrane NADPH oxidase[10]. ROS production by these latter cell types may form a part of intercellular communication pathways important in the inflammatory response[11] and perhaps an absence of this cell-signalling route in CGD patients is linked to the development of chronic granulomata in these patients. Interestingly, myeloperoxidase deficiency is not associated with disease.

Uncoupling of the xanthine dehydrogenase system

The cytosolic enzyme xanthine dehydrogenase catalyses the oxidation of hypoxanthine and xanthine to uric acid. It is thought to be located predominantly in the liver, small intestine and capillary endothelium in humans[12]. However, the distribution is different in other species. In healthy tissue most of the enzyme is present as the 'D form', which transfers electons to NAD^+:

$$\text{xanthine} + H_2O + NAD^+ \rightarrow \text{uric acid} + NADH + H^+ \tag{10}$$

However, about 10% of the enzyme is present as an oxidase ('type O') form, which transfers electrons to molecular oxygen to form $O_2^{\cdot -}$ or H_2O_2:

$$\text{xanthine} + H_2O + 2O_2 \rightarrow \text{uric acid} + 2O_2^{\cdot -} + 2H^+ \tag{11}$$

Both reactions are inhibited by oxipurinol, the principal metabolite of allopurinol and a xanthine oxidase/dehydrogenase inhibitor. In ischaemic conditions the enzyme is converted from the dehydrogenase form to the oxidase form, probably by the action of a Ca^{2+}-dependent protease activated during the ischaemia-induced influx of Ca^{2+} ions into the cell[13]. The rate of conversion from the 'D' to 'O' form is highly variable, ranging from minutes to days and, again, is species- and tissue-dependent. On restoration of blood supply the substrate of the oxidase form, molecular oxygen, is supplied and there is a burst of $O_2^{\cdot -}$ and H_2O_2 (*see below*). The concept of radical-promoted hypoxic reperfusion injury has been applied to many disease states, including regional intestinal ischaemia, myocardial ischaemia, cerebral ischaemia and ischaemic acute renal failure, as well as organ transplantation. Interestingly, xanthine oxidase also appears to contribute to *hyperoxia*-induced acute oedematous lung injury[14].

Recently, we[15,16] have provided evidence that hypoxic reperfusion injury occurs in the inflamed human joint. Joint movement in patients with rheumatoid arthritis (RA) produces intra-articular pressures in excess of the synovial capillary perfusion pressure. This phenomenon does not occur in normal joints, where the pressure remains subatmospheric throughout a movement cycle. During exercise of the inflamed joint, the intra-articular pressure is transmitted directly to the synovial membrane vasculature, producing occlusion of the superficial synovial capillary bed and ischaemia. Reperfusion of the synovial membrane occurs when exercise is stopped. Recently, ESR spectroscopy with spin trapping was employed to demonstrate that synovial membrane tissue from a patient with RA generated ROS following a transient hypoxic challenge[17]. Furthermore, exercise-induced oxidative damage to lipids and immunoglobulin G (IgG) has been demonstrated in the knee joint of patients with inflammatory synovitis[15] (Figure 6.1).

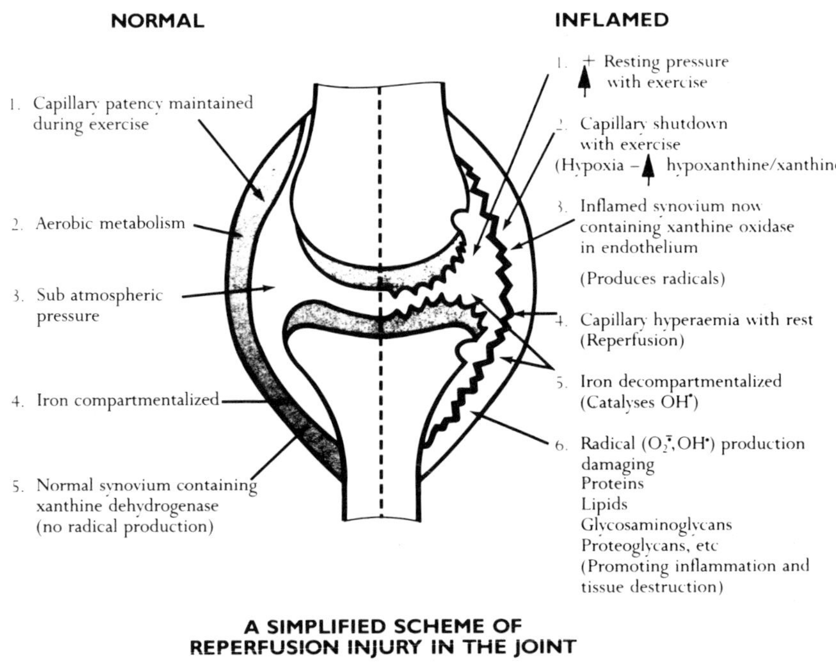

Figure 6.1 Hypoxic reperfusion injury. Reproduced with permission of the Arthritis and Rheumatism Council for Research, *Topical Reviews*, July 1990, no. 5.

Uncoupling of mitochondrial and endoplasmic reticulum electron transport chains

Most of the oxygen consumed by mammalian cells is converted to water via the mitochondrial electron transport system, in which electrons flow from NADH to sequentially reduce flavoproteins, ubiquinone (coenzyme Q), mitochondrial cytochromes and finally molecular oxygen. The final reaction of this respiratory chain, catalysed by cytochrome oxidase, consists of the donation of four electrons to each O_2 molecule to form water. Although cytochrome oxidase probably donates the four electrons to oxygen by sequential one-electron transfer, the radical intermediates are bound to the active site, so that no oxygen radicals 'leak out' into free solution[18]. However, up to about 5% of the electrons entering the electron transport chain do become uncoupled from it at several other points, especially ubiquinone[19], and singly leak out onto O_2 to form $O_2^{\cdot-}$. Recent studies on the generation of ROS in isolated perfused rat liver after hypoxic injury[20] identified xanthine oxidase as a temporary souce at the beginning of the reoxygenation period. However, damaged mitochondria represented the continuous and quantitatively dominating source of ROS in the injured liver.

The endoplasmic reticulum electron transport system (NADPH-cytochrome *P*-450 reductase)[21] can also generate $O_2^{\cdot-}$. This system, which is often responsible for the metabolism of foreign compounds, is selectively distributed in a wide variety of cell types. Its presence in hepatocytes is particularly important, since drugs are often metabolized at this site. In this system a single electron is transferred from reduced flavin to a cytochrome *P*-450–substrate complex. A second electron is then transferred through this complex to O_2. Production of $O_2^{\cdot-}$ may occur through autoxidation of the partially reduced flavin cofactor or because of uncoupling of electrons from the enzyme–substrate complex[22] to O_2.

The ability of the endoplasmic reticulum electron transport system to metabolize certain drugs is decreased in carrageenan-induced granulomatous inflammation in the rat[23]. It is conceivable that such changes are linked to increased uncoupling of this electron transport chain, with consequent ROS production leading to the observed hepatic dysfunction of certain inflammatory diseases. The metabolism of some carcinogens[24] also involves the generation of $O_2^{\cdot-}$.

Non-enzymatic reactions

Many biologically relevant molecules, such as thiol compounds, haemoglobin, flavins, quinones and catechols, will undergo autoxidation by molecular oxygen, thereby generating $O_2^{\cdot-}$. These autoxidation reactions are often stimulated by transition metal cations such as Fe^{2+} and Cu^{2+} and by $O_2^{\cdot-}$ generating systems. Adrenochrome, the oxidation product of the catechol adrenaline, has been detected in rheumatoid synovial fluid[25]. ROS are also the active agents of DNA damage produced by ionizing radiation[24].

PROTECTION AGAINST EXCESS OXYGEN RADICAL PRODUCTION

A number of intracellular enzymes protect the cell from the damaging effects of oxygen radicals by scavenging reactive oxygen species. These include SOD, which catalyses the dismutation of $O_2^{\cdot -}$ to H_2O_2 (equation 5); catalase, which catalyses the reduction of H_2O_2 to water; glutathione peroxidase, which catalyses the removal of H_2O_2 at the expense of glutathione oxidation; and glutathione lipoperoxidase, which likewise catalyses the removal of lipid peroxides.

A set of intracellular proteins, known as stress proteins or heat shock proteins, show increased synthesis *in vitro* in cells exposed to elevated temperatures. However, stress proteins are clearly necessary in helping cells survive other types of physiological stress, since they are induced by oxygen radicals, inhibitors of energy metabolism, ischaemia, hypoxic reperfusion, heavy metals such as copper and thiol-reactive agents[26]. In view of the nature of these inducers, it has been suggested that stress proteins may have antioxidant effects[27].

The stress proteins are divided into subsets or 'families' according to their molecular weight. The best studied family is the 70 kD family, which in humans consists of five structurally and immunologically related proteins; 90 kD, 60 kD and 20 kD families have also been identified. Enhanced stress protein synthesis occurs in the peripheral blood mononuclear cells from patients with systemic lupus erythematosus (SLE), and raised levels of serum antibodies to human 70 kD stress proteins have been detected in patients with RA (reviewed in ref. 28).

The modes of action of some of the stress proteins are now becoming clearer. For example, the major 32 kD stress protein (categorized into the 20 kD family) produced by a human skin fibroblast cell line, following ultraviolet irradiation or exposure to H_2O_2, has identity with the enzyme haem oxygenase[29]. This enzyme catalyses the cleavage of haem to form biliverdin, which is subsequently converted to bilirubin. Bilirubin, whether unconjugated or albumin-bound, is an efficient free radical scavenger.

In the mammalian extracellular environment, extracellular SOD (EC SOD) and caeruloplasmin serve as antioxidant enzymes. EC-SOD is a tetrameric glycoprotein containing four Cu atoms and possibly also four Zn atoms. The major part of EC SOD in the vasculature appears to be located on endothelial cell surfaces. EC SOD has an affinity for negatively charged heparin via the C-terminal end, which is hydrophilic and contains nine positively charged amino acid residues. It is believed that EC SOD binds to the vasculature via specific glycosaminoglycans – probably heparin sulphate on the endothelium. It can be released in humans by intravenous heparin injections[30]. The association of EC SOD with endothelial cell surfaces may indicate a cell-specific protective role.

Caeruloplasmin is the major copper-containing protein of human serum and is an acute phase reactant, being synthesized in increased amounts by the liver in inflammation[31]. Several groups suggested that the pool of non-caeruloplasmin-bound copper, capable of catalysing oxidative reactions, was elevated in rheumatoid extracellular fluids[32,33]. However, these reports are likely to be artifactual, since caeruloplasmin readily loses its copper during storage-induced oxidation/proteolysis[7,34].

In addition to the presence of extracellular antioxidant enzymes there appears to be a further strategy for protection against damaging oxygen radical reactions outside the cell. This involves the chelation of iron in a 'non-catalytic' form by transferrin, which has an extremely high affinity for iron. In normal human serum the concentration of low-molecular-weight chelates of iron, capable of catalysing the Haber–Weiss reaction (equation 6), is effectively zero. However, it has been shown that the intravenous infusion of iron-dextran into a rheumatoid patient results in the saturation of transferrin iron-binding capacity and the appearance of 'catalytic' iron. These changes correspond closely to an exacerbation of rheumatoid synovitis[35]. Small molecules which simply scavenge oxygen radicals have also been suggested to be important antioxidants, e.g. thiols, ascorbic acid and uric acid.

CONSEQUENCES OF UNCONTROLLED OXYGEN RADICAL PRODUCTION IN INFLAMMATION

Both oxygen radicals and proteases are thought to be involved in the tissue destruction of chronic inflammatory diseases. Interest in the tissue-destroying power of oxygen radicals was stimulated by McCord's observation[36] that free radicals would degrade hyaluronic acid, leading to a loss in its viscosity similar to that seen in rheumatoid synovial fluid. This appeared to explain the paradox of the low viscosity of rheumatoid synovial fluid in the absence of any detectable hyaluronidase. It is now known that the fibroblasts of the rheumatoid synovial membrane secrete short-chain hyaluronic acid polymers[37], so it is not clear what contribution oxygen radicals make to the depolymerization process. Nonetheless, McCord's hypothesis provided an impetus to begin a search for free-radical-oxidized biomolecules in inflammatory fluids. One important consequence of ROS production in extreme excess is cell death, giving rise to loss of intracellular contents such as ROS-damaged intracellular molecules.

Lipid peroxidation

All biological systems contain polyunsaturated lipids, which are present in membranes, in lipoproteins (e.g. low-density lipoprotein and high-density lipoprotein) and bound to albumin. The methylene-interrupted double bond of polyunsaturated lipids is particularly prone to hydrogen abstraction by $^{\bullet}OH$, resulting in the formation of a relatively stable lipid free radical. The rearrangement of the methylene-interrupted double bonds to alternate single and double bonds gives rise to a so-called 'diene conjugated' structure. In the presence of oxygen, diene conjugated lipids undergo an autocatalytic reaction to produce lipid peroxides.

The most common methods for measuring lipid peroxidation are the 'diene conjugation (DC) test', which involves the measurement of UV absorbance in chloroform extracts of biological fluids at around 234 nm, and the 'thiobarbituric acid (TBA) test', which relies on the heating of a sample with TBA under acidic conditions. The resulting TBA–lipid peroxide adduct can be measured by its absorbance at 532 nm. TBA-reactive material is present in the synovial fluid from rheumatoid patients, consistent with lipid peroxidation occurring locally, and the amount of TBA-detectable material correlates with clinical indices of inflammation[38]. Using both the conventional DC/TBA tests and modified tests, which employed second derivative spectrophotometry to give improved specificity, it was demonstrated that exercise of the inflamed human knee promotes lipid peroxidation within the joint[39].

Endothelial cells are capable of modifying low-density lipoprotein (LDL) to a form which can undergo uptake into macrophages, via a so-called 'scavenger' receptor. This process involves the production of oxygen radicals by endothelial cells, leading to the peroxidation of lipids present within the LDL molecule. It is thought that the macrophage uptake of oxidatively modified LDL is involved in the generation of lipid-laden 'foam' cells which accumulate in early atherosclerotic lesions[40]. Interestingly, such foam cells are relatively common in rheumatoid synovia, but scarce in normal synovia (C. J. Morris, personal communication).

Protein oxidation

In vitro, free radical generating systems will damage a large variety of connective tissue and plasma proteins that are of importance in inflammation. Amongst the many proteins that have been studied in this context are: collagen[41], proteoglycans[41,42], immunoglobulin G[43], caeruloplasmin[7], low-density lipoprotein[44], albumin[42], glyceraldehyde-3-phosphate dehydrogenase[45,46], and alpha-1-antitrypsin (AAT). The case of AAT is a well-documented example of the role of ROS-mediated protein inactivation in the inflammatory process and this will be discussed in detail below.

AAT is the major protease inhibitor of human serum, limiting tissue damage by the leukocyte protease, elastase[47]. AAT forms a stable 1:1 complex with elastase, in which form the protease is inactive. Elastase has a very broad substrate specificity, acting upon elastin, fibrinogen, proteoglycans, structural collagen, complement and immunoglobulins. Congenital AAT deficiency is associated with pulmonary emphysema[48] and some groups have suggested that severe rheumatoid arthritis is also associated with an abnormal AAT phenotype[49,50].

Cigarette smoking is associated with pulmonary emphysema in normal individuals, as well as those deficient in AAT. In these patients, though absolute levels of AAT are normal, elastase inhibitory activity is depressed[51]. There is strong evidence that this is due to the oxidation of a critical methionine residue (Met 358) to methionine sulphoxide[52]. Likewise, a large proportion of AAT is also inactivated in the rheumatoid joint cavity[53,54]. Again, methionine sulphoxide has been detected in AAT isolated from rheumatoid synovial fluid[55]. Because free elastase activity is not normally detectable in rheumatoid synovial fluid, it has been suggested that elastase is not important in joint destruction. This assumption neglects the effect of the microenvironment of the cartilage surface. In contrast to the 'bulk phase' synovial fluid, cartilage interferes with the interaction between AAT and elastase[56], probably because of the relative inability of alpha-1-antitrypsin to diffuse into the cartilage (charge and molecular weight considerations).

Using free radicals produced in a Fenton system (H_2O_2/Cu), Dean *et al.*[57] have shown that human neutrophil elastase is just as susceptible to inactivation as AAT. However, the oxidant species which is most likely to be important in inactivating AAT *in vivo* is hypochlorous acid, a product of the neutrophil myeloperoxidase–H_2O_2–Cl^- system[58]. Furthermore, the equal inactivation of elastase and its inhibitor was demonstrated using a high dose of H_2O_2 (5 mmol/l) – a possible differential effect at lower doses was not tested.

It has recently been demonstrated that a contribution to AAT inactivation might be made by a metalloproteinase released from neutrophils[59,60], although the *activation* of the metalloproteinase is itself dependent on myeloperoxidase-catalysed HOCl generation[59]. The above observations indicate that AAT may be inactivated, either directly or indirectly, as a result of oxygen radical generation.

These observations have provided a stimulus for pharmacological intervention: the normal human AAT cDNA has been used to transform yeast to produce AAT, known as 'Metserpin'[61]. A mutant of AAT ('Valserpin') has also been produced, where valine is substituted for the active site methionine (358 Met→Val)[61]. *In vitro*, this mutant is resistant to oxidative inactivation by neutrophils, whilst maintaining its antiprotease activity[62]. Unfortunately, the recombinant AAT molecules lack carbohydrates; consequently their plasma half-life is markedly reduced, obviating the intravenous route for their administration in inflammatory diseases such as emphysema[51]. On the other hand, *in vitro* studies[63] have shown that some anti-inflammatory drugs – e.g. penicillamine, gold sodium thiomalate, phenylbutazone and primaquine – will inhibit HOCl-mediated inactivation of AAT at physiological concentrations, suggesting that rapid scavenging of HOCl might contribute to their anti-inflammatory effects. However, sutiable *in vivo* studies to substantiate this interesting hypothesis are needed.

DNA oxidation

Single- and double-strand scission of DNA, together with hydroxylation of constituent bases, are changes characteristic of oxygen radical attack on DNA. An important mechanism is site-specific hydroxyl radical generation, catalysed by iron bound to cellular DNA[64]. For example, the reaction of the hydroxyl radical with the DNA nucleoside deoxyguanosine results in the formation of 8-hydroxydeoxyguanosine (8-OHdG)[65]. This adduct causes an increase in the frequency of misincorporation of DNA bases both at the damaged base and at the bases adjacent to it[66], suggesting that it is a mutagen.

Gas chromatography–mass spectrometry with selected ion monitoring has been applied to the analysis of the base products produced by exposure of DNA to the hypoxanthine/xanthine oxidase system in the presence of iron ions[67]. The site specificity of ˙OH generation could be altered by adding unchelated iron ions which bound to the DNA, leading to 'site-specific' ˙OH generation, or by adding Fe^{3+}–EDTA, leading to ˙OH generation in 'free' solution. Seven major products were quantitated[67], but the relative proportions of these products were dependent on whether the system was set up for site-specific ˙OH generation. For example, for site-specific ˙OH formation, 8-OHdG was the major product with no marked increase in the level of 2,6-diamino-4-hydroxy-5-formamidopyrimidine (FapyGua); for 'free' ˙OH formation FapyGua was the major product, followed by 8-OHdG. Comparative measurement of these products might allow 'fingerprinting' of the extent to which site-specific ˙OH-induced damage occurs. Within the cell nucleus, DNA exists in close association with histone and structural proteins. It is thought that copper atoms play an important role in the maintenance of this structure by linking threads of DNA to the structural proteins. Cramp *et al.*[68] have suggested that the DNA–copper–protein sites will be targets for site-specific ˙OH damage.

High-performance liquid chromatography with electrochemical detection allows the determination of 8-OHdG in femtomole amounts[69]. Using this technique, Ames' group[70] studied the oxidation state of the nuclear DNA and mitochondrial DNA of rat liver. 8-OHdG was present at a level of 1 per 130 000 bases in nuclear DNA and 1 per 8000 bases in mitochondrial DNA; it was therefore proposed that mitochondrial DNA is exposed to greater fluxes of oxygen radicals. Given our recent understanding of uncoupling events in the respiratory chain (*see above*) this is a plausible hypothesis.

Levels of 8-OHdG have also been measured in human and rodent urine. Preliminary results indicate a trend towards lower levels in CGD patients than in normal control subjects[71]. It is also reported that urinary 8-OHdG levels are higher in mice than in humans[72]. However, it is not known if this product in urine is derived exclusively from DNA via repair enzyme processes: oxidation of free guanine, normal purine metabolism and/or dietary factors might contribute to urinary 8-OHdG.

Isolated human granulocytes produce high levels of ROS after exposure to the tumour promoter tetradeconylphorbolacetate (TPA). Floyd *et al.*[69] showed that TPA-activated cells contained increased levels of 8-OHdG (about 1 8-OHdG per 600 guanine bases in their DNA) compared with non-activated cells. This increase was prevented by the presence of SOD during exposure of the cells to TPA. This observation suggests that levels of 8-OHdG might be increased in the DNA of inflammatory cells from patients with various inflammatory diseases, making this DNA oxidation product a sensitive marker of cellular activation. Recently, Perrett's group[73] measured the rate of DNA unwinding (a measure of DNA strand breaks) in circulating mononuclear cells. They found that the rate of DNA unwinding was significantly increased in RA, compared with normal control cells and osteoarthritis cells.

Many chemotherapeutic drugs, e.g. adriamycin and bleomycin, appear to exert their cytotoxic actions by virtue of their ability to redox cycle within tumour cells, thus catalysing DNA damage. Bleomycin forms a ternary complex with iron and DNA. The complex is then activated by the cytochrome P-450 system to oxidize DNA in an oxygen-dependent reaction, possibly involving ˙OH. The resulting DNA damage includes single- and double-strand breaks and release of bases[74]. It has also been shown that bleomycin will catalyse the hydroxylation of deoxyguanosine in DNA to form 8-OHdG[75]. However, we have found that although both bleomycin and gamma-irradiation induce 8-OHdG formation in isolated DNA, no increase in 8-OHdG above control levels could be detected in intact human/rat hepatocytes exposed to bleomycin *in vitro* at 4°C or 37°C[76]. Bleomycin does, however, induce unscheduled DNA synthesis in isolated, non-permeabilized hepatocytes ([^{3}H]thymidine incorporation), implying that 8-OHdG formation is not a major determinant of bleomycin-induced DNA repair[77].

Unfortunately, oxidant-generating chemotherapeutic drugs produce long-term side-effects, such as fibrosis, which may be related to extracellular generation of free radicals. Immediately following chemotherapy, patients have high plasma levels of catalytic iron, which might reflect ROS-mediated cell damage[78]. In isolated rat nuclei, SOD inhibits bleomycin-induced membrane peroxidation, but has no effect on bleomycin-catalysed DNA scission[74]. Thus, it may be possible to use iron chelators to reduce the toxic extracellular side-effects of these drugs, whilst leaving the intracellular therapeutic mode of action unaltered. In fact, it has been demonstrated that the cardiotoxicity of adriamycin can be inhibited by the chelating agent ICRF-187[78].

Relatively low levels of oxygen radicals stimulate fibroblast proliferation and collagen production[79], and may also play a role in the connective tissue disease scleroderma, which is characterized by excessive deposition of collagen and vascular damage. Several lines of evidence support this hypothesis: (1) a scleroderma-like condition can be produced in rats after repeated administration of bleomycin[80]; (2) the chromosomal aberrations seen in lymphocytes from scleroderma patients are suggested to be induced by oxygen-radical-mediated DNA damage[81]; (3) 97% of scleroderma patients have Raynaud's phenomenon (episodic digital ischaemia), a disease in which oxygen radical-mediated reperfusion injury has been implicated[82]; (4) the plasma concentration of the vascular endothelial cell-derived von Willebrand factor antigen is elevated in scleroderma, but this rise is not paralleled by an increase in von Willebrand factor functional activity[83]. A similar phenomenon has been noted in acute respiratory failure[84], possibly reflecting the oxidative inactivation of von Willebrand factor during its release from injured endothelial cells, which are putative target cells in both diseases.

Serum anti-DNA antibodies are a feature of several connective tissue diseases, including SLE. Preincubation of isolated DNA with a ROS-generating system resulted in a dose-dependent increase in binding of SLE anti-DNA antibodies[85]. This increased binding was inhibited by the ROS scavenger thiourea and the iron chelator desferrioxamine. It was suggested that oxidatively modified DNA is antigenic, stimulating the release of anti-DNA antibodies. This would be a process analogous to that proposed earlier for free-radical-modified IgG. Anti-IgG antibodies ('rheumatoid factor') are present in rheumatoid extracellular fluids and have been shown to react with free-radical-altered IgG produced *in vitro*. Oxidatively modified IgG has been detected in rheumatoid synovial fluid[43], indicating that this could be the antigenic stimulus for rheumatoid factor production.

HYPOXIC-REPERFUSION-INDUCED DNA DAMAGE AND CELLULAR ENERGY CHARGE STATE IN INFLAMMATION

The mechanism for the production of $O_2^{\cdot -}$ in ischaemic tissues appears to involve changes in purine metabolism within ischaemic cells[13]. During temporary ischaemia low oxygen concentrations cause a decline in mitochondrial oxidative phosphorylation by decreasing the capacity of the respiratory chain for coupled electron transport. This increases the dependence of the cell on ATP production via anaerobic glycolysis. Anaerobic glycolysis is an inefficient means of ATP production from glucose, and leads to raised concentrations of adenosine and of its breakdown products, including hypoxanthine and xanthine, which are substrates for the xanthine dehydrogenase enzyme system.

Cellular levels of ATP (i.e. the cell's 'energy currency') fall. It is no longer able to maintain proper ion gradients across its membranes, and this precipitates a redistribution of Ca^{2+} ions. The elevated cytosolic Ca^{2+} concentration activates a protease capable of catalysing the conversion of xanthine dehydrogenase to xanthine oxidase, in a process discussed earlier. Reperfusion of the temporarily ischaemic organ restores a supply of the remaining substrate required for xanthine oxidase activity, O_2, and $O_2^{\cdot -}$ is generated. The localization of xanthine oxidase within endothelial cells could make this cell type one of the targets for oxidant injury. Spragg *et al.*[86] have studied the effects of H_2O_2 on energy metabolism in bovine aortic endothelial cells as a model for the target cells during oxidant injury in many inflammatory conditions, e.g. adult respiratory distress syndrome.

The reperfusion-induced intracellular production of oxygen radicals and H_2O_2 will result in a sharp increase in GSH consumption, since the glutathione peroxidase-catalysed reduction of H_2O_2 to water is coupled to the oxidation of GSH to GSSG. Thus the GSSG to GSH ratio is an index of intracellular oxidant stress. The glutathione redox cycle is coupled to the hexose monophosphate shunt by NADP, which is used by glutathione reductase. Thus within seconds of the oxygen radical flux the hexose monophosphate shunt will be triggered and glutathione will be regenerated. This redox cycling system is located within the cytosol and protects the cell against oxidative damage. GSH is also necessary for maintaining membrane integrity via the gamma-glutamyl cycle.

As well as induction of the hexose monophosphate shunt, over a similar time-scale intracellular oxidant stress leads to the formation of DNA single-strand breaks[2]. Within minutes the enzyme poly(ADP-ribose) polymerase is activated as part of the DNA repair process. Poly(ADP-ribose) polymerase utilizes NAD^+, and if the degree of DNA damage exceeds a critical level then the process of NAD^+ depletion, coupled with further ATP depletion, could become irreversible; the result is cell death. Carson *et al.*[1] have suggested a role for DNA strand breakage and the programmed synthesis of poly(ADP-ribose) in the genesis of lymphocyte damage or killing induced by exposure to oxygen radicals. The latter workers have termed this process 'NAD^+-dependent programmed cell death', and have suggested that this phenomenon represents a 'suicide response' of cells with extensively damaged DNA which might prevent the early emergence of somatic mutants with maligant potential. Although this concept is attractive, perhaps it should be stressed that at the moment a role for DNA strand breaks in cell killing has not been established. Cell killing might result from oxidative damage to other critical target(s), for example cell membranes.

The fall in NAD^+ is mirrored by a further, 'second phase', decline in the energy charge state of the cell. However, the fall in NAD^+ is not the only factor thought to be involved. Two other contributory events are: (1) oxidative inactivation of the ATPase–synthase complex of mitochondria[45]; (2) oxidative inactivation of glyceraldehyde 3-phosphate dehydrogenase[45,46], the *only* enzyme of glycolysis which appears to be significantly altered by oxidants. Hyslop *et al.*[45] found that, in addition to the direct inactivation of glyceraldehyde 3-phosphate dehydrogenase, the inactivation of this step was also effected by a reduction in the intracellular concentration and redox potential of the enzyme's nicotinamide co-factors and a fall in cytosolic pH.

The loss of energy charge state will also coincide with a further accumulation of hypoxanthine, a breakdown product of ATP. Herbert *et al.*[87] demonstrated an increased concentration of hypoxanthine in rheumatoid synovial fluid, presumably the result of ATP catabolism in senescent joint cells.

The second phase loss of cellular energy charge is followed by a further increase in the free intracellular Ca^{2+} concentration, with consequent activation of Ca^{2+}-dependent endonucleases[88]. In fact, it was suggested[88] that activation of Ca^{2+}-dependent endonucleases might be an important cause of DNA strand breakage. However, this seems unlikely, since a change in the Ca^{2+} ion concentration sufficient to activate endonucleases appears to take place *after* DNA strand breakage has occurred. Even later (1–2 h post-oxidant exposure) actin polymerization and plasma membrane blebbing can be observed, leading to loss of membrane integrity.

In view of the above, Hyslop *et al.*[45] suggested that cell types which produce ATP mainly via the glycolytic pathway, with only a small pool of mitochrondria capable of increasing their compensatory rate of ADP phosphorylation, will be more susceptible to oxidant damage. It is therefore noteworthy that, in cartilage, entry of pyruvate into the citric acid cycle is possibly inhibited by acetyl-CoA derived from fat. Thus, in normal cartilage, most of the energy consumed would be produced by glycolysis[89]. Furthermore, bovine endothelial cells have a very high glycolytic activity under aerobic conditions (see ref. 45), suggesting that this cell type would also be susceptible to oxidant damage.

The metabolic disturbances described above are reminiscent of those observed in cells cultured from the rheumatoid synovium, in which the intracellular redox potential is lowered relative to normal cells[90]. Since exchange reactions take place between intracellular proteins and small molecule thiols such as glutathione, the sulphydryl:disulphide (–SH:–S–S–)

redox couple of the tissue proteins will reflect the redox potential of the cell. Butcher *et al.*[91] found that in control synoviocytes approximately 63% of the sulphur-containing amino acids were in the reduced form and 37% were in the oxidized state. This was significantly different from rheumatoid synoviocytes, in which approximately 88% of the sulphur-containing amino acids were reduced.

The relative ATP-generating capacities of glycolysis and mitochondria and/or antioxidant levels may also play a role in the observed differential susceptibility to ROS-induced cell killing of T and B lymphocytes. Using a glucose–glucose oxidase system to generate H_2O_2 in cell cultures, Farber *et al.*[92] found that B lymphocytes were more susceptible than T lymphocytes, as assessed by a dye exclusion method. In contrast, when cells were exposed to culture medium containing ROS which had been generated by prior ultraviolet irradiation[93], T cells were shown to be more susceptible than B cells. In the same study[93], it was noted that suppressor cytotoxic T cells ($CD8^+$) were more susceptible to ROS than were helper T cells ($CD4^+$). Thus the observations that, in SLE and in the rheumatoid synovium, the $CD4^+/CD8^+$ ratio is increased, might be accounted for by selective toxicity of ROS[93].

From the above it can be seen that DNA damage is an early event in cells killed by oxygen radicals. The capacity of endogenous intracellular antioxidants or of repair mechanisms for oxidative DNA damage might determine the susceptibility of different cell populations to either killing or mutation. Lawley *et al.*[94] have demonstrated that circulating lymphocytes from patients with certain autoimmune diseases, e.g. RA, SLE and Behçet's syndrome, show increased sensitivity to the toxic effects of the alkylating agent *N*-methyl-*N*-nitrosourea compared with normal subjects and patients with other disorders. The autoimmune disease cells are also relatively deficient in the DNA repair of O^6-methylguanine. Furthermore, lymphocytes from patients with a wide variety of autoimmune inflammatory conditions (for example, RA, SLE) have a higher susceptibility to X-irradiation[95]. Such ionizing radiation can damage DNA by production of $^{\bullet}OH$ radicals formed in the aqueous surroundings of the target DNA. In view of these findings it is noteworthy that there is increasing evidence that oxygen radicals may play a part in mutation induced by a wide variety of agents[96,97]. We suggest that oxygen-radical-induced somatic mutation may play a role in the aetiology of certain autoimmune diseases, for example, by producing mutant cells displaying 'altered self' antigenic determinants.

Finally, attention should be drawn to the increased incidence of malignancy found at sites of chronic inflammation. It has been suggested that the link may be oxygen radicals, since these are thought to be involved in both processes[2,98].

Acknowledgements

The authors are grateful to the Arthritis and Rheumatism Council and the British Technology Group, who have supported many of their studies cited in this review. This chapter reviews the literature up until 1989.

References

1. Carson, D. A., Seto, S., Wasson, D. B. and Carrera, C. J. (1986). DNA strand breaks, NAD metabolism, and programmed cell death. *Exp. Cell Res.*, **164**, 273–81
2. Schraufstatter, I. U., Hyslop, P. A., Jackson, J. and Cochrane, C. C. (1987). Oxidant injury of cells. *Int. J. Tiss. Reac.*, **9**, 317–24
3. Lunec, J. and Blake, D. R. (1987). Oxidative damage and its relevance to inflammatory joint disease. In Chow, C. K. (ed.), *Cellular Antioxidant Defense Mechanisms*, Vol. III, pp. 143–59 (Boca Raton, Florida: CRC Press)
4. Harris, G. (1983). DNA damage and repair in immunologically active cells. *Immunol. Today*, **4**, 109–12
5. Halliwell, B. and Gutteridge, J. M. C. (1984). Oxygen toxicity, oxygen radicals, transition metals and disease. *Biochem. J.*, **219**, 1–14
6. Aust, S. D., Morehouse, L. A. and Thomas, C. E. (1985). Role of metals in oxygen radical reactions. *J. Free Radicals Biol. Med.*, **1**, 3–25
7. Winyard, P. G., Hider, R. C., Brailsford, S., Drake, A. F., Lunec, J. and Blake, D. R. (1989). Effects of oxidative stress on some physicochemical properties of caeruloplasmin. *Biochem. J.*, **258**, 435–45
8. Forman, H. J. and Thomas, M. J. (1986). Oxidant production and bactericidal activity of phagocytes. *Ann. Rev. Physiol.*, **48**, 669–80
9. Segal, A. W. (1987). Absence of both cytochrome b_{-245} subunits from neutrophils in X-linked chronic granulomatous disease. *Nature*, **326**, 88–91
10. Hancock, J. T., Maly, F. E. and Jones, O. T. G. (1989). Properties of the superoxide-generating oxidase of B lymphocyte cell lines. Determination of Michaelis parameters. *Biochem. J.*, **262**, 373–5
11. Saran, M. and Bors, W. (1989). Oxygen radicals acting as chemical messengers: a hypothesis. *Free Radical Res. Commun.*, **7**, 213–20
12. Jarasch, E.-D., Bruder, G. and Heid, H. W. (1986). Significance of xanthine oxidase in capillary endothelial cells. *Acta Physiol. Scand.*, **548**, (Suppl.), 39–46
13. McCord, J. M. (1985). Oxygen-derived free radicals in postischemic tissue injury. *N. Engl. J. Med.*, **312**, 159–63
14. Rodell, T. C., Cheronis, J. C., Ohnemus, C. L., Piermattei, D. J. and Repine, J. E. (1987). Xanthine oxidase mediates elastase-induced injury to isolated lungs and endothelium. *J. Appl. Physiol.*, **63**, 2159–63
15. Blake, D. R., Merry, P., Unsworth, J., Kidd, B. L., Outhwaite, J. M., Ballard, R., Morris, C. J., Gray, L. and Lunec, J. (1989). Hypoxic-reperfusion injury in the inflamed human joint. *Lancet*, **1**, 289–93
16. Merry, P., Winyard, P. G., Morris, C. J., Grootveld, M. and Blake, D. R. (1989). Oxygen free radicals, inflammation, and synovitis: the current status. *Ann. Rheum. Dis.*, **48**, 864–70
17. Allen, R. E., Blake, D. R., Nazhat, N. B. and Jones, P. (1989). Superoxide radical generation by inflamed human synovium after hypoxia. *Lancet*, **1**, 282–3
18. Cadenas, E. (1989). Biochemistry of oxygen toxicity. *Ann. Rev. Biochem.*, **58**, 79–110
19. Fridovich, I. (1979). Hypoxia and oxygen toxicity. *Adv. Neurol.*, **26**, 255–9
20. Jaeschke, H. and Mitchell, J. R. (1989). Mitochondria and xanthine oxidase both generate reactive oxygen species in isolated perfused rat liver after hypoxic injury. *Biochem. Biophys. Res. Commun.*, **160**, 140–47
21. Sligar, S. G., Lipscomb, J. D., Debrunner, P. G. and Gunsalus, I. C. (1974). Superoxide anion production by the autoxidation of cytochrome $P450_{cam}$. *Biochem. Biophys. Res. Commun.*, **61**, 290–6
22. Fisher, A. B. (1988). Intracellular production of oxygen-derived free radicals. In Halliwell, B. (ed.), *Oxygen Radicals and Tissue Injury, Upjohn Symposium Proceedings*, pp. 34–39. (Bethesda, Maryland: Federation of American Societies for Experimental Biology)
23. Adolphs, M. J. P., Bonta, I. L. and Bragt, P. C. (1980). Increased lipid peroxidation and decreased hepatic aminopyrene metabolism during carrageenin-induced granulomatous inflammation in the rat. *Br. J. Pharmacol.*, **68**, 123P
24. Ames, B. N. and Saul, R. L. (1988). Cancer, ageing and oxidative DNA damage. In Iversen, O. H. (ed.), *Theories of Carcinogenesis*, pp. 203–220 (Washington, DC: Hemisphere)
25. Matthews, S. B., Hallett, M. B., Henderson, A. H. and Campbell, A. K. (1986). The

adrenochrome pathway. A potential catabolic route for adrenaline metabolism in inflammatory disease. *Adv. Myocardiol.*, **6**, 367–381

26. Rice-Evans, C., Burdon, R. H., Winrow, V. R. and Blake, D. R. (eds) (1990). *Stress Proteins in Inflammation* (London: Richelieu Press)
27. Polla, B. S. (1988). A role for heat shock proteins in inflammation? *Immunol. Today*, **9**, 134–137
28. Winrow, V. R., McLean, L., Morris, C. J. and Blake, D. R. (1990). The heat shock protein response and its role in inflammatory disease. *Ann. Rheum. Dis.* (In press)
29. Keyse, S. M. and Tyrrell, R. M. (1989). Heme oxygenase is the major 32-KDa stress protein induced in human skin fibroblasts by UVA radiation, hydrogen peroxide, and sodium arsenite. *Proc. Natl. Acad. Sci. USA*, **86**, 99–103
30. Karlsson, K. and Marklund, S. L. (1987). Heparin-induced release of extracellular superoxide dismutase to human blood plasma. *Biochem. J.*, **242**, 55–9
31. Winyard, P. G. and Blake, D. R. (1989). Caeruloplasmin and oxygen free radicals. In Beaumont, P. C., Deeble, D. J., Parsons, B. J. and Rice-Evans, C. (eds), *Free Radicals, Metal Ions and Biopolymers*, pp. 183–97 (London: Richelieu Press)
32. Gutteridge, J. M. C. (1986). Antioxidant properties of the proteins caeruloplasmin, albumin and transferrin. A study of their activity in serum and synovial fluid from patients with rheumatoid arthritis. *Biochim. Biophys. Acta*, **869**, 119–27
33. Niedermeier, W. (1965). Concentration and chemical state of copper in synovial fluid and blood serum of patients with rheumatoid arthritis. *Ann. Rheum. Dis.*, **24**, 544–548
34. Winyard, P. G., Pall, H., Lunec, J. and Blake, D. R. (1987). Non-caeruloplasmin-bound copper ('phenanthroline copper') is not detectable in fresh serum or synovial fluid from patients with rheumatoid arthritis. *Biochem. J.*, **247**, 245–247
35. Winyard, P. G., Blake, D. R., Chirico, S., Gutteridge, J. M. C. and Lunec, J. (1987). Mechanism of exacerbation of rheumatoid synovitis by total-dose iron-dextran infusion: in-vivo demonstration of iron-promoted oxidant stress. *Lancet*, **1**, 69–72
36. McCord, J. M. (1974). Free radicals and inflammation: protection of synovial fluid by superoxide dismutase. *Science*, **185**, 529–31
37. Vuorio, E., Einola, S., Hakkarainen, S. and Penttinen, R. (1982). Synthesis of underpolymerised hyaluronic acid by fibroblasts cultured from rheumatoid and non-rheumatoid synovitis. *Rheumatol. Int.*, **2**, 97–102
38. Rowley, D. A., Gutteridge, J. M. C., Blake, D. R., Farr, M. and Halliwell, B. (1984). Lipid peroxidation in rheumatoid arthritis. Thiobarbituric acid-reactive material and catalytic iron salts in synovial fluid from rheumatoid patients. *Clin. Sci.*, **66**, 691–95
39. Merry, P., Grootveld, M., Lunec, J. and Blake, D. R. (1990). Oxidative damage to lipids within the inflamed human joint provides evidence of radical-mediated hypoxic-reperfusion injury. *Am. J. Clin. Nutr.* (In press)
40. Quinn, M. T., Parthasarathy, S., Fong, L. G. and Steinberg, D. (1987). Oxidatively modified low density lipoproteins: A potential role in recruitment and retention of monocyte/macrophages during atherogenesis. *Proc. Natl. Acad. Sci. USA*, **84**, 2995–8
41. Greenwald, R. A., Moy, W. W. and Lazarus, D. (1976). Degradation of cartilage proteoglycans and collagen by superoxide anions. *Arthritis Rheum.*, **19**, 799
42. Wolff, S. P., Garner, A. and Dean, R. T. (1986). Free radicals, lipids and protein degradation. *TIBS*, **11**, 27–31
43. Lunec, J., Blake, D. R., McCleary, S. J., Brailsford, S. and Bacon, P. A. (1985). Self-perpetuating mechanisms of immunoglobulin G aggregation in rheumatoid inflammation. *J. Clin. Invest.*, **76**, 2084–90
44. Winyard, P. G., Arundell, L. A. and Blake, D. R. (1988). Lipoprotein oxidation and induction of ferroxidase activity in stored human extracellular fluids. *Free Radical Res. Commun.*, **5**, 227–35
45. Hyslop, P. A., Hinshaw, D. B., Halsey, W. A., Schraufstatter, I. U., Sauerheber, R. D., Spragg, R. G., Jackson, J. H. and Cochrane, C. G. (1988). Mechanism of oxidant-mediated cell injury. The glycolytic and mitochondrial pathways of ADP phosphorylation are major intracellular targets inactivated by hydrogen peroxide. *J. Biol. Chem.*, **263**, 1665–75
46. Baker, M. S., Feigan, J. and Lowther, D. A. (1989). The mechanism of chondrocyte hydrogen peroxide damage. Depletion of intracellular ATP due to suppression of glycolysis caused by oxidation of glyceraldehyde-3-phosphate dehydrogenase. *J. Rheumatol.*, **16**, 7–14
47. Carrell, R. W. and Travis, J. (1985). Alpha-1-antitrypsin and the serpins: variation and countervariation. *TIBS*, **10**, 20–4

48. Carrell, R. (1986). Alpha-1-antitrypsin: molecular pathology, leukocytes, and tissue damage. *J. Clin. Invest.*, **78**, 1427–31
49. Cox, D. W. and Huber, O. (1980). Association of severe rheumatoid arthritis with heterozygosity for alpha-1-antitrypsin deficiency. *Clin. Genet.*, **17**, 153–60
50. Sanders, P. A., Thomson, W., Browne, D. A., Dyer, P. A. and Grennan, D. M. (1986). Alpha-1-antitrypsin (PI) allotypes in rheumatoid arthritis. *Ann. Rheum. Dis.*, **45**, 450–3
51. Carrell, R. (1984). Therapy by instant evolution. *Nature*, **312**, 14
52. Carp, H., Miller, F., Hoidal, J. R. and Janoff, A. (1982). Potential mechanism of emphysema: alpha-1-proteinase inhibitor recovered from lungs of cigarette smokers contains oxidised methionine and has decreased elastase inhibitory capacity. *Proc. Natl. Acad. Sci. USA*, **79**, 2041–5
53. Schtacher, G., Maayan, R. and Feinstein, G. (1973). Proteinase inhibitors in human synovial fluid. *Biochim. Biophys. Acta*, **303**, 138–47
54. Lewis, D. A., Parrott, D. P., Bird, J., Cosh, J. A. and Ring, F. (1984). Inactive forms of plasma antiproteinases in arthritic synovial fluids. *IRCS Med. Sci.*, **12**, 304–5
55. Wong, P. S. and Travis, J. (1980). Isolation and properties of oxidised alpha-1-proteinase inhibitor from human rheumatoid synovial fluid. *Biochem. Biophys. Res. Commun.*, **96**, 1449–54
56. Burkhardt, H., Kasten, M., Rauls, S. and Rehkopf, E. (1987). Interference of cartilage surface with the interaction of granulocyte elastase with alpha-1-proteinase inhibitor. An in vitro model of enzyme inhibition in the joint space. *Rheumatol. Int.*, **7**, 133–8
57. Dean, R. T., Nick, H. P. and Schnebli, H. P. (1989). Free radicals inactivate human neutrophil elastase and its inhibitors with comparable efficiency. *Biochem. Biophys. Res. Commun.*, **159**, 821–7
58. Weiss, S. J. and Regiani, S. (1984). Neutrophils degrade subendothelial matrices in the presence of alpha-1-proteinase inhibitor. Cooperative use of lysosomal proteinases and oxygen metabolites. *J. Clin. Invest.*, **73**, 1297–303
59. Desrochers, P. E. and Weiss, S. J. (1988). Proteolytic inactivation of alpha-1-proteinase inhibitor by a neturophil metalloproteinase. *J. Clin. Invest.*, **81**, 1646–50
60. Vissers, M. C. M., George, P. M., Bathurst, I. C., Brennan, S. O. and Winterbourn, C. C. (1988). Cleavage and inactivation of alpha-1-antitrypsin by metalloproteinases released from neutrophils. *J. Clin. Invest.*, **82**, 706–11
61. Rosenberg, S., Barr, P. J., Najarian, R. C. and Hallewell, R. A. (1984). Synthesis in yeast of a functional, oxidation resistant active centre variant of human alpha-1-antitrypsin. *Nature*, **312**, 77–80
62. George, P. M., Vissers, M. C. M., Travis, J., Winterbourn, C. C. and Carrell, R. W. (1984). A genetically engineered mutant of alpha-1-antitrypsin protects connective tissue from neutrophil damage and may be useful in lung disease. *Lancet*, **2**, 1426–8
63. Wasil, M., Halliwell, B., Moorhouse, C. P., Hutchison, S. and Baum, H. (1987). Biologically-significant scavenging of the myeloperoxidase-derived oxidant hypochlorous acid by some anti-inflammatory drugs. *Biochem. Pharmacol.*, **36**, 3847–50
64. Loeb, L. A., James, E. A., Waltersdorph, A. M. and Klebanoff, S. J. (1988). Mutagenesis by the autoxidation of iron with isolated DNA. *Proc. Natl. Acad. Sci. USA*, **85**, 3918–22
65. Kasai, H., Crain, P. F., Kuchino, Y., Nishimura, S., Ootsuyama, A. and Tanooka, H. (1986). Formation of 8-hydroxyguanine moiety in cellular DNA by agents producing oxygen radicals and evidence for its repair. *Carcinogenesis*, **7**, 1849–51
66. Kuchino, Y., Mori, F., Kasai, H., Inoue, H., Iwai, S., Miura, K., Ohtsuka, E. and Nishimura, S. (1987). Misreading of DNA templates containing 8-hydroxydeoxyguanosine at the modified base and at adjacent residues. *Nature*, **327**, 77–9
67. Aruoma, O. I., Halliwell, B. and Dizdaroglu, M. (1989). Iron ion-dependent modification of bases in DNA by the superoxide radical-generating system hypoxanthine/xanthine oxidase. *J. Biol. Chem.*, **264**, 13024–8
68. Cramp, W. A., George, A. M., Khan, H. and Yatvin, M. B. (1989). The role of copper in radiation and drug induced changes in the quaternary structure of DNA. In Beaumont, P. C., Deeble, D. J., Parsons, B. J. and Rice-Evans, C. (eds), *Free Radicals, Metal Ions and Biopolymers*, pp. 127–141 (London: Richelieu Press)
69. Floyd, R. A., Watson, J. J., Harris, J., West, M. and Wong, P. K. (1986). Formation of 8-hydroxydeoxyguanosine, hydroxyl free radical adduct of DNA in granulocytes exposed to the tumour promotor, tetradeconylphorbolacetate. *Biochem. Biophys. Res. Commun.*, **137**, 841–6
70. Richter, C., Park, J.-W. and Ames, B. N. (1988). Normal oxidative damage to mitochondrial

and nuclear DNA is extensive. *Proc. Natl. Acad. Sci. USA*, **85**, 6465–7
71. Cundy, K. C., Kohen, R. and Ames, B. N. (1988). Determination of 8-hydroxydeoxyguanosine in human urine: a possible assay for in vivo oxidative DNA damage. In Simic, M. G., Taylor, K. A., Ward, J. F. and von Sonntag, C. (eds), *Oxygen Radicals in Biology and Medicine*, pp. 479–482 (New York: Plenum Press)
72. Bergtold, D. S., Simic, M. G., Alessio, H. and Cutler, R. G. (1988). Urine biomarkers for oxidative DNA damage. In Simic, M. G., Taylor, K. A., Ward, J. F. and von Sonntag, C. (eds), *Oxygen Radicals in Biology and Medicine*, pp. 483–489 (New York: Plenum Press)
73. Bhusate, L. L., Herbert, K. E., Scott, D. L. and Perrett, D. (1989). Increased damage to mononuclear cell DNA in rheumatoid arthritis. *Br. J. Rheumatol.*, **28**, (Suppl. 2), 28
74. Ciriolo, M. R., Peisach, J. and Magliozzo, R. S. (1989). A comparative study of the interactions of bleomycin with nuclei and purified DNA. *J. Biol. Chem.*, **264**, 1443–9
75. Kohda, K., Kasai, H., Ogawa, T., Suzuki, T. and Kawazoe, Y. (1989). Deoxyribonucleic acid (DNA) damage induced by bleomycin-Fe(II) *in vitro*: formation of 8-hydroxyguanine residues in DNA. *Chem. Pharm. Bull.*, **37**, 1028–30
76. Smith, A. J., Winyard, P. G. and Chipman, J. K. (1990). Bleomycin and gamma-radiation induced hydroxylation of deoxyguanosine in vitro. In *International Symposium on Biological Reactive Intermediates* (In press)
77. Winyard, P. G., Perrett, D., Chipman, J. K., Blake, D. R. and Harris, G. (1990). Measurement of DNA oxidation products. *Analyt. Proc.*, **27**, 224–7
78. Halliwell, B. and Bomford, A. (1989). ICRF-187 and doxorubicin-induced cardiac toxicity. *N. Engl. J. Med.*, **320**, 399–400
79. Murrell, G. A. C., Francis, M. J. O. and Bromley, L. (1987). Free radicals and Dupuytren's contracture. *Br. Med. J.*, **295**, 1373–5
80. Mountz, J. D., Downs Minor, M. B., Turner, R., Thomas, M. B., Richards, F. and Pisko, E. (1983). Bleomycin-induced cutaneous toxicity in the rat: analysis of histopathology and ultrastructure compared with progressive systemic sclerosis (scleroderma). *Br. J. Dermatol.*, **108**, 679–86
81. Emerit, I., Keck, M., Levy, A., Feingold, J. and Michelson, A. M. (1982). Activated oxygen species at the origin of chromosome breakage and sister-chromatid exchanges. *Mutat. Res.*, **103**, 165–72
82. Chopra, M., Smith, W. E., Ansell, D. and Belch, J. J. F. (1988). Free radical pathology in Raynaud's phenomenon. *Acta Chir. Scand.*, **546**, (Suppl.), 51a
83. Greaves, M., Malia, R. G., Ward, A. M., Moult, J., Holt, C. M., Lindsey, N., Hughes, P., Goodfield, M. and Rowell, N. R. (1988). Elevated von Willebrand factor antigen in systemic sclerosis: relationship to visceral disease. *Br. J. Rheumatol.*, **27**, 281–5
84. Carvalho, A. C. A., Bellman, S. M., Saullo, V. J., Quinn, D. and Zapol, W. M. (1982). Altered factor VIII in acute respiratory failure. *N. Engl. J. Med.*, **307**, 1113–19
85. Blount, S., Griffiths, H. R. and Lunec, J. (1989). Reactive oxygen species induce antigenic changes in DNA. *FEBS Lett.*, **245**, 100–4
86. Spragg, R. G., Hinshaw, D. B., Hyslop, P. A., Schraufstatter, I. U. and Cochrane, C. G. (1985). Alterations in adenosine triphosphate and energy charge in cultured endothelial and $P388D_1$ cells after oxidant injury. *J. Clin. Invest.*, **76**, 1471–6
87. Herbert, K. E., Scott, D. L. and Perrett, D. (1988). Nucleosides and bases in synovial fluid from patients with rheumatoid arthritis and osteoarthritis. *Clin. Sci.*, **74**, 97–9
88. McConkey, D. J., Hartzell, P., Nicotera, P., Wyllie, A. H. and Orrenius, S. (1988). Stimulation of endogenous endonuclease activity in hepatocytes exposed to oxidative stress. *Toxicol. Lett.*, **42**, 123–30
89. Ahlqvist, J., Osterlund, K. and Harilainen, A. (1989). Does joint cartilage require energy? *Ann. Rheum. Dis.*, **48**, 878
90. Henderson, B. (1983). The application of quantitative cytochemistry to the study of diseases of the connective tissues. *Progr. Histochem. Cytochem.*, **15**, 1–82
91. Butcher, R. G., Bitensky, L., Cashman, B. and Chayen, J. (1973). Differences in the redox balance in human rheumatoid and non-rheumatoid synovial lining cells. *Beitr. Path. Bd.*, **148**, 265–74
92. Farber, C. M., Liebes, L. F., Kanganis, D. N. and Silber, R. (1984). Human B lymphocytes show greater susceptibility to H_2O_2 toxicity than T lymphocytes. *J. Immunol.*, **132**, 2543–6
93. Allan, I. M., Lunec, J., Salmon, M. and Bacon, P. A. (1987). Reactive oxygen species selectively

deplete normal T lymphocytes via a hydroxyl radical dependent mechanism. *Scand. J. Immunol.*, **26**, 47–53

94. Lawley, P. D., Topper, R., Denman, A. M., Hylton, W., Hill, I. D. and Harris, G. (1988). Increased sensitivity of lymphocytes from patients with systemic autoimmune diseases to DNA alkylation by the methylating carcinogen *N*-methyl-*N*-nitrosourea. *Ann. Rheum. Dis.*, **47**, 445–51
95. Harris, G., Cramp, W. A., Edwards, J. C., George, A. M., Sabovljev, S. A., Hart, L., Hughes, G. R. V., Denman, A. M. and Yatvin, M. B. (1985). Radiosensitivity of peripheral blood lymphocytes in autoimmune disease. *Int. J. Radiat. Biol.*, **47**, 689–99
96. Hsie, A. W., Recio, L., Katz, D. S., Lee, C. Q., Wagner, M. and Schenley, R. L. (1986). Evidence for reactive oxygen species inducing mutations in mammalian cells. *Proc. Natl. Acad. Sci. USA*, **83**, 9616–20
97. Fiala, E. S., Conaway, C. C. and Mathis, J. E. (1989). Oxidative DNA and RNA damage in the livers of Sprague-Dawley rats treated with the hepatocarcinogen 2-nitropropane. *Cancer Res.*, **49**, 5518–22
98. Trush, M. A., Seed, J. L. and Kensler, T. W. (1985). Oxidant-dependent metabolic activation of polycyclic aromatic hydrocarbons by phorbol ester-stimulated human polymorphonuclear leukocytes: possible link between inflammation and cancer. *Proc. Natl. Acad. Sci. USA*, **82**, 5194–8

7
Glucocorticoids and lipocortin

S. H. PEERS and R. J. FLOWER

INTRODUCTION

Glucocorticoids and inflammation

One of the responses of an animal to injury, infection or other stresses is the release from the adrenal cortex of glucocorticosteroids (GCs). In humans this is predominantly hydrocortisone (cortisol), but other animals may release different but related steroids. For a long while it was believed that steroids were in some way involved in the mounting of the response to stress (such as an inflammatory response), but it has only recently become clear that in fact steroids are actually part of the system which prevents our 'defence mechanisms' from running out of control and threatening homeostasis. Glucocorticosteroids are thus part of the normal regulation of the immune system, which explains why adrenalectomized animals tend to produce exaggerated responses to environmental trauma such as infection or injury.

The glucocorticoids influence many systems within the body including the immune system, carbohydrate metabolizing enzymes and bone, leading to osteoporosis. Suppressive actions on the hypothalamus and pituitary may lead to adrenal insufficiency. The glucocorticoids are potent and effective anti-inflammatory agents, used in the treatment of a wide range of conditions, from skin irritation to asthma, multiple sclerosis and rheumatoid arthiritis.

The glucocorticosteroids used clinically are naturally occurring steroids (hydrocortisone) or related synthetic analogues, and hence have a very similar wide range of biological activities. This means that when used as anti-inflammatory agents they possess the range of unwanted side-effects associated with over-production of endogenous corticosteroids seen in Cushing's syndrome. Much work has attempted to discover the mechanism by which steroids cause their various effects in the hope that it might be possible to develop analogues with specific, desirable actions and minimal side-effects.

Mechanism of action of GCs

One of the most important findings in the study of GC action was the discovery of the steroid receptor and the elucidation of the mechanism by which occupation of the soluble receptor causes translocation of the steroid–receptor complex to the cell nucleus, interaction with certain sites on chromosomes ('hormone responsive elements' (HREs) of steroid-sensitive genes) and regulation of transcription of those genes. Most mammalian cells have up to 100 000 glucocorticoid steroid receptors per cell. These receptors are members of a gene 'superfamily' whose products are ligand-sensitive transcription factors, and includes receptors for thyroid hormone, vitamin D and retinoic acid. The steroid receptors (and other members of the superfamily) are large proteins (MW 30–70 kD) organized structurally into functional domains. They have a variable N-terminal region (which modulates transactivation), a short and well-conserved central domain (responsible for DNA binding via so-called zinc fingers) next to a short sequence which appears to be partly responsible for intranuclear localization of the receptor. This region is also important for interaction with the 90 kD heat shock protein, which dissociates from the receptor upon steroid binding. The C-terminal domain is relatively well conserved and has complex functions since, as well as being involved in hormone binding and nuclear translocation, it may have transactivation and dimerization functions. For further information, see reviews by Beato[1] or Rousseau[2].

Interaction of the steroid hormone with the receptor leads to dissociation of the heat shock protein and a change in receptor conformation which allows it to bind to chromatin. The hormone–receptor complex binds to specific structures on certain genes (HREs) and stimulates transactivation by a mechanism not yet fully understood. Some genes are repressed by steroid hormones, and these have an HRE distinct from genes whose transcription is enhanced by steroids. The mechanism by which transcription is repressed has also yet to be described.

Since steroid action requires mRNA and protein synthesis, drugs such as actinomycin D or cycloheximide can block steroid effects. The actions of steroids depend upon either induction or inhibition of protein synthesis, and it is these steroid-regulated proteins which mediate the actions of the drug or hormone. In some cases, for example interleukin 1, the actions of the protein are well known; in other cases the steroid-regulated protein may be an enzyme (e.g. tyrosine aminotransferase) and steroid action depends upon changes in enzyme activity. In other cases the protein which mediates steroid action may be as yet unidentified.

ANTI-INFLAMMATORY ACTIONS OF STEROIDS

Glucocorticoids inhibit both acute and chronic inflammation, caused by infection by pathogens, chemical or physical trauma, or by the immune response itself such as hypersensitivity reactions or autoimmune disease. In acute inflammation, steroids inhibit oedema development, partly due to a vasoconstrictor effect on small blood vessels, and partly due to inhibition of synthesis of vasodilator prostaglandins. Corticosteroids also inhibit accumulation of neutrophils and monocytes, and this may be due to either an inhibition of synthesis of chemotactic factors such as leukotrienes, a direct effect upon the leukocytes themselves, or both. Corticosteroids cause a neutrophilia, due to increased release of neutrophils from bone marrow and reduced margination of circulating neutrophils, but a monocytopenia due to decreased monocyte release from bone marrow.

Glucocorticoids also affect neutrophil and monocyte behaviour, for example inhibition of release of active oxygen species and hence reduced microbiocidal activity. This may be a direct effect, or may be due to a general reduction in leukocyte activation following inhibition of synthesis of certain cytokines. Steroids have so far been shown to inhibit synthesis of interferon γ, interleukin 1 and interleukin 2, and various leukocyte-activating substances such as interluekins 6 and 8, and hence may have a wide-ranging and complicated mechanism of immune suppression. Glucocorticoids also affect cells of the immune system, causing lympholysis of T and B cells in 'steroid-sensitive' species such as rabbits or rats, and decreased responsiveness of T and B cells in steroid-insensitive species such as humans or guinea pig. This may also be the result of inhibition of synthesis of cytokines such as the interleukins.

LIPOCORTIN, A SECOND MESSENGER PROTEIN

As mentioned above, some of the anti-inflammatory actions of the glucocorticoids may depend upon their inhibition of cytokine synthesis, with consequent effects depending upon this. A distinct 'second messenger' protein has been proposed to mediate the acute inhibition of prostaglandin, leukotriene and PAF synthesis by glucocorticoids, where corticosteroid action appears to result following inhibition of phospholipase A_2 activity. Corticosteroids do not directly inhibit phospholipase A_2, but their inhibitory action requires mRNA and protein synthesis. They induce synthesis and release of a protein which in turn inhibits phospholipase A_2 activity. This protein has been named 'lipocortin'.

Lipocortin is a member of a family of glucocorticoid-inducible proteins with phospholipase A_2 inhibitory activity originally purified from a variety of biological sources. One member of the family, lipocortin 1, has been produced using recombinant technology, and work has begun to characterize its biological activities.

The lipocortin family

Lipocortin 1 appears to be a member of a group of structurally related proteins whose exact function remain to be clarified. The lipocortin family (to date) is listed in Table 7.1. Some of the proteins classified here as lipocortin have been isolated and purified in contexts other than as potentially

Table 7.1 Members of the lipocortin family

Name	*MW (kD)*	*Other names*
Lipocortin 1	38	calpactin II p35 chromobindin 9
Lipocortin 2	38	calpactin I heavy chain p36 chromobindin 8 protein I
Lipocortins 3 & 4	35	chromobindin 4 endonexin 35 kD – calelectrin protein II
Lipocortin 5	35	renocortin chromobindin 5 endonexin II anticoagulant protein (PAP)
Lipocortin 6	68	p68 chromobindin – 20 protein III 67 kD – calcimedin 67 kD – calelectrin

Data taken from Pepinsky *et al.*[11]

anti-inflammatory proteins, and some of their alternative names are also listed. As yet, the complete sequences of all of the proteins have not been published, but it is clear that they have substantial structural similarities, and high sequence homologies.

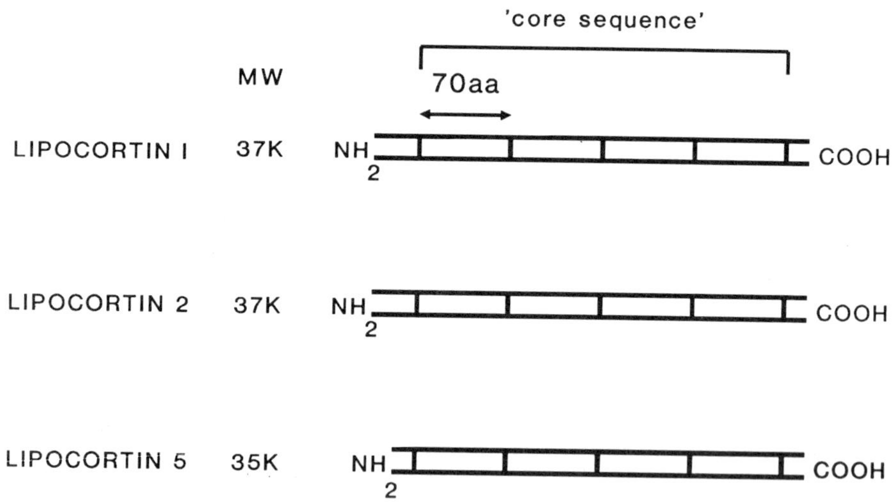

Figure 7.1 Lipocortin structure.

A common feature of all the proteins is a 'core sequence' represented diagrammatically in Figure 7.1. This 'core sequence', which makes up the bulk of the protein, contains four repeating segments which have a high degree of homology with each other, and each begin with a 17-amino acid 'consensus sequence' which is a characteristic of a group of Ca^{2+}-binding proteins. This core region appears to be responsible for the ability of the lipocortins to bind Ca^{2+} and negatively charged phospholipids. The proteins so far sequenced (lipocortins 1, 2, 4, 5) all have unique N-termini, ranging from just a few amino acid residues in the case of lipocortin 5 to 30 or so in the case of lipocortin 1. It is this N-terminus which appears to confer different biological activities upon each protein. For example lipocortin 2 (also known as calpactin 1 heavy chain) interacts with a smaller 10 kD protein (calpactin 1 light chain) via this N-terminus, and the resulting complex can then bind actin. However, the study of the molecular properties and functions of all these proteins is still in its infancy.

The discovery of lipocortin

It was discovered during the 1970s, by a group working with John Vane at the Wellcome Research Foundation, that the actions of non-steroidal anti-inflammatory drugs such as aspirin depend upon their inhibition of the enzyme cyclooxygenase and hence inhibition of prostaglandin synthesis. As mentioned above, glucocorticoids, although they have no direct action upon cyclooxygenase, were found also to inhibit prostaglandin, leukotriene and platelet activating factor synthesis in intact tissues. Their action depends on inhbition of the release of the substrates for eicosanoid or PAF generation, a step catalysed by the membrane-bound enzyme phospholipase A_2; moreover, their effect required a time lag, and mRNA and protein synthesis. It was proposed that their action might depend upon the synthesis of a 'second messenger' protein which then inhibited phospholipase A_2. The Wellcome group showed with elegant experiments illustrated in Figure 7.2 that if the guinea pig lung was perfused with a corticosteroid, then the effluent contained a protein which could inhibit generation of eicosanoids in a second perfused lung. While inhibition of eicosanoid generation by the first lung required a lag phase and could be inhibited by actinomycin D or cycloheximide, the protein from the perfusate from steroid-treated lungs had an immediate effect, and inhibitors of protein or RNA synthesis did not affect its action. The Wellcome group collaborated with a group working at Naples University, and discovered that a protein with the same effects and essentially similar properties could be obtained from the peritoneal lavage fluid of corticosteroid-treated rats. They named the protein 'macrocortin' in order to describe both its size (15 kD) and its probable source (the macrophage) as well as its corticosteroid-like effects.

Around the same time, proteins with similar properties were isolated from corticosteroid-treated rabbit neutrophils ('lipomodulin') and rat renomedullary cells ('renocortin') by groups working respectively with Hirata at the NIH and with Russo-Marie at the Pasteur Institute, Paris. It was soon discovered

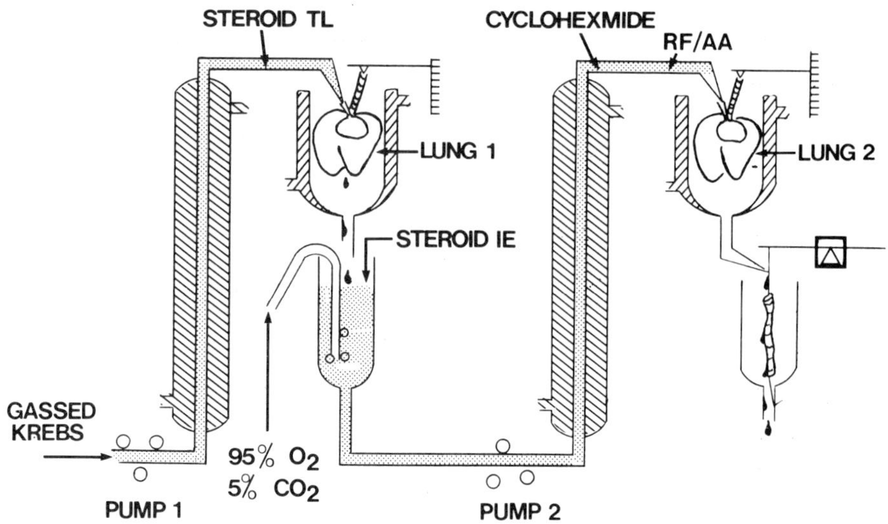

Figure 7.2 Serial perfusion experiments. In this experiment two guinea pig isolated lungs were perfused in series. The effluent from the first lung was reoxygenated and pumped into the second lung. Eicosanoids released by this lung in response to releasing factors or arachidonic acid were measured by bioassay using a rabbit aortic strip to detect thromboxane A_2. The second lung received a constant infusion of cycloheximide to render it insensitive to the direct actions of glucocorticoids infused either through the pulmonary circulation of the first lung (TL) or into the effluent draining the tissue (IE). If dexamethasone given TL induced a soluble inhibitor of phospholipase A_2 activity, then it should pass from the first ('generator') lung to the second ('target') lung and there inhibit eicosanoid release in response to phospholipase A_2-dependent releasing factors but not to arachidonic acid. Dexamethasone given IE does not affect eicosanoid generation by the second lung because of the presence of cycloheximide.

that these proteins, despite their different molecular weights, were similar to the extent that antibodies which recognized one protein would recognize the others. Table 7.2 describes various properties of these proteins. The proteins were renamed collectively 'lipocortins'. 'Macrocortin' from rat peritoneal lavage fluid was found to comprise at least four similar proteins. One of these was purified using gel, ion exchange and affinity (phospholipase A_2) chromatography and a single protein of molecular weight approx 38 kD isolated. A group working at Biogen, USA, used this material to develop oligonucleotide probes, and these in turn were used to search for the human gene. A single gene was found which gave rise to a unique 37 kD protein which has been expressed in *E. coli*[3]. It can be phosphorylated by several different kinases, as described later (for further information, see Flower[4]). The molecule is now referred to as lipocortin 1, and is by definition analogous to the peptide I fraction of crude 'macrocortin'. However, as it was apparent that 'macrocortin' itself was possibly a mixture of several closely related proteins, it has yet to be shown definitively whether lipocortin 1 is identical to lipomodulin or renocortin. Renocortin has been tentatively identified as lipocortin 5 (see Table 7.1).

Table 7.2 Properties of purified lipocortins

Name	*MW (kD)*	*Source*	*Properties*
Macrocortin	40 and 15	rat peritoneal lavage fluid guinea-pig perfused lung	PLA_2 inhibition inhibition of eiocosanoid and PAF generation anti-inflammatory
Lipomodulin	40	rabbit neutrophils	PLA_2 inhibition inhibition of chemotaxis inhibition of antibody production
Renocortin	30 and 15	rat mesangial cells	PLA_2 inhibition inhibition of eiocosanoid generation

Biological actions of lipocortin(s)

This section will outline what is known concerning the biological activities of lipocortins, both the proteins purified from animal sources and the recombinant material lipocortin 1 (r-LC1). Work is still underway to discover whether all the activities possessed by 'macrocortin', 'lipomodulin' and 'renocortin' are represented by r-LC1. The 'biological' names (macrocortin, lipomodulin, etc.) will be used to refer to the purified natural proteins; so far only r-LC1 is available in recombinant form. In addition this section will attempt to link the relevance of the biological actions of lipocortin to the anti-inflammatory effects of corticosteroids.

Steroid induction of lipocortin

The proteins macrocortin, lipomodulin and renocortin were all initially purified from glucocorticoid-treated cells, and according to the 1984 statement[5], lipocortins are by definition steroid-inducible proteins. It was soon discovered that macrocortin levels appeared to be tonically controlled by steroids: steroid injection caused macrocortin synthesis in control animals, and in addition adrenalectomized animals possessed little detectable macrocortin. Since adrenalectomized animals show greatly enhanced inflammatory responses associated with enhanced levels of eicosanoid synthesis, which can be normalized by corticosteroid injection, it was proposed that at least part of this was due to absence of 'tonic' levels of macrocortin. Hence macrocortin, as well as being of importance during inflammation, actually has a tonic role related to normal corticosteroid levels. Changes in macrocortin levels could also be detected *in vitro* (of course lipomodulin and renocortin were collected from cells treated with steroids in culture). Rat peritoneal macrophages release macrocortin following a time lag when treated with corticosteroids *in vitro*. Interestingly, it was found that, following the initial release of macrocortin (associated with reduced eicosanoid generation by the cells), the cells showed a period of 'steroid resistance' which was associated with low macrocortin levels. It is possible that GCs have one action to quickly release macrocortin but then have a secondary effect when macrocortin is resynthesized by a slower process. These findings have yet to be confirmed using probes against recombinant LC1. The Wellcome group also made the very interesting observation that the actions of steroids to inhibit eicosanoid generation could be prevented by a neutralizing antibody against macrocortin. This suggested very strongly that macrocortin acted from the exterior of the cells, and could therefore act upon the cell which produced the material as well as upon other cells, confirming the action of a large molecular weight protein to act extracellularly. A phospholipase A_2 is believed to be located on the plasma membrane of cells, and presumably is accessible to extracellular lipocortin.

When the gene for lipocortin 1 was identified it was found to be steroid-sensitive, in that sites associated with steroid receptor binding were detected. Steroid treatment of the U937 cell line was also reported to cause a modest rise in lipocortin 1 mRNA. However, only recently has the protein itself been shown unequivocally to be induced following steroid treatment. Increase in immunodetectable LC1 has been shown in the rat and in the human. Steroid treatment *in vivo* causes an increase in levels of LC1 in resident peritoneal macrophages of the rat as detected by SDS-PAGE and Western blotting. Dexamethasone and hydrocortisone are both effective, and moreover pretreatment of the animal with the steroid receptor antagonist RU 486 prevents steroid induction. Using antibodies raised against highly purified lipocortins 2 and 5, it has been shown that lipocortin 2 is steroid-inducible under the same conditions but, interestingly, that lipocortin is not. Lipocortin 1 synthesis has also been shown in the human circulating monocyte following hydrocortisone injection using an ELISA technique. An increase in serum LC was not detected[14]. Other groups, however, have failed to detect increases in lipocortin 1 levels in other cell types, for example the endothelial cells, despite observing a decrease in eicosanoid generation following steroid treatment. These differences have yet to be reconciled, although the finding in Swiss 3T3 cells that only in the presence of fetal calf serum would the cells respond to GCs (and show lipocortin 1 induction) may suggest some co-factor essential for steroid induction of lipocortin(s).

However, the increase in lipocortins following steroid injection, and the absence of lipocortin in adrenalectomized animals, suggests that lipocortins may have an important role to play in the control of inflammation, which is associated with an increase in circulating GC levels.

PHOSPHOLIPASE A_2

Lipocortins were defined as a group of proteins which possess the ability to inhibit phospholipase A_2 activity, and were originally discovered as the second messenger protein for steroids responsible for this action. Before continuing, however, it is necessary to briefly outline the nature of phospholipases A_2, and to explain the potential importance of these enzymes in inflammation. For a more in-depth survey of this huge topic the reader is referred to excellent reviews by Van den Bosch[7] and Vadas and Pruzanski[8].

Phospholipases A_2 (PLA_2) are defined as such on the basis of their ability to cleave the acyl linkage between the glyceryl backbone and the 2′ position fatty acid of a phospholipid. They are a diverse group of enzymes, with different pH optima, different Ca^{2+} requirements, different preferred substrates and so on. The enzymes which have been most studied have been the soluble and readily obtainable forms found typically in pancreatic secretions or in the venom of the bee or various snakes. These enzymes typically have a molecular weight of 13–14 kD, an alkaline optimum of pH 8–9 and require the presence of Ca^{2+} for activity. The activity of these enzymes is critically dependent upon the physical state of their phospholipid substrate which (as a broad generalization) must be in at least a partially disrupted state to allow the soluble enzyme first to bind at the water–lipid interface and then to lyse the substrate.

These enzymes have been classified into two broad groups based upon distinct characteristics in their primary structure, apparently leading to differences in their mechanism of interaction with the substrate. Group I is typified by soluble pancreatic PLA_2, and much is known concerning these enzymes. Group II PLA_2s are those of the crotalid or vipera venom type, but secretory PLA_2s from inflammatory cells which have recently been isolated and purified appear also to be of this type.

It is only very recently that information concerning the structure of mammalian phospholipases A_2 has been obtained and, to date, examples have been found which seem to fall into both groups of PLA_2. The important difference between PLA_2s involved, for example, in generation of eicosanoids and enzymes from venoms of pancreatic juices is that in this former case the PLA_2 is known to be membrane-bound, and hence in effect actually embedded within its substrate. Although this PLA_2 is known to require Ca^{2+} for activation, it is not known how, or indeed if, the physical state of its substrate is important for its activity. PLA_2s are secreted from inflammatory cells such as neutrophils, and identical enzymes have been isolated from inflammatory exudate. Thus PLA_2s present in cell membrane may be important for eicosanoid and PAF generation, whereas enzymes released from cells may be important in causing damage to other cells.

Inhibition of phospholipase A_2 by lipocortin

Lipocortins are, by definition, inhibitors of phospholipase A_2. Since they can be purified using PLA_2 affinity columns it was assumed that their activity in assays such as hydrolysis of phosphatidyl choline vesicles or autoclaved *E. coli* lipids was due to an interaction with the enzyme. This type of assay was used to show that rabbit neutrophil-derived lipomodulin could inhibit phospholipases A_2 from porcine pancreas, bee and snake (*Naja*) venoms. Lipomodulin could also inhibit phospholipases C from bacterial sources, and phospholipase D from cabbage, but was much less effective. Equilibrium dialysis showed that lipomodulin binds Ca^{2+}, a possible explanation for its enzyme inhibitory action. Kinetic studies showed that lipomodulin reduced that V_{max} of the reaction, but did not affect the K_m for the substrate. It was suggested that a stoichiometric enzyme–lipomodulin complex is formed.

This conclusion has been questioned since publication of the structure of the lipocortins; see Davidson and Dennis[9] for some of the arguments.

The ability of the highly purified or recombinant lipocortin to inhibit phospholipase A_2 was tested by several groups including the authors: Peers *et al.*[10], using a novel assay procedure, demonstrated that the recombinant lipocortin 1 molecule seemed to block the interaction of phospholipase A_2 with its substrate. Other groups examined further the mechanism of inhibition, concluding that the action of the protein was, in the case of the well-known *E. coli* assay, to inhibit phospholipase activity by a mechanism involving binding of the inhibitor to lipids on the *E. coli* membrane. An effect of substrate binding was also held to be accountable for the ability of the protein to inhibit hydrolysis in the micelle assay in which *E. coli* lipids were used as a substrate. The term 'substrate depletion' was coined to identify this type of inhibitory activity. Different assays using a variety of substrates appear to yield different results, and it is clear that the question of 'substrate depletion' requires address.

Whilst the balance of evidence at the moment suggests that the inhibition of phospholipase A_2 by lipocortin in cell-free enzyme assays occurs by some type of interaction with the substrate it should not be construed as being 'non-specific'. For example, Pepinsky *et al.*[11] quote data in which inhibition by lipocortin of the pancreatic PLA_2-catalyzed hydrolysis of deoxycholate–phosphatidylcholine mixed vesicles can occur at 1000–10 000-fold molar excess of lipid over lipcortin, and that in the same system the human platelet enzyme was completely unaffected.

In summary, there is evidence to suggest that lipocortins bind weakly to (at least) one PLA_2; that they bind strongly to some but not all phospholipid substrates and also that they bind calcium. It is clear that these proteins have the ability to complex or interact with all the components of the *in vitro* assay system, explaining why the results are so difficult to interpret. Nevertheless, despite the many vicissitudes of this type of assay, it has proved an immensely useful technique for following lipocortins through purification protocols and for screening samples for the protein, and is still widely used for this purpose by many investigators.

Inhibition of mediator production *in vitro*

The search for the lipocortins began with the discovery that corticosteroids could inhibit prostaglandin release from cells. Lipocortins – both purified macrocortin and recombinant lipocortin 1 – mimic this action of steroids, although of course without a lag phase, and without being affected by inhibitors of protein or RNA synthesis. Macrocortin was first identified due to its ability to inhibit generation of 'rabbit aorta contracting substance'

(TXA_2) by the perfused guinea pig lung, as illustrated in Figure 7.2. Recombinant lipocortin 1 has been shown to have the same activity, inhibiting release of TXA_2 (as measured by bioassay) from the perfused guinea pig lung in response to histamine and LTC_4 but not arachidonic acid[12]. Interestingly r-LC mimicked the action of steroids completely, in that TXA_2 release in response to bradykinin was not affected. It is possible that bradykinin-induced eicosanoid release from the lung may involve a PLA_2-independent pathway. Lipocortin 1 and the purified proteins inhibit release of other eicosanoids (e.g. PGI_2, PGE_2) and, as expected from an inhibitor of PLA_2 activity, leukotriene and platelet-activating factor (PAF) release in response to various stimuli. It seems likely that this action of lipocortin occurs from the outside of the cell membrane. In the guinea pig perfused lung system, for example, inhibition of eicosanoid generation occurs very rapidly following infusion of lipocortin, and it seems unlikely that a large molecular weight protein could gain access to the cell interior so quickly. In addition, it was found that the neutralizing antibody Rm23 raised against 'macrocortin' could inhibit the action not only of purified macrocortin but also of hydrocortisone[13], suggesting that endogenous macrocortin is released from cells. Another antibody raised against lipomodulin has been shown to stain proteins on the surface of mouse thymocytes. More recently, the presence of saturable binding sites on the surface of circulating leukocytes (monocytes, neutrophils and thymocytes) has been shown using FACS (fluorescence activated cell sorter) analysis[6]. This finding has yet to be extended to discover the nature of these sites.

Anti-inflammatory activity *in vivo*

If the inhibition of eicosanoid generation explains part of the anti-inflammatory activity of corticosteroids, then clearly the lipocortins should possess some anti-inflammatory activity *in vivo*. The purified proteins were tested on models such as carrageenan-induced rat paw oedema or pleurisy, and shown to be effective. In this model a suspension of carrageenan is injected into the paw or pleural cavity of the rat, and either paw volume measured plethysmographically, or after a certain interval the animal is killed and the pleural cavity washed. The volume of exudate is calculated, and the number of infiltrating leukocytes (predominantly neutrophils after 4–6 h) counted. These models are sensitive to corticosteroid or indomethacin treatment, suggesting that prostaglandin synthesis is important for the inflammatory response. Recombinant lipocortin 1 mimics the steroids in that co-injection of lipocortin 1 with carrageenan inhibits the development of paw oedema[25]. The effect is dose-dependent, but reaches a maximum at about 70% inhibition of the oedema. The authors conducted a series of experiments to discover whether lipocortin exerted its effects through actions on kinin generation inhibition, mast cell amine release or effects on neutrophils, but concluded that the most likely mechanism of action of lipocortin injected locally was through inhibition of eicosanoid generation, since co-treatment with the dual cyclooxygenase/lipoxygenase inhibitor BW755c masked inhibitory activity of lipocortin.

Systemically administered lipocortin from mouse thymus or lungs, identical to a lipocortin from human mononuclear cells, has been shown to inhibit neutrophil infiltration into polyacrylamide gel injected subcutaneously in the mouse[15]. This was associated with reduced production of PGE_2 and LTB_4 at the inflammatory sites. The authors suggested that lipocortin may inhibit neutrophil activation *in vivo*, since *in vitro* chemotaxis of neutrophils was inhibited by lipocortin, confirming previous findings with lipomodulin.

There are, however, models of inflammation in which lipocortin does not mimic steroid effects. It was discovered that macrocortin did not inhibit pleurisy caused by dextran administration, and recombinant lipocortin 1 also lacks this activity. This model is dependent upon degranulation of mast cells, and a second 'steroid second messenger' was proposed to mediate this action of steroids. This mediator was named 'vasocortin', and we will return to this later. Recombinant lipocortin does not inhibit paw oedema induced by mediators such as PAF, bradykinin or 5-HT, although corticosteroids are effective, and it is possible in these cases that vasocortin or a different mechanism of action is involved.

Clearly, more studies are required, testing the anti-inflammatory actions of the other lipocortins and vasocortin in order to assign 'second messenger' status for the various acute anti-inflammatory actions of steroids. Lipocortins have yet to be tested in more chronic models of inflammation, although recently it has been observed that rats with the model experimental allergic encephalomyelitis ('EAE') of the disease multiple sclerosis show increased levels of lipocortin 1[16].

Another potential anti-inflammatory effect of lipocortins is their ability to inhibit active oxygen metabolite production by leukocytes. Leukocytes such as neutrophils, monocytes, macrophages and eosinophils are able to produce a range of active oxygen species such as superoxide ion or the hydroxyl radical which are involved in killing of ingested microorganisms, but have also been implicated in cell damage at sites of inflammation. Neutrophils from patients with chronic granulomatous disease show normal phagocytosis of bacteria, but are unable to kill them – neutrophils lack the ability to produce active oxygen metabolites. Corticosteroid treatment is also associated with reduced oxygen metabolite production, and this may at least in part explain the increased susceptibility to infection seen with steroid therapy. It has been found that recombinant lipocortin and lipocortin from mouse monocytes can inhibit oxygen metabolite production from human neutrophils and mouse bronchial macrophages respectively[17,18]. Interestingly, both groups found that lipocortin inhibited oxygen metabolite production to certain stimuli only, suggesting that only some of the pathways of activation involve phospholipase A_2.

AUTOANTIBODIES TO LIPOCORTIN ASSOCIATED WITH CHRONIC INFLAMMATORY DISEASE

In some diseases, for example myasthenia gravis or insulin-dependent diabetes, autoantibodies for cell surface molecules are believed to be related to the pathogenesis of the disease. In 1981, Hirata's group[26] reported that sera from patients with the chronic inflammatory diseases rheumatoid arthritis and systemic lupus erythematosus contained IgM antibodies which inhibited the activity of lipomodulin, and which could precipitate the radiolabelled protein. They observed that sera from patients with active SLE contained higher titres than that from patients with inactive disease, and also found that a strain of mice which spontaneously develop SLE-like illnesses also had anti-lipomodulin antibodies.

These findings have been confirmed and extended using recombinant lipocortin 1 as antigen in an ELISA method[20]. The group have shown that in rheumatoid arthritis (RA), the antibody titre is highest in patients who are classed clinically as 'steroid-resistant', i.e. who require high dose maintenance therapy with steroids, whereas in SLE, high antibody titre is associated with active disease. Both IgM and IgG levels are raised, although the former is more striking. Patients with polymyalgia rheumatica (PMR), even those receiving high-dose steroid treatment, did not show elevated antibody titres, suggesting that the nature of the autoimmune disorder is important in the generation of autoantibodies.

The authors suggest that, in the case of RA, steroid therapy might be important in the generation of the antibodies, and speculate that chronic oral steroids and hence repetitive antigen (lipocortin) challenge in the gut may predispose to autoantibody generation. In SLE, however, high titres were found to be independent of steroid therapy but associated with active inflammatory disease. They suggest that the antibodies may actually play a role in the disease in this case. Clearly the involvement of lipocortin autoantibody formation in inflammatory diseases requires further study, especially since corticosteroids are widely used in the treatment of these diseases.

PHOSPHORYLATION OF LIPOCORTIN

An important discovery in the story of lipocortin was the finding that lipomodulin (purified from rabbit neutrophils) could be phosphorylated by cAMP-dependent kinase (protein kinase A) and that this phosphorylation decreased its inhibitory activity on phospholipase A_2[19]. This might allow a finer control mechanism for PLA_2 activity other than lipocortin synthesis – namely phosphorylation–dephosphorylation associated with a change in its activity. Hirata also showed that, in rabbit neutrophil, chemoattractant peptides increased phosphorylation of lipomodulin when the cells were incubated with ^{32}P. A similar finding was made with mouse thymocytes stimulated with concanavalin Z, Ca^{2+} ionophore or phorbol 12-myristoyl-13-acetate. In the latter case Hirata suggested that protein kinase C might be responsible for the phosphorylation.

Upon publication of the sequence of lipocortin 1 it was quickly realized that lipocortin 1 is identical to that protein which was phosphorylated by the epidermal growth factor (EGF) receptor/kinase in A431 cells. Lipocortin 1 is phosphorylated by this kinase near its N-terminus, at Tyr-21. The same residue can be phosphorylated by several $pp60^{v-src}$ oncogene products. In addition, protein kinase C phosphorylates lipocortin 1 near its N-terminus at ser-27 and Thr-41. cAMP-dependent kinase phosphorylates lipocortin 1 at it C-terminus, at Thr-216. The significance of these multiple phosphorylations is unclear, although it has been reported that tyrosine phosphorylation reduces the Ca^{2+} requirement for association of lipocortin with membrane vesicles. This would not, however, explain the reported diminution of anti-phospholipase A_2 activity by phosphorylation.

Lipocortin 2 is also phosphorylated near its N-terminus at Tyr-23 by $pp60^{v-src}$, although little sequence similarity exists between lipocortin 1 and 2 in this region. The N-terminus of lipocortin 2 is important for its association with p10, and its phosphorylation, as well as its affinity for Ca^{2+}, may be influenced by the interaction with p10[21].

OTHER ANTI-INFLAMMATORY STEROID 'SECOND MESSENGERS'

Vasocortin

As described above, lipocortin does not mediate all the anti-inflammatory actions of corticosteroids. Another steroid-inducible protein has been described, and named 'Vasocortin'[22]. This protein is distinct from the lipocortins – it has a molecular weight of approximately 100 kD, and different physical properties. It is released into the peritoneal cavity of rats following corticosteroid treatment, or by aortic rings following incubation with dexamethasone *in vitro*. Vasocortin mimics steroids in that it is effective against dextran-induced oedema development, a model in which lipocortin is without effect. Vasocortin inhibits mast cell degranulation in response to dextran or concanavalin A, but not in response to compound 48/80 or calcium ionophore $A_2$3187, and this may explain part of its anti-inflammatory action.

The structure of vasocortin has yet to be described.

Uteroglobin and antiflammins

Uteroglobin is a small (16 kD) protein originally identified as being secreted from rabbit uterus in response to progesterone during early pregnancy. It has since been shown that in other tissues (rabbit trachea and bronchus) it may be induced by corticosteroids. The structure of uteroglobin is known, and it has been shown to consist of two identical subunits of 70 amino acids each, which show strong similarity to the third repeat of lipocortin 1. Uteroglobin inhibits phospholipase A_2 activity in a macrophage line, and also inhibits rabbit neutrophil and monocyte chemotaxis. It is interesting to speculate upon the physiological function of this protein. For further information, see Miele *et al.*[23]

The similarity between uteroglobin and lipocortin has been exploited to produce short peptides corresponding to the highest regions of similarity[24]. These peptides, the 'antiflammins', dose-dependently inhibit phospholipase A_2, and have been reported to inhibit carrageenan paw oedema in the rat. We await further reports of their activity.

SUMMARY

In this chapter we have attempted to review the 'history' of lipocortins, and to describe some of the areas of research which are of interest in the field of inflammation. The area has become an extraordinarily complex one, with many conflicting claims in the literature. However, there are enough interesting discoveries in the work already published to encourage further research into this family of membrane-associated regulatory molecues. Future research will no doubt clarify points which at present remain uncertain.

References

1. Beato, M. (1989). Gene regulation by steroid hormones. *Cell*, **56**, 335–44
2. Rousseau, G. G. (1984). Control of gene expression by glucocorticoid hormones. *Biochem. J.*, **224**, 1–12
3. Wallner, B. P., Mattaliano, R. J., Hession, C. *et al.* (1986). Cloning and expression of human lipocortin, a phospholipase A_2 inhibitor with potential anti-inflammatory activity. *Nature*, **320**, 77–81
4. Flower, R. J. (1988). Lipocortin and the mechanism of action of the glucocorticoids. *Br. J. Pharmacol.*, **94**, 987–1015
5. Di Rosa, M., Flower, R. J., Hirata, F. *et al.* (1984). Nomenclature announcement: Anti-phospholipase proteins. *Prostaglandins*, **28**, 441–2
6. Goulding, N. J., Iuying, P. and Guyre, P. M. (1990). Characteristics of lipocortin 1 binding to the surface of human peripheral blood leukocytes. *Biochem. Soc. Trans.*, **18**, 1237–8
7. Van den Bosch, H. (1980). Intracellular phospholipases A. *Biochim. Biophys. Acta*, **604**, 191–246
8. Vadas, P. and Pruzanski, W. (1984). Role of extracellular phospholipase A_2 in inflammation. In Otterness, I. *et al.* (eds), *Advances in Inflammation Research*, vol. 17, pp. 51–9 (New York: Raven Press)
9. Davidson, F. F. and Dennis, E. A. (1989). Biological relevance of lipocortins and related proteins as inhibitors of phospholipase A_2. *Biochem. Pharmacol.*, **38**, 3645–51
10. Peers, S. H., Taylor, R. D. and Flower, R. J. (1987). A novel binding assay for phospholipase A_2. *Biochem. Pharmacol.*, **36**, 4287–91
11. Pepinsky, R. B., Sinclair, L. K., Chow, E. P. and O'Brine-Greco, B. (1989). A dimeric form of lipocortin 1 in human placenta. *Biochem. J.*, **263**, 97–103
12. Cirino, G., Flower, R. J., Browning, J. L. *et al.* (1987). Recombinant human lipocortin 1 inhibits thromboxane release from guinea pig isolated perfused lung. *Nature*, **328**, 270–2
13. Flower, R. J., Wood, J. N. and Parente, L. (1984). Macrocortin and the mechanism of action of the glucocorticoids. In Otterness, I. *et al.* (eds), Advances in Inflammation Research, vol. 7, pp. 61–70 (New York: Raven Press)
14. Goulding, N. J., Godolphin, J. L., Sampson, M. B. *et al.* (1990). Hydrocortisone induces lipocortin 1 production by peripheral blood mononuclear cells *in vivo* in man. *Lancet*, **335**, 1416–18
15. Errasfa, M. and Russo-Marie, F. (1989). A purified lipocortin shares the anti-inflammatory effect of glucocorticosteroids *in vivo* in mice. *Br. J. Pharmacol.*, **97**, 1051–8
16. Bolton, C. T., Elderfield, A. J. and Flower, R. J. (1990). The detection of lipocortins 1, 2 and 5 in central nervous system tissues from Lewis rats with acute EAE. *J. Neuroimmunol.* (In press)
17. Stevens, T. R. J., Drasdo, A. L., Peers, S. H. *et al.* (1988). Stimulus-specific inhibition of human neutrophil H202 production by human recombinant lipocortin 1. *Br. J. Pharmacol.*, **93**, 139P
18. Maridonneau-Parini, I., Errasfa, M. and Russo-Marie, F. (1989). Inhibition of O_2-generation by dexamethasone is mimicked by lipocortin 1 in alveolar macrophages. *J. Clin. Invest.*, **83**, 1936–40
19. Hirata, F. (1981). The regulation of lipomodulin, a phospholipase inhibitory protein, in rabbit neutrophils by phosphorylation. *J. Biol. Chem.*, **256**, 7730–3

20. Goulding, N. J., Podgorski, M. R., Hall, N. D. *et al.* (1989). Autoantibodies to recombinant lipocortin 1 in rheumatoid arthritis and systemic lupus erythematosis. *Ann. Rheum. Dis.*, **48**, 843–50
21. Davidson, F. F., Dennis, E. A., Powell, M. and Glenney, J. R. (1987). Inhibition of phospholipase A_2 by 'lipocortins' and calpactins. *J. Biol. Chem.*, **262**, 1698–705
22. Carnuccio, R., Di Rosa, M., Guerrassio, B. *et al.* (1987). Vasocortin: a novel glucocorticoid-induced anti-inflammatory protein. *Br. J. Pharmacol.*, **90**, 443–5
23. Miele, L., Cordella-Miele, E. and Mulcherjee, A. B. (1987). Uteroglobin: structure, molecular biology and new perspectives on its function as a phospholipase A_2 inhibitor. *Endocrine Rev.*, **8**, 474–90
24. Miele, L., Cordella-Miele, E., Facchiano, A. and Mulcherjee, A. B. (1988). Novel anti-inflammatory peptides from the region of highest similarity between uteroglobin and lipocortin 1. *Nature*, **335**, 726–30
25. Cirino, G., Peers, S. H., Flower, R. J., Browning, J. L. and Pepinsky, R. B. (1989). Human recombinant lipocortin 1 has acute local anti-inflammatory properties in the rat paw oedema test. *Proc. Natl. Acad. Sci. USA*, **86**, 3428–32
26. Hirata, F., Del Carmine, R., Nelson, C. A., Axelrod, J., Schiffmann, E., Warabi, A., De Blas, A. L., Nirenberg, M., Manganiello, V., Vaughan, M., Kumagi, S., Green, I., Decker, J. L. and Steinberg, A. D. (1981). *Proc. Natl. Acad. Sci. USA*, **78**, 3190–4

8
Platelet activating factor and cytokine feedback regulation of endothelial integrity; implications for the treatment of inflammatory disease

D. HOSFORD, M. PAUBERT-BRAQUET and P. BRAQUET

INTRODUCTION

The inflammatory process is an essential response of the body to injury. Viewed very simply, inflammation confines tissue damage and assists in repair, while immune functions prevent invasion by foreign organisms. These two processes are closely linked as many of the same cells and molecules are operative in both. In a normal controlled response following injury, polymorphonuclear leukocytes (PMNL) leave the flowing blood and adhere to the endothelial cells lining the blood vessels. The endothelial cells undergo structural modification and PMNL infiltrate into the damaged tissue to destroy microbes that may be present in the wound. The PMNL are soon joined by macrophages and, concomitantly with the infiltration processes, thromboformation occurs to limit the insult and the inflammatory reaction. Lymphocyte activation occurs, controlling infection, and eventually connective tissue cells begin to effect repair mechanisms. Usually this response is strictly regulated; however, if the process becomes uncontrolled this normally beneficial local event may escalate into a wider malignant activity, characterized by endothelial injury, excessive cell infiltration and vascular leakage. Such a phenomenon may underlie the microcirculatory damage observed in pathologies such as shock, sepsis, asthma, ischaemia and graft rejection[1].

It is clear even from this extremely brief synopsis of the inflammatory process that the crucial physiological event involved is an interaction or 'cross-talk' between circulating cells and endothelial cells. Indeed, endothelial integrity is the key determinant of the degree of cellular traffic from the blood stream to the surrounding tissues, and thus of the extent and severity of the inflammatory response. We feel that the importance of this process cannot be overemphasized as it constitutes the fundamental event which unifies a diverse range of immuno-inflammatory diseases, even though the cause and evolution of the various pathologies up to this point may be different. It also gives a focal point for the development of potential therapeutic agents for the treatment of inflammatory diseases such as those mentioned above. As we will discuss in this review, numerous drugs effective in the treatment of immuno-inflammatory conditions may basically act as stabilizers of endothelial integrity, although the actual mechanisms of action that lead to this end-result are diverse.

Obviously, in order to develop drugs effective in counteracting inflammation it is essential to have an understanding of the vectors which regulate endothelial/blood cell cross-talk and immuno-inflammatory responses. Indeed, these processes are coordinated by a vast array of mediators. Generally these may be divided into two broad groups. Substances such as serotonin, histamine, kinins, leukotrienes, prostaglandins, thromboxane, neuropeptides, proteases, complement and other various chemotactic factors appear to be primarily involved in the early events of acute allergic and inflammatory reactions. A second group of mediators, which may also include some of the former but more importantly cytokines such as growth factors, tumour necrosis factor (TNF) and the interleukins, which are essential vectors in the cellular communication system, may be involved in long-term tissue alterations in inflammatory diseases. Platelet-activating factor (PAF) appears to be a member of both these groups, and in this review we will focus our attention on its relationship with the latter group of substances.

PAF is a potent autacoid mediator implicated in a diverse range of human pathologies including asthma, shock, cardiac and systemic anaphylaxis, myocardial and cerebral ischaemia, immune and renal disorders and a variety of inflammatory conditions[1,2]. Originally isolated from antigen-stimulated rabbit basophils and characterized structurally as 1-*O*-alkyl-2(*R*)-acetyl-glycero-3-phosphocholine, the alkyl phospholipid is now known to be produced by, and act on, a variety of cell types including neutrophils (PMN), eosinophils, monocytes, macrophages, platelets and endothelial cells[1,2]. Pertinent to this review is the marked effect of PAF on the microcirculation, where the mediator induces an intensive leakage of plasma. This appears to result from both a direct PAF effect on the vessel wall and, by destabiliation of the endothelium by the generation and release of leukotrienes, thromboxane, free radicals and other toxic products, from various blood cells stimulated by the agonist[1,3].

Studies on the pathophysiological role of PAF have been facilitated by a variety of compounds which can specifically inhibit the binding of PAF to its receptors in various cells and tissues[4,5]. PAF antagonists can be broadly divided into two groups. Synthetic inhibitors include SRI 63-441, SRI 63-119, CV-3988 and BN 52111, which are related to the PAF framework and compounds such as the triazolothienodiazepine, WEB 2086, which are unrelated to the PAF structure. Many natural compounds and their synthetic derivatives are also potent PAF antagonists[5]. This group includes the 20 carbon terpene, BN 52021, lignans such as kadsurenone and its synthetic derivative L-652,731 and gliotoxin-related compounds produced by various fungi and bacteria. Indeed, studies with PAF antagonists have suggested an interaction between PAF release from various cell types and protease activity. PAF antagonists inhibit the increase in plasma trypsin-like activity induced by administration of PAF or endotoxin[6], while protease inhibitors reduce PAF production[7].

Recently, we and other research groups have utilized PAF antagonists in an attempt to elucidate the relationship between PAF and various cytokines involved in immuno-inflammatory processes. These studies have led to a new understanding of the role of PAF in health and disease. As discussed in this review, it is becoming increasingly apparent that PAF is an important amplifier of biological processes, a role conferred on the mediator by its ability to 'prime' the responses of various cell types participating in allergic and inflammatory responses. It is also now clear that PAF occupies an important position in the cytokine network which usually safeguards the body against injury and infection, but which in some instances destroys the host it is designed to defend.

In this chapter we will consider the importance of PAF and various cytokines in the mediation of the inflammatory process. We will focus particular attention on the role of PAF and cytokines as participants in feedback networks deleterious to endothelial integrity. In addition, starting from the theoretical considerations developed by Thom[8] and Zeeman[9], we will propose a model describing the control and dysfunction of immuno-inflammatory responses based on the 'singularity' of PAF and certain cytokines as expressed by their ability to elicit their autogeneration and the consequent 'catastrophic' microvascular events which occur when there is a loss of control of the feedback system. Finally, we will consider how PAF antagonists in combination with other drugs may constitute valuable therapeutic agents in the treatment of inflammatory conditions due to their ability to decouple the deleterious feedback cycles. Such beneficial effects may account for the protective effects of PAF antagonists against bronchial hyperreactivity, shock, myocardial and cerebral ischaemia, and graft rejection.

PAF/CYTOKINE INTERACTIONS AND BLOOD CELLS

PAF and IL 1 production

Several recent studies have examined the relationship between PAF and the generation of interleukin 1 (IL 1). For example, PAF markedly altered in a dose-dependent fashion the IL 1 production by rat monocytes stimulated with lipopolysaccharide (LPS)[10]. When added at concentrations ranging from 1 fmol/L to 1 nmol/L to LPS-stimulated adherent monocytes, PAF enhanced the release of IL 1, whereas concentrations above 10 nmol/L decreased it. These alterations in IL 1 release from monocytes by PAF were noted regardless of whether either phytohaemagglutinin (PHA) or concanavalin A (Con A) was used as the mitogenic agent in the proliferation assay on thymocytes. BN 52021 (10 μmol/L) reversed the increase in LPS-induced IL

1 release evoked by 1 pmol/L PAF by 95%. In addition, the decrease in IL 1 release by 0.1 μmol/L PAF was markedly reduced in the presence of the antagonist at a concentration of 10 μmol/L, cell viability remaining unaffected.

Similar data have been obtained with guinea pig keratinocytes[11]. Although no effect of PAF on IL 1 production by guinea pig keratinocytes was observed, simultaneous addition of 1 pmol/L of the autacoid with 1 μg/ml LPS increased IL 1 production, compared to that observed with LPS alone. When 1 pmol/L PAF was added 1 h before or 1 h after LPS, no effect on IL 1 production by keratinocytes was noted. Addition of 10 fmol/L PAF to keratinocytes 1 h before stimulation with LPS induced a significant increase in IL 1 production. In contrast, when 10 fmol/L of the autacoid was added simultaneously or after LPS, no significant alteration of IL 1 production was observed.

Furthermore, Westwick and colleagues[12,13] have demonstrated that (R) PAF and a less hydrolysable synthetic racemic analogue, PR1501, can induce IL 1-like activity from LPS-stimulated and unstimulated human monocyte–macrophage cell cultures, as determined by the mouse thymocyte assay. This effect occurred in the dose range of 3 pmol/L to 30 nmol/L, with optimum production of IL 1-like activity being observed at a concentration of 30–300 pmol/L PAF. The effect of (R) PAF was stereospecific since the unnatural enantiomer (S) PAF and lyso (R) PAF in the same concentration range were inactive. PAF has also been demonstrated to increase IL 1 production by human monocytes stimulated with muramyl dipeptide (MDP), higher concentrations of PAF inducing the maximum responses[14].

Studies by Rola-Pleszczynski *et al.*[15] also indicate a positive effect of PAF on IL 1 production by human monocytes stimulated with MDP or LPS. Using platelet-free, elutriated monocytes these workers found that PAF dose-dependently augmented IL 1 production characterized by two peaks, one at high (10 nmol/L–1 μmol/L) and another at low (1–10 fmol/L) concentrations of PAF. Failure to remove platelets following isolation of monocytes by adherence resulted in varied responses to PAF, with predominant inhibition of IL 1 production at higher concentrations. BN 52021 abrogated the PAF effects, mainly in the higher concentration range. It should be noted that PAF can also synergize with interferon gamma (IFN-γ) or TNF to induce higher levels of IL 1 production by human monocytes[16]. This may be part of an amplification loop since cytokines (IL 1, TNF, IFN-γ) stimulate a biphasic synthesis of PAF by human monocytes[17].

Finally, *ex vivo* experiments using minipumps loaded with PAF or solvent alone, placed under the back skin of rats and connected to the jugular vein, have shown that monocytes from animals receiving 1, 4.5, or 9 μg PAF for 7 days exhibited increased capacity to produce IL 1[18]. In contrast, with 28 μg PAF per day for 7 days, IL 1 production by the monocytes was markedly decreased.

PAF and IL 2 production

There is also considerable evidence indicating that PAF is a potent modulator of lymphocyte proliferation and interleukin 2 (IL 2) production[19,20]. *In vitro*,

PAF has been shown to either inhibit[18,21] or stimulate[22] both these processes. In either case the effect of PAF is reversed by various antagonists of the mediator.

Pignol and colleagues[18,21] measured the production of IL 2 by peripheral blood mononuclear leukocytes (PBML) following 24 h stimulation with PHA in the presence or absence of PAF. A concentration-dependent inhibition of IL 2 production was observed with an IC_{50} of 10 pmol/L. This suppressive effect was fully reversed by BN 52021. In this system PAF needed to be present in the first hour of the 24 h culture period for the inhibition to be detected. In contrast to these data, PAF and two non-hydrolysable PAF analogues have been shown to increase the proliferation of IL 2-stimulated human lymphoblasts, whereas some antagonists (CV-3988 and L-652,-731, but not WEB 2086 and BN 52021) are inhibitory[22]. This effect of the antagonists was observed even when the drugs were added 48 h after the beginning of a 72 h culture period, suggesting interference with a late event in T cell activation. Furthermore, it is possible that endogenously produced PAF may be involved in some step(s) of IL 2-induced proliferation of T lymphoblasts. This is indicated by the inhibition of this process by the PAF synthesis inhibitor, L-648,611[22].

An important corrobation of some of the *in vitro* observations outlined above has been provided by the *in vivo* instillation of PAF into rats via subcutaneously implanted osmotic minipumps connected to the jugular vein[23]. In these experiments, using rats implanted for 7 days with minipumps containing up to 9 μg PAF, lymphocytes, withdrawn from the animals and cultured, showed increased capacity to produce IL 2 compared to those from rats receiving solvent alone. Thus although the relationship between IL 2 and PAF is poorly defined, an interaction between the two clearly exists.

PAF and TNF production

Apart from its ability to mimic the effects of endotoxic shock in a variety of species[24], TNF is known to exert several specific immunomodulatory effects. For example, it can activate macrophages for the production of IL 1, granulocyte–monocyte colony stimulating factors (GM-CSF) and prostaglandins and modulate generation of IFN-γ by lymphocytes. The exposure of PMN to both TNF-α and TNF-β stimulates the production of superoxide radicals, induces a phagocytic response and enhances antibody-dependent cell cytotoxicity[25,26].

However, while it appears that TNF possesses interesting properties *per se*, recent studies suggest that the relationship between TNF and PAF is of particular importance in mediating the inflammatory response. Recent investigations[27] have demonstrated that PAF activates peripheral blood-derived monocytes to produce and secrete TNF as assessed by a sensitive radioimmunoassay. In these studies the addition of various concentrations of PAF (1–30 μmol/l) to monocyte cultures for 24 h initially resulted in a significant enhancement of cytotoxicity. The supernatant contained TNF in concentrations that were dependent on the dose of PAF added, and reached levels equivalent to those derived from IFN-γ-stimulated monocytes. TNF was produced within 2 h following exposure of the cells to PAF, an effect that was completely inhibited by BN 52021[27].

Cytotoxic activity, as measured by the release of cytotoxic factors in the supernatant, was present initially but declined after 24 h. These results suggest that PAF induces TNF release from monocytes but that the cytotoxic activity is subsequently masked by the presence of an inhibitor or is partially denatured. Further experiments[28,29] have also demonstrated that PAF at very low doses (1 pmol/L to 10 nmol/L) significantly amplifies the IFN-γ-, IL 1-, MDP- or LPS-induced production of TNF. All these data suggest that priming of monocytes by PAF may constitute an important step in amplification of inflammatory and immune responses.

This concept is further substantiated by the fact that human monocytes stimulated with IL-1β, TNF or IFN-γ are able to produce PAF in a biphasic fashion[30]. The autacoid in the early peak (1–2 h) is largely retained intracellularly, whereas the majority of PAF in the late peak (6–8 h), is released into the culture medium. In the following section we will consider more fully the role of PAF in priming and amplification processes, and their importance in endothelial/blood cell cross-talk.

PAF and cytokine priming of blood cell responses

Effect of PAF and TNF on PMN and eosinophil function

In the preceding discussion we have considered how PAF can directly induce the production of various cytokines from different circulating cell types. In this section we will review the evidence showing that extremely low concentrations of PAF and cytokines can 'prime' certain blood cells to respond in an enhanced manner to subsequent antagonistic stimuli that would otherwise be ineffectual. Firstly it is important to briefly consider the role of two of the most important circulating cell types in inflammation and their response to the mediators released in the inflammatory microenvironment.

PMN appear to play a particularly important role in inflammation[31]. During this process PMN become activated by various agonists, adhere to the endothelial surface and release lysosomal proteases. Activated PMN also undergo a 'respiratory burst', which results in the reduction of molecular oxygen to superoxide. This latter product is rapidly converted to hydrogen peroxide and toxic free radicals which damage the endothelium[31].

PAF is a potent chemotactic agent for PMN, inducing superoxide release, aggregation and degranulation in this cell type[1]. *In vivo* the mediator evokes pulmonary sequestration of PMN, hypotension and bronchoconstriction, PAF is also one of the most active chemotactic factors for eosinophils, cells from which it elicits the release of major basic protein (MBP), free radicals and leukotriene C_4 (LTC_4), products extremely damaging to microvascular integrity[1,2].

Eosinophils are another cell type intimately involved in inflammatory processes. PAF is now recognized as an important activator of eosinophil functions. Indeed, the autacoid is one of the most potent chemotactic agents for human eosinophils[32]. This effect is receptor-mediated and BN 52021 dose-dependently inhibits eosinophil locomotion[3,32]. In experimental animals, PAF or antigen administration is associated with an extravascular recruitment of eosinophils and platelets in the airways[32,34]. For example, exposure of conscious guinea pigs to either an aerosol of PAF or ovalbumin in sensitized animals results in a selective accumulation of eosinophils as assessed by bronchoalveolar lavage after 24 h. This eosinophil accumulation, in addition to the associated bronchial hyperreactivity, is reduced by pretreatment with BN 52021 or WEB 2086[34,35]. Furthermore, recent evidence suggests that PAF enhances eosinophil IgE receptor expression and primes IgE-dependent cytotoxicity against schistosomula of *Schistosoma mansoni* and leukotriene generation[36].

Eosinophil infiltration is a crucial factor in microvascular damage and this cell type is a prominent feature of inflammatory lesions, particularly in asthma and graft rejection. The granules of these cells contain cationic proteins including MBP, which is released by marginated eosinophils and causes endothelial damage[37,38]. LTC_4 and $O_2^{\cdot -}$, two other toxic agents for endothelial integrity, are also generated by this cell type. In combination, these components are capable of causing severe impairment to the microvascular wall, and appear to be largely responsible for inflicting the pulmonary damage observed in asthmatic patients. With regard to the system of cellular 'cross-talk' in inflammatory processes, it is of particular interest to note that PAF induces release of both MBP (P. Braquet, unpublished), and LTC_4 and $O_2^{\cdot -}$ from eosinophils, these phenomena being inhibited by BN 52021[39].

Similarly to PAF, TNF enhances neutrophil superoxide production and adherence[40]. TNF may also indirectly regulate eosinophil cytotoxicity via its effect on the release of other cytokines and growth factors.

PAF and TNF as priming agents

At adequate concentrations both PAF and TNF can directly evoke these cellular responses; however, exposure of the cells to extremely low concentrations of these mediators, which are ineffective in their own right, produces enhanced responses to subsequent stimulation by agonists such as thrombin and chemotactic peptides. Vercelotti *et al.*[41] have demonstrated that minuscule quantities of PAF (10^{-12} mol/l) markedly enhanced neutrophil responses to subsequent activation by the agonists *N*-formylmethionylleucyl phenylalanine (FMLP) and PMA. The primed neutrophil responses included respiratory burst as evidenced by enhanced superoxide release, degranulation as measured by elastase release, and adhesion as measured by adherence of PMN to human endothelium as well as PMN aggregation. Concomitantly, these PAF-primed neutrophils were excessively damaging to cultured endothelial cells. These PAF-primed PMN responses and subsequent PMN-mediated endothelial damage were completely inhibited by the PAF antagonists, BN 52021, L-652,731 and kadsurenone. Similarly, TNF has also been shown to prime PMN to various agonists[42].

Priming human PMN for 18 h with various concentrations of PAF (0.1 fmol/L–1 μmol/L) markedly enhances their subsequent TNF production in response to IL 1[29]. Maximum priming activity is observed at 10 fmol/L–0.1 nmol/L PAF, resulting in a 2–3-fold increase in TNF production. Furthermore, we have recently demonstrated that PAF can amplify TNF-induced superoxide generation by human PMN[43,44]. When PMN are incubated for 3 h at 37°C with various concentrations of TNF (1–1000 ng/ml), a significant dose-dependent generation of superoxide is observed. The response is maximal with 10 ng/ml TNF and after 60–90 min of incubation, $O_2^{\cdot -}$ production declining after this time. PAF alone (0.1 pmol/L–0.1 nmol/L) fails to elicit any superoxide production; however, when PAF is added for 10 min to cells previously incubated for 50 min with 10 ng/ml TNF, superoxide production is enhanced relative to that induced by TNF alone. Maximum amplification (+30%) is obtained with 10 fmol/L PAF, and the enhancing effect of the mediator is completely abolished by four structurally unrelated PAF antagonists (BN 52021, kadsurenone, BN 52111 and WEB 2086), added either simultaneously with the TNF or the PAF. In addition, the PAF antagonists also decrease by 50% the superoxide production elicited solely by TNF, indicating that TNF-induced superoxide generation is partially mediated by a mechanism involving endogenous PAF. We have also recently established that a preincubation of the PMN for 30 min with a low concentration of LPS or TNF prior to stimulation with FMLP primed the cells so that superoxide production was increased by 120% and 180%, respectively, relative to that induced by FMLP alone[45].

GM-CSF and TNF prime PAF-induced responses

In addition to their role in stem cell proliferation GM-CSF and TNF appear to play an important role in host defence by priming the functional activities of mature effector cells such as PMN, monocytes and eosinophils. GM-CSF, granulocyte-colony stimulating factor (G-CSF) and TNF are, by themselves, essentially devoid of detectable activity toward PMN[46]. However, pretreatment of PMN with GM-CSF enhances their chemotactic, phagocytic, cytotoxic and oxidative responses to various stimuli such as leukotriene B_4 (LTB_4) and the complement-derived C5a[47]. GM-CSF, which also augments phagocytosis by PMN[48], increases expression of the major surface adhesive proteins[49] and receptor expression[50], primes eosinophils for enhanced killing of *Schistosoma mansoni* and enhanced synthesis and extracellular export[51] of LTC_4. PMN pretreatment with GM-CSF also results in increased arachidonic acid release[52] and LTB_4 synthesis in response to FMLP, C5a and the calcium ionophore A 23187[53]. Similarly, pretreatment of human PMN with TNF enhances their superoxide production induced by FMLP[42,54].

With regard to PAF, recent studies have established that PAF/cytokine (GM-CSF, TNF) interactions appear to be vital in the enhancement of PMN responses to various stimuli: interestingly, in PMN where PAF *per se* at low doses is not able to produce superoxide generation, a preincubation of the cells with TNF[43,44] or GM-CSF[55] results in a significant amplification of free radical production. This phenomenon is inhibited by various PAF antagonists such as BN 52021 or BN 50741, and appears to be impaired after thermal injury. Interestingly PAF antagonists also partially inhibited the TNF-induced superoxide production, suggesting that an endogenous production of the autacoid is involved in this process[43,44]. PMN priming by the two cytokines is not limited to superoxide production. Preincubation of PBML with recombinant human GM-CSF primes the cells so that PAF (1 μmol/L)-induced LTB_4 production is increased by 10-fold relative to non-primed cells.[56] Furthermore, leukotriene synthesis is induced by a PAF concentration of 10 nmol/L in GM-CSF-primed cells, whereas in untreated cells the same concentration of PAF is unable to elicit a response. Similarly, TNF also induces significant leukotriene production, a phenomenon inhibited by PAF antagonists[43].

Putative function and mechanism of cytokine priming

The physiological function and mechanism of action of GM-CSF and TNF in priming neutrophil responses to inflammatory stimuli remains unknown. Studies by English[57] have demonstrated that priming results from an irreversible induction of temperature-dependent cellular processes, and that receptor expression on the surface of PMNL is markedly accelerated by cytokine priming. Receptor expression confers functional responsiveness on circulating 'end-stage' PMNL which may be hyporesponsive to metabolic antagonists. Deployment of surface receptors, which is accompanied by a dramatic increase in cell responsiveness, normally occurs after the cell has left the circulation, thus priming may be crucial for an efficient host defence system.

With regard to the precise mechanism of GM-CSF and TNF priming, very recent data suggest that some pertussis toxin-sensitive G-proteins are probably involved in the process. Indeed, pretreatment of PMNL with the toxin abolishes the amplification of superoxide production induced by low doses of PAF in TNF-pretreated PMNL[43]. GM-CSF has recently been shown to modulate the activity of guanylate and adenylate cyclases in human PMNL[58], more specifically, the cytokine inhibits adenylate cyclase and stimulates guanylate cyclase. Furthermore, studies on human monocytes have demonstrated that GM-CSF-induced sodium influx involves activation of a pertussis toxin-sensitive GTP-binding protein[59].

In addition, TNF induces an increase in GTP binding and GTPase activity in HL-60 promyelocytic leukaemic cells, the latter of these processes being sensitive to pertussis toxin[60]. The toxin also inhibits the TNF-induced cytotoxicity in mouse L296 fibroblasts, suggesting the presence of a GTP-binding protein which couples TNF-induced signalling to the biological effect[60].

In view of the inhibitory effect of increased levels of cAMP on human neutrophil responses[61], one can speculate that a part of the effect of GM-CSF is mediated via this response. In addition, incubation of human PMNL with GM-CSF inhibits the alkalinization response to various stimuli including PAF, LTB_4 and FMLP[62], while preincubation with GM-CSF results in an increase in the magnitude of the calcium transients that follows the stimulation of the cells with chemotactic factors[62]. Taken together these findings suggest that the priming phenomenon may result from:

1. a modification of the functional state of certain pertussis toxin-sensitive G proteins;
2. a decrease in calcium signal threshold;
3. an uncoupling between the increase in calcium transient and the activation of Na^+/H^+ antiport – the action site of the G proteins involved in the process may be located between the cytokine receptor and the mechanism activating the Na^+/H^+ exchange.

Similar priming phenomena have also been found with LPS[63]. Indeed, it has been shown that LPS primes PMNL for enhanced production of superoxide upon subsequent stimulation and that LPS priming induces a small but significant increase in intracellular PAF. Further stimulation of the primed PMN also produces a marked increase in cell-associated PAF as compared to non-LPS treated controls[63].

The pathophysiological importance of these priming processes by cytokines has also been assessed *in vivo*. Heuer and Letts[64] have shown that pretreatment of mice with either *S. typhosa* endotoxin or TNF significantly enhanced the mortality induced by PAF. This effect occurred at doses at which PAF, endotoxin or TNF given alone did not significantly affect these parameters. Similar to the situation observed *in vitro* with PMN responses[43,44], the enhancing effect was not recorded when PAF was given prior to TNF.

In addition, in studies where rats received an injection of TNF prior the injection of a low and non-active dose of PAF, a marked amplification of the vascular escape was recorded, mainly in the trachea, bronchi, lung parenchyma, pancreas, kidneys and duodenum[65]. A similar potentiation of cytokine/PAF effects has also been observed in models of cartilage breakdown where the combination of non-active individual doses of TNF and PAF caused a significant loss of glycosaminoglycans[66].

Relationship between PAF and other cytokines

The relationship between PAF and other cytokines apart from IL 1, IL 2 and TNF, is presently unknown, although it would seem likely that interactions occur considering the complex network of cellular growth signals required for proliferation of immuno-competent cells. For example, various synergistic and antagonistic effects have been noted between IL 3, IL 4 and IFN-γ[67,68] and between IL 3, IL 1, G-CSF and M-CSF[69] on the growth of different cell lines.

In addition to PAF, the newly described lymphokine, interleukin 5 (IL 5), which is generated by T helper lymphocytes, is a potent eosinophil activating agent[70]. Indeed, apart from influencing stem cell differentiation, IL 5 appears to exert a direct effect on preformed eosinophils and activate mature cells[71].

We have recently investigated the mechanisms of *in vivo* eosinophil activation by comparing the mobilization of this cell type induced by PAF or antigen injection in the peritoneal cavity of hypereosinophilic rats and the effects of the PAF antagonist, BN 52021, the somatostatin analogue, BIM 23014, and cyclosporin A (CsA) on this process[72]. PAF induced a significant increase of both peritoneal and circulating eosinophil count. CsA almost totally abrogated these variations, whereas BN 52021 reduced the peritoneal increase. Similarly to PAF, peritoneal antigen challenge in actively sensitized animals increased peritoneal and circulating eosinophil infiltration. BIM 23014 reduced the circulating eosinophils and cell infiltration. In contrast, BN 52021 primarily decreased peritoneal eosinophil recruitment, while having little effect on circulating cells[72].

This study indicates that the mechanism by which CsA and BIM 23014 inhibit eosinophil mobilization appears to be different from that of the PAF antagonist. Both CsA and somatostatin are known to affect T cell proliferation which, via the production of IL 3, IL 5 and GM-CSF, is involved in the differentiation of haematopoietic cells into eosinophils[73]. Thus CsA and BIM 23014 probably decrease cell availability for recruitment. In contrast, the PAF antagonist appears primarily to act by inhibiting PAF-induced eosinophil chemotaxis. Thus control of eosinophil recruitment at inflammatory sites appears to be regulated by PAF and various cytokines, particularly IL 5.

Interleukin 6 (IL 6) may be of particular importance in the inflammatory response. Initially thought to be derived from T cells, IL 6 is now known to be produced by various other cell types including monocytes, fibroblasts, hepatocytes, cardia myxoma and glial cells, and of particular interest, vascular endothelial cells[74]. In addition to playing an essential role in B cell growth processes and regulating the proliferation of fibroblasts[75], thymocytes[76], lymph node T cells[77] and peripheral blood T lymphocytes[74], this lymphokine displays other interesting properties. IL 6 has been reported to be active against viruses[78] and is a major inducer of acute phase protein synthesis in cultured liver cells[79].

Indeed, this lymphokine may play an important role in acute pathological responses such as those observed in shock, sepsis and ischaemia. Increases in IL 6 of up to a 100-fold have been observed in serum from severe burn patients within hours following thermal injury[80]. Levels of the lymphokine were closely correlated with body temperature and were maximal immediately prior to an increase in acute phase proteins, suggesting that the cytokine may act as an endogenous thermoregulator. Increased IL 6 activity has also been detected in the cerebrospinal fluid of patients suffering from acute viral, bacterial or tuberculous infections[81]. Similarly, elevated levels of IL 6 have been observed in serum and urine of renal transplant recipients[82], and various reports suggest that the cytokine may be associated with the pathology of rheumatoid arthritis[83].

Many of the biological properties currently being ascribed to IL 6 are similar to those exhibited by IL 1, and a close relationship appears to exist between these two cytokines. Indeed IL 1 is a potent inducer of IL 6 expression in many cell types[84]. As previously discussed, PAF can influence IL 1 synthesis and thus, via this effect, may modulate IL 6 activity.

PAF/CYTOKINE INTERACTIONS AND ENDOTHELIAL CELLS

Effect of cytokines on PAF synthesis by the endothelium

In the preceding section we have considered how PAF and various cytokines can prime, amplify and directly elicit the release of toxic products from circulating cells which can diminish endothelial integrity.We will now focus attention on the role of the endothelium in inflammatory processes. Indeed, this tissue cannot simply be considered as a passive victim of the damaging effects of blood cell responses provoked by PAF and cytokines. Numerous studies have shown that, under certain conditions, endothelial cells generate PAF and certain cytokines, and thus eventually contribute to their own destabilization.

When vascular endothelial cells are exposed to perturbing stimuli a number of cellular haemostatic properties are altered, including increased synthesis of PAF, which is released into the medium. Initially, it was shown that both hormones (angiotension II and vasopressin) and antibodies reacting with antigens expressed on the surface of endothelial cells induced a rapid and transient release of PAF from cultured human umbilical vein endothelial cells[85]. Subsequent studies revealed that, although thrombin was unable to induce PAF release, it was capable of eliciting its synthesis, the PAF remaining associated with the cells and being partially expressed on the outer membrane[86]. Indeed, other investigations demonstrated that thrombin can induce an increase in both intracellular calcium and subsequent phosphatidylinositol (PI) turnover in human endothelial cell monolayers[87]. Associated with these perturbations, thrombin-treated endothelial cell monolayers increased superoxide generation by FMLP (0.1 μmol/L)-stimulated PMN, this enhancement being completely inhibited by BN 52021. Thrombin stimulation of endothelial cells would seem, therefore, to initiate a sequence of events involving PMN/endothelial cell 'cross-talk' which leads to contact activation of marginated PMN by endothelial-derived PAF. In addition to thrombin, cultured endothelial cells produce PAF rapidly in response to diverse stimuli such as leukotrienes, histamine, hydrogen peroxide, ATP and bradykinin[88-90]. Indeed, PAF production by endothelial cells appears to be a general phenomenon since endothelium derived from bovine aorta, pulmonary artery, coronary vasculature and inferior vena cava accumulates PAF in response to various stimuli[91].

In contrast to the above-mentioned stimuli that cause a virtually immediate production of PAF, Bussolino and co-workers have recently elucidated a new pathway of PAF production that requires protein synthesis and is primed by IL 1 and TNF[91-94]. Studies by this latter group have shown that human endothelial cells synthesize large amounts of PAF following 20 min treatment with recombinant TNF or IL 1. With TNF, synthesis of PAF peaks at 4–6 h, whereas in endothelial cells treated with IL 1 it peaks at 8–12 h. More than twice as much PAF is synthesized in response to optimal concentrations of TNF than in response to IL 1, although PAF synthesis is stimulated by lower concentrations of IL 1 than TNF. About 30% of PAF produced in response to either TNF or IL 1 is released into the medium, whereas 70% remains cell-associated.

In this experimental system[92–94], studies with labelled precursors demonstrated that PAF is synthesized *de novo* in response to TNF. This effect of TNF is inhibited by treating endothelial cells with inhibitors of protein or RNA synthesis such as cycloheximide or actinomycin D. This finding may be explained by the observation that, in endothelial cells, TNF induces an acetyltransferase required for PAF synthesis. The induction of this enzymatic activity precedes the peak of PAF synthesis in TNF-treated cells. After prolonged incubation with either TNF or IL 1, endothelial cells no longer respond to the same monokine, but are still capable of producing PAF when treated with the other monokine. The finding that these monokines do not show reciprocal tachyphylaxis in endothelial cells may be accounted for by their binding to different receptors. In cells treated simultaneously with different concentrations of TNF and IL 1, PAF synthesis is stimulated in an additive rather than synergistic way, suggesting that PAF is synthesized by the same pathway in response to either of the two cytokines[92–94]. Finally, very recent data indicate that lymphotoxin also induces PAF synthesis in a way similar to that of TNF[95]. Other cytokines such as interleukins 1 to 6, interferons and colony-stimulating factors are inactive[95,96]. However, IFN-γ primes endothelial cells to produce more PAF after challenge with TNF and IL 1[95].

Relationship between protease activity and PAF synthesis by the endothelium

In addition to the previously described mediators and cytokines that induce PAF synthesis by the endothelium, recent evidence suggests that in inflammation a close relationship exists between protease activity and PAF production. It has been widely demonstrated that serum inhibits PAF production even after inactivation of an acetylhydrolase that degrades PAF. In addition, PAF or endotoxin injection in the rat induces a rapid increase in serum protease activity and this increase is inhibited by BN 52021[6]. Phospholipase A_2 can be activated by various proteases leading to PAF production, which in turn may induce increased protease activity. Part of the protective effects of PAF antagonists in inflammatory pathologies may be attributable to the inhibition of this deleterious feedback cycle.

Recently, human plasma subjected to gel filtration chromatography has been shown to contain two inhibitory fractions, one containing PAF-acetylhydrolase activity and the other an α_1-protease inhibitor[7]. Low concentrations of this antiprotease and of human plasma α_1-antichymotrypsin inhibited TNF-induced PAF synthesis in PMN, macrophages and vascular endothelial cells. Both antiproteases also inhibited PAF production stimulated by phagocytosis in macrophages and induced with IL 1 in PMN or with TNF in vascular endothelial cells. These results suggest that a protease activated on the plasma membrane or secreted by these cells is involved in promoting PAF synthesis.

Indeed, addition of elastase to macrophages, PMN and endothelial cells stimulated synthesis and relase of PAF much faster than TNF. A similar stimulation was observed in incubations with cathepsin G. To identify the protease activated in TNF-treated cells, PMN and endothelial cells were incubated with specific chloromethyl ketone inhibitors of elastase and cathepsin G[7]. Synthesis of PAF was significantly inhibited by low concentrations of the cathepsin G inhibitor. The finding that antiproteases are inhibitory at concentrations 100-fold lower than those present in plasma raises questions as to the ability of TNF and IL 1 to stimulate PMN in circulation or endothelial cells to synthesize PAF. Indeed, these results suggest that PAF production may be limited to zones of close contact between cells which exclude antiproteases.

The biological significance of endothelial-derived PAF

The importance of PAF released by endothelial cells is evident in several inflammatory conditions. For example, transplantation of a renal allograft into a rabbit presensitized with rabbit skin allograft results in immediate binding of antibodies and complement to glomerular and peritubular capillary endothelium. PAF is detected within a few minutes in the venous effluent, which is followed by an influx of platelets and PMN[97]. In addition, the recent observation that PAF is produced during endotoxaemia[98,99] and is released in the plasma of patients affected by sepsis[100] suggests that the clinical manifestations of sepsis may be caused by the release of PAF by endothelial cells stimulated with TNF and IL 1. Furthermore, since PAF antagonists afford significant protection against various forms of ischaemia[101] and graft rejection[1], this suggests that PAF also plays an important role in these pathologies.

As previously mentioned, the majority of PAF produced by the endothelium remains associated with the cells, where it could play an intracellular role, or in the outer plasma membrane where it may interact with circulating cells[102]. Indeed, in addition to PMN, PAF increases the adherence of other cell types such as leukocytes[103], basophils[104] and eosinophils[105,106] to the endothelial surface. There is a marked similarity between the stimuli which induce neutrophil adhesion to the endothelium and those which induce synthesis of PAF by endothelial cells. Thrombin[86] and leukotrienes C_4 (LTC_4) and D_4 (LTD_4)[88] make EC adhesive to PMN in a way which is compatible with the time-course and dose-dependency of PAF generation by these cells. In addition, PMN made refractory to PAF are less adherent to stimulated endothelial cells[107].

Apart from inducing PAF synthesis, both TNF and IL 1 exert direct effects on endothelial adhesive properties[108] and induce procoagulant activity[109]. Furthermore, IL 1 reduces the fibrinolytic activity of endothelial cells[110] and TNF suppresses the activity of a co-factor for the anticoagulant protein C[111]. These responses result in a change of the endothelial cell surface from antithrombotic to thrombotic. Both monokines induce transient expression of specific antigens recognized by monoclonal antibodies raised against endothelial cells treated with IL 1, increase the expression of an intercellular adhesion molecule[112], and cause endothelial cells to become markedly adhesive for PMN, monocytes, and lymphocytes[113]. The morphology of endothelial cells is converted from epithelioid to fibroblastoid by treatment with TNF or IFN-γ, singly or in combination, but not by IL 1 alone[114].

Recently, several investigators have studied the possibility that the endothelial changes induced by TNF and IL 1 may be partially mediated by PAF. In a recent study[115], when four selective PAF antagonists (BN 52021, BN 53013, CV 3988 and RP 47130) were added to IL 1-stimulated endothelial cells during the PMN adhesion assay, adhesion was reduced in a dose-dependent manner. Similarly, pretreatment of PMN with PAF before the adhesion assay induced desensitization to the phospholipid and reduced PMN adhesion to IL 1-treated endothelial cells. However, comparing the time-course and the concentration–response curve of IL 1-induced endothelial adhesivity and PAF synthesis, it was found that this increased adhesivity to PMN required a shorter incubation time and lower concentration of IL 1 than that needed for PAF production. When acetyl-CoA was added to endothelial cell cultures at a concentration that raised PAF synthesis by 60%, no significant increase in PMN adhesion was observed. In addition, after nine or 10 divisions the ability of endothelial cells to synthesize PAF decreased by 85–90%, while IL 1-induced adhesivity to PMN was only slightly diminished. When IL 1 α and β were tested on EC, both were equally active in promoting PMN adhesion to endothelial cells, but only the α form was able to stimulate PAF production[116].

These observations do not support the hypothesis that IL 1-induced PAF production could completely mediate PMN adhesion and distinguish IL 1 from other stimuli such as thrombin or LTs. However, the IL 1-induced increase of PMN adhesion to the endothelium is partially inhibited by PAF antagonists and, similarly to that caused by thrombin and leukotrienes, by desensitization of PMN to PAF. Thus, the possibility was investigated that PMN themselves, and not endothelial cells, might be the source of PAF during the adhesion assay. When PMN were seeded on IL 1-treated endothelial cells, increased amounts of PAF were detected in the total extract of the cells and PMN adhering to them. This was also the case when endothelial cells were fixed with paraformaldehyde after treatment with IL 1 to block their ability to synthesize PAF during the adhesion assay.

Increased amounts of PAF were detected only when PMN were seeded on IL 1-treated endothelial cells. In contrast, PAF was undetectable when PMN were seeded on plastic dishes or on untreated cells[117]. Thus, when PMN adhere to IL 1-treated endothelial cells they seem to be activated to synthesize PAF, which in turn acts synergistically to promote more PMN adhesion and activation. This could explain the inhibitory activity of PAF antagonists and PAF desensitization on PMN adhesion to IL 1-treated endothelial cells.

IL 1 has been shown to induce expression of endothelial surface proteins not detectable in unstimulated cells[118]. Some of these antigens have been characterized by monoclonal antibodies, and a complex of two glycoproteins of 120 000 and 100 000 MW has been described, which appears to be involved in leukocyte adhesion. Monoclonal antibodies to this complex inhibit PMN adhesion to IL 1-stimulated endothelial cells[119]. An attractive hypothesis is that IL 1-inducible endothelial cell membrane antigens could specifically interact with PMN receptors and promote their adhesion and activation. Activation of PMN would then lead to synthesis of synergistic agonists such as PAF, which could then contribute to the PMN response[115].

Recently, we have shown that adhesion of PMN to TNF-treated endothelial cells was inhibited by up to 36% by three structurally unrelated PAF antagonists, BN 52021, BN 50741 and BN 50726[116]. This suggests that PAF may play a role in the TNF-induced adhesion process, but as with the case of IL 1-induced cell adhesivity, the origin of PAF remains to be clarified.

Effect of PAF and cytokines on microvascular integrity

As emphasized in the introduction, the control of microvascular permeability is a crucial factor in the regulation of the inflammatory response. While limited cell infiltration is essential for efficient defence of the host, loss of control of endothelial integrity and PMNL traffic from the blood stream can lead to vascular collapse. The activity of PAF as an inducer of increased microvascular permeability has been widely documented[1]. A direct agonistic activity of the mediator on endothelial cells has been suggested by experiments showing that PAF stimulates Ca^{2+} influx–efflux in cultured human endothelial cells[120]. Indeed, in a recent study[121], we have shown that PAF, but not its deacetylated and biologically inactive metabolite lyso-PAF, dose-dependently (0.1 to 10 nmol/L), induces cultured human endothelial cells to change their shape. In this study, when the endothelium was treated with PAF the cells retracted and tended to lose reciprocal contact, while the distribution of stress fibres was changed and the cells assumed a migratory phenotype. Further studies using endothelial cells grown on fibronectin-coated polycarbonate filters, which restrict the diffusion of [^{125}I]-albumin, revealed that PAF promoted [^{125}I]-albumin diffusion with a dose-dependency similar to that observed for PAF-induced cytoskeleton changes. Three chemically unrelated PAF antagonists, CV-3988, BN 52021 and 48740 RP, prevented the alterations induced by PAF[121]. These findings, coupled with the lack of effect of (S) PAF, support the existence of a specific mechanism of PAF-induced activation of endothelial cells, most probably receptor-mediated. Thus these results may explain, at least in part, the mechanism by which PAF induces increased vascular permeability *in vivo*.

Impairment of endothelial cells by PAF has also been observed *in vivo*. Following 5–10 min superfusion with the autacoid (10^{-7} mol/L) in the mesenteric bed of anaesthetized guinea pigs, retraction of endothelial cells occurred in the area corresponding to the site of application of PAF[122]. This retraction resulted in exposure of the sub-intimal tissue to the blood stream and substantial thrombus formation involving platelets, monocytes and eosinophils, cell infiltration and diapedesis. Bleb formation and interstitial oedema clearly indicated that fluid penetrated the vascular wall as the result of the application of PAF. Administration of prostacylin, inhibitors of phospholipase A_2 or acetyl transferase (ketotifene) or calcium-entry blockers disaggregated the thrombus; however, after discontinuing superfusion of these drugs, thrombus formation recurred immediately[122]. This was not the case if specific PAF antagonists such as BN 52021, RP 48740, WEB 2086 or kadsurenone were injected[123]; when these compounds were applied not only was the thrombus rapidly disaggregated but no new thromboformation was recorded. This very important finding suggests that exogenous mediator superfusion induces the generation of an endogenous PAF-like substance which in a positive-feedback mechanism perpetuates the thrombotic phenomenon and its related processes.

Interestingly, in the same model, superfusion of TNF and subsequent injection of a low dose of PAF in the mesenteric bed dramatically enhanced thrombosis. This enhanced activity of PAF induced by pretreatment with TNF occurred at doses at which PAF and TNF given alone did not significantly affect thrombogenesis. BN 52021 or anti-TNF antibodies inhibited this synergism (R. Bourgain and P. Braquet, in preparation). This result suggests that TNF primes the effect of PAF on the endothelial cell wall. Furthermore, superfusion of the mesenteric bed with a non-thrombogenic dose of LPS, followed by injection of a low dose of PAF (which did not induce a thrombogenic effect *per se*) produced an extensive thrombus. PAF antagonists inhibited this synergism in a dose-dependent fashion (R. Bourgain and P. Braquet, in preparation).

Such endothelial injury, excessive blood cell infiltration and bleb and oedema formation are characteristic of the microvascular alterations observed in diverse immuno-inflammatory pathologies such as ischaemia[101], shock and sepsis[124], graft rejection[125] and asthma[126]. PAF influsion mimics these microvascular impairments and thus may be one of the important mediators involved in such conditions.

While PAF, TNF and IL 1 induce direct effects on endothelial integrity, other cytokines may exert indirect effects. For example, in patients receiving immunotherapy with IL 2, this cytokine induces vascular leakage via indirect activation of endothelial cells[127]. As IL 2 fails to induce the same antigens on cultured endothelial cells, the latter authors speculated that IL 2 acts *in vivo* by inducing production of other cytokines such as lymphotoxin, IL 1, TNF, and IFN-γ. As previously discussed, these three latter cytokines may in turn interact with PAF to produce amplified cell responses. It is known that in endothelial cells, expression of intercellular adhesion complexes, which may confer adhesivity for lymphocytes, is induced by IL 1, TNF, lymphotoxin and IFN-γ[128]. It has been recently reported that IL 2 increases *in vitro* production of IFN-γ[129], TNF and lymphotoxin[130], while, as previously mentioned, PAF can modulate the production of IL 2. Indeed, the notion that IL 2 indirectly induces vascular leak via the induction of other lymphokines and monokines is supported by the fact that, in mice, infusion of IL 2 can elicit endothelial damage only in the presence of T lymphocytes[131].

APPLICATION OF THE CATASTROPHE THEORY TO PAF/CYTOKINE INTERACTIONS IN INFLAMMATION

From the preceding discussion it seems that complex interactions may exist between PAF and various cytokines during inflammation. During this process it appears that a 'cross-talk' becomes established between platelets, macrophages, PMN, eosinophils and endothelial cells, with PAF, proteases, TNF, IL 1 and other cytokines, thrombin and ATP serving as important vectors in this system.

Some of the potential feedback processes that may arise can be illustrated by considering possible mediator interactions in the inflammatory microenvironment. As discussed, PAF is a potent amplifier of platelet and leukocyte responses. At very low concentrations it not only primes the release of IL 1 and TNF by monocytes/macrophages activated by IFN-γ, LPS, MDP, but also the production of leukotrienes[56] and free radicals[41] from activated PMN. Furthermore, PAF induces platelets to form thrombin and ATP, which in turn, as IL 1 and TNF, may act on the endothelium to produce more PAF, resulting in increased PMN chemotaxis. These cells may then be primed by TNF for PAF-induced superoxide generation. In addition, PAF generated by endothelial cells may amplify the TNF- and IL 1-activated production of GM-CSF and IL 6 from the endothelium[132]. GM-CSF, which is also produced by stimulated monocytes, potently enhances release of superoxide and LTC_4 by eosinophils[133]. Furthermore, in combination with IL 3, it elicits monocyte cytotoxity by inducing TNF secretion from this cell type[134].

The priming ability of these mediators indicates the extreme sensitivity of the inflammatory process and the rigid controls which must usually operate to stop excessive inflammatory responses. We propose that an equilibrium may exist between the mediators involved in the priming and feedback processes and internal mechanisms which down-regulate these loops. An important component of this regulatory system appears to include desensitization processes and endogenous suppressive factors which under normal conditions confine immuno-inflammatory reactions to a specific site; for example, the localized response to an antigen.

An important component of this regulatory system appears to include desensitization mechanisms and endogenous suppressive factors which under normal conditions confine cytotoxic reactions to a specific site; for example the localized response to an antigen. Indeed, several inhibitors to the inflammatory vectors have been partially characterized. Lignans such as enterolactone and related compounds with PAF antagonistic activity[135] have been identified in mammalian urine, with elevated levels being observed during early pregnancy[136]. Endogenous lipid-like PAF inhibitors have been detected in rat hepatocytes[137] and uterus[138], and also in renal venous blood of patients suffering from renovascular hypotension[139]. Furthermore, various endogenous protease inhibitors have been detected in humans[140], dogs and rats[141]. The concentration and activity of the endogenous protease inhibitor, alpha-1-antiprotease, has also been shown to be reduced in patients with adult respiratory distress syndrome[142].

A considerable number of endogenous inhibitors of IL 1 and IL 2 have been reported. The neuropeptide, alpha-melanocyte-stimulating hormone[143] and catecholamines[144] depress IL 1 activity. Suppressive factors have also been identified in PBML from patients with rheumatoid arthritis[145] and in urine from patients with monocytic leukaemia[146].

Various serum inhibitors of IL 2 which have identified have been recently reviewed[147]. Several reports indicate that both human and murine serum contains a T cell-derived heat-labile protein (or protein–glycolipid complex) which acts in a homeostatic mechanism to restrict IL 2 action in the vicinity of the activated T cells. Changes in inhibitory activity have been found in various pathophysiological states such as during ontogeny, systemic lupus erythematosus, rheumatoid arthritis and systemic infections. There are also suggestions that some tumour cells generate IL 2 inhibitors which diminish killer cell activity against the tumour. Potential endogenous inhibitors of TNF are less well documented, although fibroblasts and monocytes have been reported to release factors which respectively either suppress the release[27] or cytotoxicity[148] of TNF. It has also been recently proposed that glucocorticoids may serve as modulators of TNF activity[149].

Under normal physiological conditions an equilibrium may be maintained between cytotoxic and inhibitory mechanisms, which would strictly control the inflammatory process and prevent endothelial cell injury. In contrast, if there is either an overloading of the system by excessive mediator production or a critical reduction in inhibitory factors, the feedback cycles would become unregulated and the toxicity would be converted into a systemic process, resulting in endothelial cell damage, cell infiltration, vascular leakage and microcirculatory collapse. Such a phenomenon may underlie the endothelial damage and vascular leakage observed in shock, asthma, sepsis, ischaemia and graft rejection. Indeed, endothelium that has been previously damaged may be particularly prone to such injury. Recently, it has been shown that the recovery of balloon-denuded pig endothelium is not complete as the cells lose the ability to produce endothelium-derived relaxing factor (EDRF) and possibly other relaxant agents[150]. EDRF also reduces platelet aggregation, and the inability of previously damaged endothelial cells to produce such factors suppressive to the activity of the feedback mediators makes regenerated endothelium markedly more susceptible to further inflammatory injury.

This fine balance between the protection and destruction of the processes maintaining life is reminiscent of the catastrophe theory proposed by René Thom[8] and Christopher Zeeman[9] in the early 1970s, which proposes a mathematical definition for the sudden changes that can occur in normally well-ordered and smooth-running systems. Such an event or ‘catastrophe’ can be defined as an abrupt change arising as a sudden response of a system to a smooth change in external conditions, and occurs as a result of the expression of a ‘singularity’ by the system. Defined mathematically as a point on a graphic curve where the direction or quality of curvature changes, expression of this characteristic can lead to a catastrophic change. The fact that PAF[122,151] and certain cytokines[152] possess the unique property of being able to induce their own production *in vivo* can be regarded as a singularity inherent to these mediators. In certain pathological conditions one can consider this phenomenon as the generation of a ‘fold’ in the feedback loops controlling the microvascular defence system, and thus an expression of the singularity characteristic of the catastrophe theory. We are currently examining this biological feedback system by mathematical modelling, in order to gain further insight into its relationship with the catastrophe hypothesis.

CONCLUSION: IMPLICATIONS OF PAF/CYTOKINE INTERACTIONS FOR THE TREATMENT OF INFLAMMATORY DISEASE

The fact that the inflammatory response is a complex, multicomponent system has important implications for the treatment of diverse inflammatory disorders. In conditions such as shock, graft rejection and ischaemia where control of this system may be lost and has to be reinstated therapeutically, specific antagonists of the feedback vectors would be indicated and a mixture of different antagonists may be required depending on the complexity of the feedback network. However, if because of their priming ability, vectors such as PAF and TNF are initial loop generators which recruit and sustain other feedback components, then a combination of a PAF antagonist, antiprotease and anti-TNF antibodies may be effective in preventing formation of the deleterious feedback circuit. Indeed, to some extent this has been demonstrated experimentally by studies showing that PAF antagonists can prevent TNF-induced bowel necrosis in the rat[153]. Presumably a similar effect could also be obtained by treatments inducing enhanced release of suppressive factors, although these are currently unknown.

In contrast, in certain pathologies such as cancer or AIDS, it may be advantageous to initiate this feedback network to assist specific immune processes. This could be achieved by reducing suppressor levels which may be elevated, or by increasing the concentration of a primary network component to levels high enough to activate the feedback loops. With regard to this it is of interest to note that in leukopenic patients with AIDS, GM-CSF has been successfully administered to increase the number of circulating leukocytes, PMN, eosinophils and monocytes[154]. In other pathologies such as cancer a more specific targeting of the feedback component may be required, for example to initiate tumour destruction. Indeed, TNF given systemically to patients with various types of cancer has yielded low response rates of less than 5%[155]. Higher rates of remission of up to 40%, however, have been reported after direct injection of TNF into the tumour[156].

In conclusion, it appears that there are complex interactions between PAF, proteases and cytokines in the control of the inflammatory response. The fact that PAF is part of a multicomponent system may explain why PAF antagonists, which inhibit both the direct and amplification effects of the mediator, are effective in diverse pathological models such as shock, airway hyperreactivity, graft rejection and ischaemic diseases. Indeed, PAF antagonists are currently being evaluated clinically and may constitute valuable drugs in asthma and other human diseases, where control of the inflammatory response has to be reinstated therapeutically. In common with the numerous other drugs already employed for the treatment of inflammation, the end-result of PAF antagonist action is protection of vascular integrity. While PAF inhibitors probably achieve this result by inhibiting the priming, amplification and feedback processes described in this review, other anti-inflammatory or immunodepressant drugs may produce a similar vascular protection via their own individual mechanisms of action.

However, it should be emphasized that PAF antagonists alone are only capable of blocking the pathological processes directly or indirectly dependent on PAF, no matter how diverse these may be. The vast majority of other anti-inflammatory drugs also only act through inhibition of a single mediator, synthetic pathway or process. As proposed in this chapter, the complex multicomponent nature of the deleterious processes operating in inflammatory conditions suggests that more successful therapeutic regimes may consist of a combination of drugs, possibly including protease inhibitors, calcium antagonists, prostacyclin analogues, inhibitors of interleukins and growth factors, anti-TNF antibodies and PAF antagonists.

The other possible pharamacological approach to the treatment of such conditions is the design of compounds which possess a dual or multi-inhibitory activity. Our laboratory is currently developing such drugs, and studies on animal models with compounds acting as PAF antagonists/antiproteases or PAF antagonists/5-lipoxygenase inhibitors have produced very encouraging results. Despite the technical difficulties of combining various inhibitory properties in one molecule, we believe that this approach offers great potential for the therapy of inflammatory disease.

References

1. Braquet, P., Touqui, L., Shen, T. S. and Vargaftig, B. B. (1987). Perspectives in platelet-activating factor research. *Pharmacol. Rev.*, **39**, 97–145
2. Sturk, A., Ten-Cate, J. W., Hosford, D., Mencia-Huerta, J. M. and Braquet, P. (1989). Synthesis, catalobism and pathophysiological role of platelet-activating factor. In Paoletti, R. and Kritchevsky, D. (eds), *Advances in Lipid Research*, vol. 23, pp. 219–76. (London: Academic Press)
3. Vargaftig, B. B. and Braquet, P. (1987). PAF-acether today: relevance for acute experimental anaphylaxis. *Br. Med. Bull.*, **43**, 312–35
4. Braquet, P., Chabrier, P. E. and Mencia-Huerta, J. M. (1987). The promise of PAF antagonists. *Adv. Inflammation Res.*, **16**, 179–98
5. Hosford, D., Mencia-Huerta, J. M., Page, C. and Braquet, P. (1988). Natural antagonists of platelet-activating factor. *Phytotherapy Res.*, **2**, 1–24
6. Etienne, A., Hecquect, F., Guilmard, C., Soulard, C. and Braquet, P. (1987). Inhibition of rat endotoxin-induced lethality by BN 52021 and BN 52063 compounds with PAF-acether antagonistic effect and prostease-inhibitory activity, *Int. J. Tiss. Reac.*, **9**, 19–26
7. Camussi, G., Tetta, C., Bussolino, F. and Baglioni, C. (1988). Synthesis and release of platelet-activating factor is inhibited by plasma α_1-proteinase inhibitor or α_1-antichymotrypsin and is stimulated by proteinases. *J. Exp. Med.*, **168**, 1293–306
8. Thom, R. (1975). *Structural Stability and Morphogenesis* (trans. D. H. Fowler) (New York: Benjamin–Addison Wesley)
9. Zeeman, E. C. (1972). 1072, A catastrophe machine. In Waddington, C. H. (ed.), *Towards a Theoretical Biology*, vol. 4, pp. 276–82 (Edinburgh: Edinburgh University Press)
10. Pignol, B., Henane, S., Mencia-Huerta, J. M., Rola-Pleszczynski, M. and Braquet, P. (1987). Effect of PAF-acether (platelet-activating factor) and its specific antagonist, BN 52021, on interleukin 1 (IL 1) synthesis and release by rat monocytes. *Prostaglandins*, **33**, 931–9
11. Pignol, B., Lonchampt, M. O., Chabrier, P. E., Mencia-Huerta, J. M. and Braquet, P. (1989). Platelet-activating factor (PAF) potentiates interleukin 1/ETAF production by guinea-pig keratinocytes stimulated with lipopolysaccharide (LPS). *J. Lipid Mediators* (in press)
12. Barett, M. L., Lewis, G. P., Ward, S. and Westwick, J. (1987). Platelet-activating factor induces Interleukin-1 production from human adherent macrophages. *Br. J. Pharmacol.*, **90**, 113P
13. Ward, S. G., Lewis, G. P. and Westwick, J. (1988). Platelet-activating factor stimulates interleukin I production from human adherent monocyte–macrophages. In Braquet, P. (ed.), *New Trends in Lipid Mediator Research*, vol. 1, pp. 6–15 (Basel: Karger)

14. Salem, P., Dulioust, A., Derickz, S., Vivier, E., Benveniste, J. and Thomas, Y. (1987). PAF-acether (platelet-activating factor) increases interleukin 1 (IL 1) secretion by human monocytes. *Fed. Proc.*, **46**, 922–6
15. Rola-Pleszczynski, M., Gingras, D. and Poubelle, P. (1988a). PAF-acether enhances the production of tumor necrosis factor (TNF) and interleukin 1 (IL 1) by human monocytes. *J. Immunol.* (In press)
16. Barthelson, R., Valone, F. H., Debs, R. and Philip, R. (1988). Synergy in interleukin 1 (IL 1) release by human monocytes stimulated with platelet-activating factor (PAF) plus gamma interferon (IFN gamma) or tumor necrosis factor (TNF). *FASEB J.*, **2**, A1228
17. Valone, F. H. and Epstein, L. B. (1988). Biphasic platelet-activating factor (PAF) synthesis by human monocytes stimulated with interleukin 1 beta (IL 1), tumor necrosis factor (TNF). *FASEB J.*, **2**, A878
18. Pignol, B., Henane, S., Sorlin, B., Rola-Pleszczynski, M., Mencia-Huerta, J. M. and Braquet, P. (1988). Long-term *in vivo* treatment with platelet-activating factor on interleukin 1 and interleukin 2 production by rat splenocytes. In Braquet, P. (ed.), *New Trends in Lipid Mediators Research*, vol. 1, pp. 38–43 (Basel: Karger)
19. Braquet, P. and Rola-Pleszczynski, M. (1987). Platelet-activating factor and cellular immune responses. *Immunol. Today*, **8**, 345–52
20. Hosford, D., Mencia-Huerta, J. M. and Braquet, P. (1988). The role of platelet-activating factor and structurally related alkyl phospholipids in immune and cytotoxic processes. In Nigham, S. and Slater, T. F. (eds), *Eicosanoids, Lipid Peroxidation and Cancer*, pp. 53–5 (Heidelberg: Springer Verlag)
21. Rola-Pleszczynski, M., Pignol, B., Pouliot, C. and Braquet, P. (1987). Inhibition of human lymphocyte proliferation and interleukin 2 production by platelet-activating factor (PAF-acether): reversal by a specific antagonist, BN 52021. *Biochem. Biophys. Res. Commun.*, **142**, 754–60
22. Barrett, M. L., Lewis, G. P., Ward, S., Westwick, J. (1986). Platelet-activating factor modulates interleukin 2 induced proliferation of human T-lymphoblasts. *Br. J. Pharmacol.*, **89**, 505P
23. Pignol, B., Henane, S., Mencia-Huerta, J. M. and Braquet, P. (1989). Effect of long-term treatment with platelet-activating factor on cytokine production by rat spleen cells. *Int. Arch. Allergy Appl. Immunol.*, **88**, 161–3
24. Tracey, K. J., Beutler, B., Lowry, S. F., Merryweather, J., Wolpe, S., Milsark, I. W., Hariri, R. J., Fahey, T. J., Zentella, A., Albert, J. D., Shires, T. and Cerami, A. (1986). Shock and tissue injury induced by recombinant human cachectin. *Science*, **234**, 470–4
25. Aggarwal, B. B. (1987). Tumor necrosis factors, TNF-α and TNF-β: their structure and pleiotropic biological effects. *Drugs of the Future*, **12**, 891–8
26. Cerami, A. and Beutler, B. (1988). The role of cachectin/TNF in endotoxic shock and cachexia. *Immunol. Today*, **9**, 28–31
27. Bonavida, B., Mencia-Huerta, J. M. and Braquet, P. (1989). Effect of platelet-activating factor (PAF) on monocyte activation and production of tumour necrosis factor (TNF). *Int. Arch. Allergy Appl. Immunol.*, **88**, 157–60
28. Bonavida, B., Mencia-Huerta, J. M. and Braquet, P. (1990). Effect of platelet-activating factor on peripheral blood monocytes: induction and priming for TNF secretion. *J. Lipid Mediators*, **2**, S65–S76
29. Rola-Pleszczynski, M. (1989). Priming of human monocytes with PAF augments their production of tumor necrosis factor. *J. Lipid Mediators*, **2**, 577–82
30. Valone, F. H. and Epstein, L. B. (1988). Biphasic platelet-activating factor synthesis by human monocytes stimulated with IL-1-β, tumor necrosis factor, or IFN-γ. *J. Immunol.*, **11**, 3945–50
31. Malech, H. L. and Gallin, J. I. (1987). Neutrophils in human diseases. *N. Engl. J. Med.*, **11**, 687–94
32. Wardlaw, A. J. and Kay, A. B. (1986). PAF-acether is a potent chemotactic factor for human eosinophils. *J. Allergy Clin. Immunol.*, **77**, 236–42
33. Coyle, A. J., Urwin, S. C., Page, C. P., Touvay, C., Vilain, B. and Braquet, P. (1988). The effect of the selective PAF antagonist BN 52021 on PAF an antigen-induced bronchial hyperreactivity and eosinophil accumulation. *Eur. J. Pharmacol.*, **148**, 51–8
34. Lellouch-Tubiana, A., Lefort, J., Simon, M. T., Pfister, A. and Vargaftig, B. B. (1988). Eosinophil recruitment into guinea-pig lungs after PAF-acether and allergen administration;

modulation by prostacyclin, platelet depletion and selective antagonists. *Am. Rev. Resp. Dis.*, **137**, 948–54

35. Lellouch-Tubiana, A., Lefort, J., Pirotzky, E., Vargaftig, B. B. and Pfister, A. (1985). Ultrastructural evidence for extra-vascular platelet recruitment in the lung upon intravenous injection of PAF-acether to guinea-pigs. *Br. J. Exp. Pathol.*, **66**, 345–55
36. Walsh, G. M., Moqbel, R., Nagakura, T., Iikura, Y. and Kay, A. B. (1989). Enhancement of the expression of eosinophil IgE receptor ($Fc_{\varepsilon}R2$) and its function by platelet activating factor. *J. Lipid Mediators*, **2**, S177–S186
37. Gleich, G. L., Loegering, D. A., Kueppers, F., Bajaj, S. P. and Mann, K. G., (1974). Physio-chemical and biological properties of the major basic protein from guinea-pig eosinophil granules. *J. Exp. Med.*, **140**, 313–32
38. Firgas, E., Loegering, D. A., Solley, G. O., Farrow, G. M. and Gleich, G. J. (1981). Elevated levels of the eosinophil granule major basic protein in the sputum of patients with bronchial asthma. *Mayo Clin. Proc.*, **56**, 345–53
39. Bruijnzeel, P. L. M., Koenderman, L., Kok, P. T. M., Hamelin, M. L. and Verhagne, J. L. (1986). Platelet-activating factor (PAF-acether) induced release of leukotriene C_4 formation and luminol-dependent chemiluminescence by human eosinophils. *Pharmacol. Res. Commun.*, **18**, 61–9
40. Ozaki, Y., Ohashi, T., Niwa, Y. and Kume, S. (1987). Effect of recombinant DNA-produced tumor necrosis factor on various parameters of neutrophil function. *Inflammation*, **12**, 297–309
41. Vercellotti, G. M., Yin, H. Q., Gustafson, K. S., Nelson, P. O. and Jacob, H. S. (1988). Platelet activating factor primes neutrophil responses to agonists: role in promoting neutrophil-mediated endothelial damage. *Blood*, **71**, 1100–6
42. Berkow, R. L., Wang, D., Larrich, J. W., Dodson, R. W. and Howard, T. H. (1987). Enhancement of neutrophil superoxide production by preincubation with recombinant human tumor necrosis factor. *J. Immunol.*, **139**, 3783–91
43. Paubert-Braquet, M., Koltz, P., Longchamp, M. O., Guilbaud, J., Hosford, D. and Braquet, P. (1989). TNF primes the PAF-induced superoxide production by human neutrophils: possible involvement of G proteins. *J. Lipid Mediators*, **2**, S1–S14
44. Paubert-Braquet, M., Koltz, P., Guilbaud, J., Hosford, D. and Braquet, P. (1990). Platelet-activating factor amplifies tumour necrosis factor-induced superoxide generation by human neutrophils. In Emerit, I., Packer, L. and Auclair, C. (eds), *Antioxidants in Therapy and Preventive Medicine* (London: Plenum Press) pp. 275–82
45. Paubert-Braquet, M., Hosford, D., Koltz, P. K., Guilbaud, J. and Braquet, P. (1990). Two structurally unrelated PAF antagonists, BN 52021 and BN 52111, partially inhibit TNF-induced superoxide release by human neutrophils. In a Crastes de Paulet, L. Douste Blazy and Paoletti, R. (eds), *Free Radicals, Lipoproteins and Membrane Lipids* (London: Plenum Press) pp. 45–53
46. Sullivan, R., Griffin, J. D., Simons, E. R., Schafer, A. I., Meshulam, T., Fredette, J. P., Maas, A. K., Gadenne, A. S., Leavitt, J. L. and Melnick, D. A. (1987). Effects of recombinant human granulocyte and macrophage colony-stimulating factors on signal transduction pathways in human granulocytes. *J. Immunol.*, **139**, 3422–30
47. Weisbart, R. H., Kwan, L., Golde, E. W. and Gasson, J. C. (1987). Human GM-CSF primes neutrophils for enhanced oxidative metabolism in response to the major physiological chemoattractants. *Blood*, **69**, 18–21
48. Fleischmann, J., Golde, D. W., Weisbart, R. H. and Gasson, J. C. (1986). Granulocyte-macrophage colony-stimulating factor enhances phagocytosis of bacteria by human neutrophils. *Blood*, **68**, 708–11
49. Arnaout, M. A., Wang, E. A., Clark, S. C. and Sieff, C. A. (1986). Human recombinant granulocyte-macrophage colony-stimulating factor increases cell-to-cell adhesion and surface expression of adhesion-promoting surface glycoproteins on mature granulocytes, *Clin. Invest.*, **78**, 597–601
50. Lopez, A. F., Williamson, D. J., Gamble, J. R., Begley, C. G., Harlan, J. M., Klebanoff, S. J., Walterdorph, A., Wong, C., Clarka, S. C. and Vadas, M. A. (1986). Recombinant human granulocyte-macrophage colony-stimulating factor stimulates in vitro mature human neutrophil and eosinophil function, surface receptor expression and survival. *J. Clin. Invest.*, **78**, 1220 – 8
51. Silberstein, D. J., Owen, M. F., Gasson, J. C., DiPersio, J. F., Golde, D. W., Bina, J. C.,

Soberman, R., Austen, K. F. and David, J. R. (1986). Enhancement of human eosinophil cytotoxicity and leukotriene synthesis by biosynthetic (recombinant) granulocyte–macrophage colony stimulating factor. *J. Immunol.*, **137**, 3290–4

52. DiPersio, J. F., Billing, P., Williams, R. and Gasson, J. C. (1988). Human granulocyte–macrophage colony-stimulating factor and other cytokines primes human neutrophils for enhanced arachidonic acid release and leukotriene B_4 synthesis. *J. Immunol.*, **140**, 4315–22
53. Dahinden, C. A., Zirgg, I., Malif, F. E. and de Weck, A. L. (1988). Leukotriene production in human neutrophils primed by recombinant human granulocyte/macrophage colony-stimulating factor and stimulated with the complement component C5A and FMLP as second signals. *Exp. Med.*, **167**, 1281–95
54. English, D., Broxmeyer, H. E., Gabig, T. G., Akard, L. P., Williams, D. E., Hoffman, R. (1988). Temporal adaptation of neutrophil oxidative responsiveness to n-formyl-methionyl-leucyl-phenylalanine. *J. Immunol.*, **4**, 2400–6
55. Braquet, P., Paubert-Braquet, M. and Hosford, D. (1990). PAF/cytokine networks in microvascular immune injury. *Am. Chem. Soc.*, **199**, 1–2
56. McColl, S. H., Krump, E., Naccache, P. H., Poubelle, P. E., Braquet, P. and Borgeat, P. (1989). Granulocyte–macrophage colony-stimulating factor enhances the synthesis of leukotriene B_4 by human neutrophils in response to PAF-acether. *Blood J. Immunol.*, **146**, 1204–11
57. Mock, B. H. and English, D. (1989). GM-CSF enhances exudation of neutrophils to sites of inflammatory challenge in vivo. *J. Lipid Mediators*, **2**, S137–S142
58. Coffey, R. G., Davis, J. S. and Djeu, J. Y. (1988). Stimulation of guanylate cyclase activity and reduction of adenylate cyclase activity by granulocyte–macrophage colony stimulating factor in human blood neutrophils. *J. Immunol.*, **140**, 2695–701
59. Imamura, K. and Kufe, D. (1988). Colony-stimulating factor 1-induced Na^+ influx into human monocytes involves activation of a pertussis toxin-sensitive GTP-binding protein. *J. Biol. Chem.*, **263**, 14093–8
60. Imamura, K., Sherman, M. L., Spriggs, D. and Kufe, D. (1988). Effect of tumor necrosis factor on GTP binding and GTPase activity in HL-60 and L929 cells. *J. Biol. Chem.*, **263**, 10247–53
61. Weissmann, G., Dukor, P. and Zurier, R. B. (1971). Effects of cyclic AMP on release of lysosomal enzymes from phagocytes. *Nature New Biol.*, **231**, 131–5
62. Naccache, P. H., Faucher, N., Borgeat, P., Gasson, J. C. and Dipersio, J. F. (1988). Granulocyte–macrophage colony-stimulating factor modulates the excitation–response coupling sequence in human neutrophils, *J. Immunol.*, **140**, 3541–6
63. Worthen, G. S., Seccombe, J. F., Clay, K. L., Guthrie, L. A. and Johnston, R. B. (1988). The priming of neutrophils by lipopolysaccharide for production of intracellular platelet-activation factor. *J. Immunol.*, **140**, 3553–9
64. Heuer, H., Letts, G. and Meade, C. (1989). Tumor necrosis factor (TNF) and endotoxin prime effects of PAF n vivo. *J. Lipid Mediators*, **2**, S101–S108
65. Sirois, M. G., Plante, G. E., Braquet, P. and Sirois, P. (1989). Tumor necrosis factor primes the effects of platelet activating factor on rat vascular permeability. *J. Lipid Mediators*, **2**, S109–S118
66. Howat, D., Desa, F., Chander, C., Moore, A. and Willoughby, D. A. (1989). The synergism between PAF and interleukin-1 in cartilage breakdown. *J. Lipid Mediators*, **2**, S143–S150
67. Rennick, D., Yang, G., Muller Sieburg, C., Smith, C., Arai, N., Takabe, Y. and Gemmell, L. (1987). Interleukin 4 (B-cell stimulatory factor 1) can enhance or antagonize the factor-dependent growth of hemopoietic progenitor cells. *Proc. Natl. Acad. Sci. USA*, **84**, 6889–93
68. Ransom, J., Fischer, M., Mosmann, T., Yokota, T., DeLuca, D., Schumacher, J. and Zlotnik, A. (1987). Interferon-gamma is produced by activated immature mouse thymocytes and inhibits the interleukin 4-induced proliferation of immature thymocytes. *J. Immunol.*, **139**, 4102–8
69. Santoli, D., Yang, Y. C., Clark, S. C., Kreider, B. L., Caracciolo, D. and Rovera, G. (1987). Synergistic and antagonistic effects of recombinant human interleukin (IL) 3, IL 1 alpha, granulocyte and macrophage colony-stimulating factors (G-CSF and M-CSF) on the growth of GM-CSF-dependent leukemic cell lines. *J. Immunol.*, **139**, 3348–54

70. Campbell, H. D., Tucker, W. Q. J., Hort, Y., Martinson, M. E., Mayo, G., Clutterbuck, E. J., Sanderson, C. J. and Young, I. G. (1987). Molecular cloning and expression of the gene encoding human eosinophil differentiation factor (interleukin-5). *Proc. Natl. Acad. Sci.*, **84**, 6629–34
71. Yamaguchi, Y., Suda, T., Suda, J., Eguchi, M., Miura, Y., Harada, N., Tominaga, ?. and Takatsu, K. (1988). Purified interleukin 5 supports the terminal differentiation and proliferation of murine eosinophilic precursors. *J. Exp. Med.*, **167**, 43–56
72. Etienne, A., Soulard, C., Thonier, F. and Braquet, P. (1989). Modulation by drugs of eosinophil recruitment induced by immune challenge in the rat. *Int. Arch. Allergy Appl. Immunol.*, **88**, 71–9
73. Warren, D. J. and Moore, M. A. (1988). Synergism among interleukin 1, interleukin 3, and interleukin 5 in the production of eosinophils from primitive hemopoietic stem cells. *J. Immunol.*, **140**, 94–9
74. Wong, G. C. and Clark, S. C. (1988). Multiple actions of interleukin 6 within a cytokine network. *Immunol. Today*, **9**, 137–9
75. Murasuchi, A., Hirano, T., Tana, B., Matsuda, T., Horii, Y., Nakajima, K. and Kishimoto, T. (1988). The essential role of B cell stimulatory factor 2 (BSF-2/IL-6) for the terminal differentiation of B cells. *J. Exp. Med.*, **167**, 332–44
76. Lotz, M., Jirik, F., Kabouridis, P., Tsoukas, C., Hirano, T., Kishimoto, T. and Carson, A. (1988). B Cells stimulating factor 2/interleukin 6 is a costimulant for human thymocytes and T lymphocytes. *J. Exp. Med.*, **167**, 1253–8
77. Garman, R. D., Jacobs, K. A., Clark, S. C. and Raulet, D. H. (1987). B-cell stimulatory factor 2 (β_2 interferon) functions as a second signal for interleukin 2 production by mature murine T cells. *Proc. Natl. Acad. Sci. USA*, **84**, 7629–33
78. Zilberstein, A., Ruggieri, R., Korn, J. H. and Revel, M. (1986). Structure and expression of cDNA and genes for human interferon-beta-2, a distinct species inducible by growth-stimulatory cytokines. *EMBO*, **5**, 2519–37
79. Gauldie, J., Richards, C., Harnish, D., Landsdorp, P. and Baumann, H. (1987). Interferon beta-2/B cell stimulatory factor type 2 shares identity with monocyte-derived hepatocyte-stimulating factor and regulates the major acute phase protein response in liver cells. *Proc. Natl. Acad. Sci.*, **84**, 7251–5
80. Nijsten, M. W. N., Degroot, E. R., Tenduis, H. J., Klasen, H. J., Hack, C. E. and Aarden, L. A. (1987). Serum level of interleukin-6 and acute phase responses. *Lancet*, **2**, 921
81. Houssiau, F. A., Bukasa, K., Sindic, C. J. M., Vandamme, J. and Vansnick, J. (1988). Elevated levels of the 26K human hybridoma growth-factor (interleukin-6) in cerebrospinal fluid of patients with acute infection of the central nervous system. *Clin. Exp. Immunol.*, **71**, 320–3
82. Vanders, M. H. J., Vanderheyden, A. A. and Aarden, L. (1988). Interleukin 6 (IL 6) in serum and urine of renal-transplant recipients. *Clin. Exp. Immunol.*, **71**, 314–9
83. Hirano, T., Matsuda, T., Turner, M., Feldmann, M., Tang, B., Miyasaka, N., Shimizy, M. and Kishimoto, T. (1987). B-cell stimulatory factor II (BSF2/IL-6) and rheumatoid arthritis. *Proc. Japan Acad. Ser.*, **63**, 281–3
84. Van Damme, J., Opdenakker, G., Simpson, R. J., Rubira, M. R., Cayphas, S., Vink, A., Billiau, A. and Van Snick, J. (1987). Identification of the human 26-kD protein, interferon-$\beta 2$, as a B cell hybridoma plasmacytoma growth factor inducible by interleukin 1 and tumor necrosis factor. *J. Exp. Med.*, **165**, 914–19
85. Camussi, G., Aglietta, M., Malavasi, F., Tetta, C., Piacibello, F., Sanavio, F. and Bussolino, F. (1983). The release of platelet-activating factor from human endothelial cells in culture. *J. Immunol.*, **131**, 2397–403
86. Prescott, S. M., Zimmerman, G. A. and McIntyre, T. M. (1984). Human endothelial cells in culture produce platelet-activating factor (1-alkyl-2-acetyl-*sn*-glyceryl-3-phosphocholine) when stimulated with thrombin. *Proc. Natl. Acad. Sci.*, **81**, 3934–8
87. Wickham, N. W. R., Vercellotti, G. M., Yin, H. Q., Moldow, C. F. and Jacob, H. S. (1987). Neutrophils are primed to release toxic oxidants by contact with thrombin-stimulated endothelium: role of endothelial cell-generated platelet-activating factor. *Clin. Res.*, **35**, 603A
88. McIntyre, T. M., Zimmerman, G. A., Satoh, K. and Prescott, S. M. (1985). Cultured endothelial cells synthesize both platelet-activating factor and prostacyclin in response to histamine, bradykinin and ATP. *J. Clin. Invest.*, **76**, 271–80
89. McIntyre, T. M., Zimmerman, G. A. and Prescott, S. M. (1986). Luekotriene C_4 and D_4

stimulate human endothelial cells to synthesize platelet-activating factor and bind neutrophils. *Proc. Natl. Acad. Sci. USA*, **83**, 2204–6
90. Lewis, M. S., Whatley, R. E., Cain, P., McIntyre, T. M., Prescott, S. M. and Zimmerman, G. A. (1988). Hydrogen peroxide stimulates the synthesis of platelet-activating factor by endothelium and induces endothelial cell-dependent neutrophil adhesion. *J. Clin. Invest.*, **82**, 2045–55
91. Whatley, R. E., Zimmerman, G. A., McIntyre, T. M. and Prescott, S. M. (1988). Endothelium from diverse vascular sources synthesizes platelet-activating factor. *Arteriosclerosis*, **8**, 321–31
92. Bussolino, F., Breviario, F., Tetta, C., Aglietta, M., Mantovani, A. and Dejana, E. (1986). Interleukin 1 stimulates platelet-activating factor production in cultured human endothelial cells. *J. Clin. Invest.*, **77**, 2027–33
93. Bussolino, F., Camussi, G. and Baglioni, C. (1988). Synthesis and release of platelet-activating factor by human vascular endothelial cells treated with tumor necrosis factor or unterleukin 1α. *J. Biol. Chem.*, **263**, 11856–61
94. Camussi, G., Bussolino, F., Salvidio, G. and Baglioni, C. (1987). Tumor necrosis factor/cachectin stimulates peritoneal macrophages, polymorphonuclear neutrophils, and vascular endothelial cells to synthesize and release platelet-activating factor. *J. Exp. Med.*, **166**, 1390–404
95. Bussolino, F., Camussi, G., Tetta, C., Bosia, A. and Baglioni, C. (1989). Selected cytokines stimulate endothelial cells to produce platelet-activating factor. *J. Lipid Mediators*, **2**, S15–S22
96. Braquet, P., Paubert-Braquet, M., Bourgain, R., Bussolisno, F. and Hosford, D. (1989). PAF/cytokine auto-generated feedback networks in microvascular immune injury: consequences in shock, ischemia and graft rejection. *J. Lipid Mediators*, **10**, 1–38
97. Ito, S., Camussi, G., Tetta, G., Mibrou, F. and Andres, G. (1984). Hyperacute renal allograft rejection in the rabbit. The role of platelet activating factor and of cationic proteins derived from polymorphonuclear leukocytes and from platelets. *Lab. Invest.*, **51**, 148–61
98. Inarrea, P., Gomez-Cambronero, J., Pacual, J., del Carmen Ponte, M., Hernando, P. and Sanchez Crespo, M. (1985). Synthesis of PAF-acether and blood volume changes in gram-negative sepsis. *Immunopharmacology*, **9**, 45–53
99. Chang, S. W., Feddersen, C. O. and Henson, P. M. (1987). Platelet-activating factor mediates hemodynamic changes and lung injury in endotoxin-treated rats. *J. Clin. Invest.*, **79**, 1496–506
100. Bussolino, F., Porcellini, M. G., Varese, L. and Bosia, A. (1987). Intravascular release of platelet-activating factor in children with sepsis. *Thromb. Res.*, **48**, 619–20
101. Braquet, P., Paubert-Braquet, M., Koltai, M., Bourgain, R., Bussolino, F. and Hosford, D. (1989). Is there a case for PAF antagonists in the treatment of ischemic states? *Trends Pharmacol. Sci.*, **10**, 23–30
102. Henson, P. M. (1987). Extracellular and intracellular activities of platelet-activating factor. In Winslow, C. M. and Lee, M. L. (eds), *New Horizons in Platelet-activating Factor Research*, pp. 3–10 (Chichester: John Wiley & Sons)
103. Dillon, P. K., Fitzpatrick, M. F., Ritter, A. B. and Duran, W. N. (1988). Effect of platelet-activating factor on leukocyte adhesion to microvascular endothelium. *Inflammation*, **12**, 563–73
104. Bochner, B. S., Peachell, P. T., Brown, K. E. and Schleimer, R. P. (1988). Adherence of human basophils to cultured umbilical vein endothelial cells. *J. Clin. Invest.*, **81**, 1355–64
105. Kimani, G., Tonnesen, M. G. and Henson, P. M. (1988). Stimulation of eosinophil adherence to human vascular endothelial cells in vitro by platelet-activating factor. *J. Immunol.*, **140**, 3161–6
106. Lamas, A. M., Mulroney, C. M. and Schleimer, R. P. (1988). Studies on the adhesive interaction between purified human eosinophils and cultured vascular endothelial cells. *J. Immunol.*, **140**, 1500–5
107. Zimmerman, G. A., McIntyre, T. M. and Prescott, S. M. (1985). Thrombin stimulates the adherence of neutrophils to human endothelial cells *in vitro*. *J. Clin. Invest.*, **76**, 2235–46
108. Bevilacqua, M. P., Pober, J. S., Wheeler, M. E., Contran, R. S. and Gimbrone, M. A. (1985). Interleukin 1 acts on cultured human vascular endothelium to increase the adhesion of polymorphonuclear leukocytes, monocytes and related leukocyte cell lines. *J. Clin. Invest.*, **76**, 2003–11
109. Bevilacqua, M. P., Pober, J. S., Wheeler, M. E., Cotran, R. S. and Gimbrone, M. A. (1985). Interleukin 1 activation of vascular endothelium. Effects on procoagulant activity and leukocyte adhesion. *Am. J. Pathol.*, **121**, 393–403
110. Bevilacqua, P. M., Schleff, R. R., Gimbrone, M. A. and Loskutoff, D. L. (1986). Regulation

of the fibrinolytic system of cultured human vascular endothelium by interleukin 1. *J. Clin. Invest.*, **78**, 587–91

111. Nawroth, P. P. and Stern, D. M. (1986). Modulation of endothelial cell hemostatic properties by tumor necrosis factor. *J. Exp. Med.*, **163**, 740–9
112. Pober, J. S., Gimbrone, M. A., Lapierre, L. A., Mendrick, D. L., Fiers, W., Rothlein, R. and Springer, T. A. (1986). Overlapping patterns of activity of activation of human endothelial cells by interleukin 1 and tumor necrosis factor. *J. Immunol.*, **137**, 1893–6
113. Gamble, J. R., Harlan, J. M., Klebanoff, S. J. and Vadas, M. A. (1985). Stimulation of the adherence of neutrophils to umbilical vein endothelium by human recombinant tumor necrosis factor. *Proc. Natl. Acad. Sci. USA*, **82**, 8667–71
114. Stolpen, A. H., Guinan, E. C., Fiers, W. and Pober, J. S. (1986). Recombinant tumor necrosis factor and immune interferon act singly and in combination to reorganize human vascular endothelial cell monolayers. *Am. J. Pathol.*, **123**, 16–24
115. Breviario, F., Bertocch, F., Dejana, E. and Bussolino, F. (1988). Interleukin-1 induced adhesion of polymorphonuclear leukocytes to cultured human endothelial cells. Role of platelet-activating factor. *J. Immunol.*, **141**, 3391–7
116. Dejana, E., Breviario, F., Erroi, A., Bussolino, F., Mussoni, L., Gramse, M., Pintucci, G., Casali, B., Dinarello, C. A., Van Dame, J. and Mantovani, A. (1987). Modulation of endothelial cell functions by different molecular species of interleukin 1. *Blood*, **69**, 695–9
117. Bussolino, F., Camussi, G., Breviario, F., Bertocchi, F., Ghigo, D., Pescarmona, G., Aglietta, M., Garbarino, G., Bosia, A. and Dejana, E. (1988). Endothelial cells and inflammation: the role of platelet-activating factor, interleukin 1, tumor necrosis factor, and circulating neutrophils. In Braquet, P. (ed.), *New Trends in Lipid Mediator Research*, vol. 1, pp. 135–43 (Karger: Basel)
118. Pober, J. S., Bevilacqua, M. P., Mendrick, D. L., Lapierre, L. A., Fiers, W. and Gimbrone, M. A. (1986). Two distinct monokines, interleukin 1 and tumor necrosis factor, each independently induce biosynthesis and transient expression of the same antigen on the surface of cultured human endothelial cells. *J. Immunol.*, **136**, 1680–4
119. Gimbrone, M. A., Bevilacqua, M. P. and Wheeler, M. E. (1987). Endothelial-dependent mechanism of leukocyte adhesion: role of monokines. *Thromb. Haemostas.*, **1164**, 325
120. Bussolino, F., Aglietta, M., Sanavio, F., Stacchini, A., Lauri, D. and Cammusi, G. (1985). Alkyl-ether phosphaglycerides influence calcium fluxes into human endothelial cells. *J. Immunol.*, **135**, 2748–55
121. Bussolino, F., Camussi, G., Aglietta, M., Braquet, P., Bosia, A., Pescarmona, G., Sanavio, F., d'Urso, N. and Marchisio, P. C. (1987). Human endothelial cells are a target for platelet-activating factor. *J. Immunol.*, **139**, 2439–46
122. Bourgain, R. H., Maes, L., Braquet, P., Andries, R., Touqui, L. and Braquet, M. (1985). The effect of 1-*O*-alkyl-2-acetyl-sn-glycero-3-phosphocholine (PAF-acether) on the arterial wall. *Prostaglandins*, **30**, 185–97
123. Bourgain, R. H., Andries, R. and Bourgain, C. (1988). Arterial thrombosis induced by PAF-acether (1-*O*-alkyl-sn-glycero-3-phosphorylcholine) and its inhibition by Ginkgolides. In Braquet, P. (ed.), *The Ginkgolides: Chemistry, Pharmacology and Clinical Perspective*, pp. 137–50 (Barcelona: J. R. Prous Science Publishers)
124. Nordstoga, K. and Aasen, A. O. (1979). Hepatic changes in late canine endotoxin shock. A light and electron microscopic investigation. *Acta Pathol. Microbiol. Scand.*, **87**, 335–46
125. Nonomura, A., Kono, N., Yoshida, K., Nakanuma, Y. and Ohtag, G. (1988). Histological changes of bile duct in experimental graft-versus-host disease across minor histocompatibility barriers. II: Electron microscopic observations. *Liver*, **8**, 32–41
126. Beasley, R. C., Roche, W. and Holgate, S. T. (1989). Inflammatory processes in bronchial asthma. *Drugs*, **37**, 117–22
127. Cotran, R. S., Pober, J. S., Gimbrone, M. A., Spriner, A. G., Wiebke, E. A., Gaspari, A. A., Rosenberg, S. A. and Lotze, M. T. (1988). Endothelial activation during interleukin 2 immunotherapy. A possible mechanism for the vascular leak syndrome. *J. Immunol.*, **139**, 1883–8
128. Pober, J. S., Lapierre, L. A., Stolpen, A. H., Brock, T. A., Springer, T. A., Fiers, W., Bevilacqua, M. P., Mendrick, D. L. and Gimbrone, M. A. (1987). Activation of cultured human endothelial cells by recombinant lymphotoxin: comparison with tumor necrosis factor and interleukin species. *J. Immunol.*, **318**, 3319–24

129. Grabstein, K., Dower, S., Gillis, S., Urdal, D. and Larsen, A. (1986). Expression of interleukin 2, interferon γ, and the IL 2 receptor by human peripheral blood lymphocytes. *J. Immunol.*, **136**, 4503–8
130. Nedwin, G. E., Svedersky, L. P., Bringman, T. S., Palladino, M. A. Jr and Goeddel, D. V. (1965). Effect of interleukin 2, interferon γ, and mitogens on the production of tumor necrosis factors α and β. *J. Immunol.*, **135**, 2492–7
131. Rosenstein, M., Ettinghausen, S. A. and Rosenberg, S. A. (1986). Extravasation of intravascular fluid mediated by systemic administration of recombinant IL 2. *J. Immunol.*, **137**, 1735–42
132. Braquet, P., Hosford, D., Paubert-Braquet, M., Bourgain, R. and Bussolino, F. (1989). Role of cytokines and platelet-activating factor in microvascular immune injury. *Int. Arch. Allergy Appl. Immunol.*, **88**, 89–100
133. Silberstein, D. J., Owen, W. F., Gasson, J. C., DiPersio, J. F., Golde, D. W., Bina, J. C., Soberman, R., Austen, K. F. and David, J. R. (1986). Enhancement of human eosinophil cytotoxicity and leukotriene synthesis by biosynthetic (recombinant) granulocyte–macrophage colony stimulating factor. *J. Immunol.*, **137**, 3290–4
134. Cannistra, S. A., Vellenga, E., Groshek, P., Rambaldi, A. and Griffin, J. D. (1988). Human granulocyte–monocyte colony-stimulating factor and interleukin 3 stimulate monocyte cytotoxicity through a tumor necrosis factor-dependent mechanism. *Blood*, **71**, 672–6
135. Braquet, P., Esanu, A., Etienne, A. and Robin, J. P. (1987). Endogenous mammalian lignans: a dual action on PAF-acether receptors and the Na^+, K^+-pump. In Winslow, C. M. and Lee, M. L. (eds), Proceedings of the First Sandoz Research Symposium, *New Horizons in Platelet-activating Factor Research*, pp. 28–39 (London: John Wiley)
136. Setchel, K. D., Lawson, A. M., Mitchel, F. L., Adlercreutz, H., Kirk, D. N. and Axelson, M. (1980). Lignans in man and in animal species. *Nature*, **287**, 740–2
137. Miwa, M., Hill, C., Kumar, R., Sugatani, J., Olson, M. S. and Hanahan, D. J. (1987). Occurrence of an endogenous inhibitor of platelet-activating factor in rat liver. *J. Biol. Chem.*, **262**, 527–30
138. Najayala, R., Yasuda, K. and Saito, K. (1987). Existence of endogenous inhibitors of platelet-activating factor (PAF) with PAF in rat uterus. *J. Biol. Chem.*, **262**, 13174–9
139. Masugi, F., Ogihara, T., Saaki, S., Sakaguchi, K., Kumahara, Y., Satouchi, K., Oda, M., Saito, K. and Tokunaga, K. (1988). Endogenous platelet-activating factor and anti-platelet-activating factor in patients with renovascular hypertenson. *Life Sci.*, **42**, 455–60
140. Fraki, J. E. and Hopsu-Havu, V. K. (1972). Human skin proteases. Differential extraction of proteases and of endogenous protease inhibitors. *Arch. Dermatol Forsch.*, **242**, 329–42
141. Osmond, D. H., Wilczynski, E. A. and Loh, A. Y. (1982). Peculiarities of plasma 'prorenin' measurements in man, dog and rat and their theoretical implications. *Clin. Exp. Hypertens.*, **4**, 2213–30
142. Lee, C. T., Fein, A. M., Lippmann, M., Holtzman, H., Kimbel, P. and Weinbaum, G. (1981). Elastolytic activity in pulmonary lavage fluid from patients with adult respiratory-distress syndrome. *N. Engl. J. Med.*, **304**, 192–6
143. Daynes, R. A., Robertson, B. A., Cho, B. H., Burnham, D. K. and Newton, R. (1987). Alpha-melanocyte stimulating hormone exhibits target cell selectivity in its capacity to affect interleukin 1-inducible responses *in vivo* and *in vitro*. *J. Immunol.*, **139**, 103–9
144. Koff, W. C., Fann, A. V., Dunegan, M. A. and Lachman, L. B. (1986). Catecholamine-induced suppression of interleukin-1 production. *Lymphokine Res.*, **5**, 239–47
145. Lotz, M., Tsoukas, C. D., Fong, S., Dinarello, C. A., Carson, D. A. and Vaughan, J. H. (1986). Release of lymphokines after infection with Epstein Barr virus *in vitro*. II. A monocyte-dependent inhibitor of interleukin 1 downregulates the production of interleukin 2 and interferon-gamma in rheumatoid arthritis. *J. Immunol.*, **136**, 3643–8
146. Seckinger, P., Williamson, K., Balavoine, J. F., Mach, B., Mazzei, G., Shaw, A. and Dayer, J. M. (1987). A urine inhibitor of interleukin 1 activity affects both interleukin 1 alpha and 1 beta but not tumor necrosis factor alpha. *J. Immunol.*, **139**, 1541–5
147. Kucharz, E. J. and Goodwin, J. S. (1988). Serum inhibitors of interleukin-2. *Life Sci.*, **42**, 1485–91
148. Gifford, G. E., Loewenstein, J., Yamin, A. and Gallily, R. (1988). Correlation of macrophage-mediated tumor-cell lysis with the production of macrophage cytolytic factor (CF). Preliminary characterization of a factor inhibiting CF production. *Int. J. Cancer*, **37**, 73–9
149. Abe, S., Yamamoto, T., Inagawa, H., Oshima, H., Soma, G. I., Yamazaki, M. and Mizuno,

D. (1987). A possible role of glucocorticoids a natural and endogenous inhibitor to tumor necrosis factor. *Immunobiology*, **175**, 124
150. Shimokawa, H., Aarhus, L. L. and Vanhoutte, P. M. (1987). Porcine coronary arteries with regenerated endothelium have a reduced endothelium-dependent responsiveness to aggregating platelets and serotonin. *Circ. Res.*, **61**, 256–70
151. Doebber, T. W. and Wu, M. S. (1987). Platelet-activating factor (PAF) stimulates the PAF-synthesizing enzyme acetyl-CoA: 1-alkyl-sn-glycero-3-phosphocholine acetyltransferase and PAF synthesis in neutrophils. *Proc. Natl. Acad. Sci. USA*, **84**, 7557–61
152. Ghezzi, P. and Dinarello, C. A. (1988). IL-1 induces IL-1. III. Specific inhibition of IL-1 production by IFN-gamma. *Immunology*, **140**, 4238–44
153. Sun, X. and Hsueh, W. (1988). Bowel necrosis induced by tumor necrosis factor in rats is mediated by platelet-activating factor. *J. Clin. Invest.*, **81**, 1328–31
154. Groopman, J. E., Ronald, M. D., Mitsuyasu, T., Deleo, M. J., Oette, D. H. and Golde, D. W. (1987). Effect of recombinant human granulocyte–macrophage colony-stimulating factor on myelopoiesis in the acquired immunodeficiency syndrome. *N. Engl. J. Med.*, **317**, 593–8
155. Blick, M., Shervin, S. A., Rosenblum, M. and Gutterman, J. (1987). Phase I Study of recombinant tumor necrosis factor in cancer patients. *Cancer Res.*, **47**, 1986–9
156. Taguchi, T. (1987). Clinical studies on recombinant human tumour necrosis factor. *Immunobiology*, **175**, 37–9

9
A role for neuropeptides in inflammation

C. W. DENKO

INTRODUCTION

Inflammation, the process by which animal organisms combat noxious stimuli, is a complex cascade of events leading to homeostasis. Uncontrolled inflammation is undesirable because its reversible features, such as pain, redness, heat and swelling, are joined by a fifth and less transient feature, namely, loss of function of involved organs. Therefore, control of inflammation is sought to protect bodily function. Inflammation-inducing modalities include chemical and physical agents, immunological stimuli, as well as viruses, bacteria and neoplasms. Inflammation is initiated by blood-borne biochemicals, interactive cytokines and hormones, elaborated by diverse surveillance cells. These mediators, in turn, induce altered metabolic functions in other parts of the body such as the liver which produces acute-phase reactants, multipotent proteins with overlapping functions[1,2]. The list of active agents keeps growing as research continues.

Experimental models of inflammation demonstrate numerous physiological changes that find a parallel in human disorders, especially in various forms of arthritis. These responses to inflammation include variation in temperature, leukocyte count, sedimentation rate and haematocrit. In addition, serum levels of acute-phase proteins are altered, including proteinases and carrier proteins such as transferrin, albumin, α_1-antitrypsin, α_1-acid glycoprotein, ceruloplasmin, fibrinogen, and the proteinase inhibitor, thiostatin, precursor of bradykinin[3]. Clinical studies of patients afflicted by one of several inflammatory disorders, such as rheumatoid arthritis, systemic lupus erythematosus, osteoarthritis, pseudogout and gout, show biochemical changes similar to those seen in experimental models involving acute-phase proteins[4]. In addition to these changes, decreased levels of the regulatory neuropeptide, β-endorphin, have been noted[5].

MECHANISMS (PRO-INFLAMMOGENIC, ANTI-INFLAMMOGENIC)

These variations in acute-phase proteins induced by regulatory cytokines, especially interleukin-6 (IL-6), are important protective mechanisms in mammalian systems[1,2]. Studies of the actions of individual acute-phase proteins elucidate their general response in inflammation. α_1-Antitrypsin[6] and ceruloplasmin[7] are shown to be antiphlogistic. Acid glycoprotein also exhibits anti-inflammatory action[8]. The carrier proteins, transferrin and albumin, on the other hand, are pro-inflammogens; therefore, inflammation improves when their levels decrease[9]. A study of patients with rheumatic disorders entailing concomitant assays of acute-phase reactants, immunoglobulins and β-endorphin, in serum and synovial fluid suggests that β-endorphin demonstrates anti-inflammatory properties[10]. Obviously, the regulatory compounds must balance each other to maintain homeostasis. The studies herein reported are incomplete examples as research in inflammation continues.

This hypothesis, that variations in acute-phase proteins are protective in the same way as are variations in the peptides[3], was subjected to experimental evaluation in animal models of rheumatoid arthritis (adjuvant disease) and gout (urate crystal-induced inflammation). The findings demonstrated that regulatory neuropeptides, like the acute-phase proteins, are of two contrasting types, anti-inflammatory and pro-inflammogenic[11]. Previous reports document that growth hormone, prolactin, and substance P aggravate both inflammation and arthritis, while adrenocorticotropin and calcitonin inhibit inflammation and arthritis[12–15] (Table 9.1).

Growth hormone induces a form of arthritis with features of osteoarthritis and rheumatoid arthritis in rats[12]. In patients treated for the human disorder, acromegaly, serum growth hormone levels correlate with manifestations of arthritis, especially joint pain and stiffness[16,17]. When patients with arthritic symptoms received treatment that reduced serum levels of growth hormone, the arthritis was ameliorated. When blood levels of growth hormone showed no reduction with treatment arthritis symptoms did not improve.

Interaction between peptides and prostaglandins (PG), both regulators of local physiological activity, demonstrates interrelated pharmacological actions,

Table 9.1 Effects of neuropeptides in inflammation

		Action on inflammation		
Peptide	*No. of amino acids*	*Anti-inflammatory*	*Pro-inflammatory*	*Reference*
Growth hormone	191		+	12, 14
Prolactin	199		+	14
Adrenocorticotropin	39	+		14
Calcitonin	32	+		13, 11
β-Endorphin	31	+		11
Somatostatin	14	+		11
α-MSH	13	+		11
Neurotensin	13		+	11
Substance P	11		+	11, 15

e.g. between bradykinin and several prostaglandins[18]. The phlogistic effects of several prostaglandins were established in an experimental model using urate-crystal-induced inflammation in a rat deficient in essential fatty acids (EFA), the nutritional precursors of prostaglandins[19,20]. Assays of tissues from animals eating an EFA-deficient diet demonstrated[21] markedly reduced levels of PGE_2. Rigid exclusion of fat from the diet resulted in EFA-deficiency characterized by dermatitis of the feet and tail of the rat[22]. This animal is sensitive to minute amounts of prostaglandins and serves as a sensitive model for inflammation evaluation.

The optimal effective anti-inflammatory dose of β-endorphin in a study of urate-crystal inflammation was determined to be 1.5 ng. Too little (0.15 ng) or too much (15 ng) β-endorphin was ineffective. In similar experimental EFA-deficient rats, β-endorphin reduced inflammation, while PGE_2 aggravated inflammation; when β-endorphin was given with PGE_2, the pro-inflammogenic effect of prostaglandin was nullified[23] (Table 9.2).

In contrast to β-endorphin, substance P exerts a pro-inflammogenic effect[11]. Elegant studies by Lotz and co-workers[24] demonstrate substance P and substance K interacting with monocyte-derived cytokines in the neural regulation of immunological and inflammatory responses. The neuropeptides induce release of interleukin-1, tumour necrosis factor-α, and interleukin-6 from human blood monocytes. Since monocyte-derived cytokines regulate multiple cellular functions in inflammation, neuropeptides should also demonstrate multiple cellular effects. They help repair the tissue damage of inflammation with new growth. In this way, neuropeptides exhibit growth-stimulating activity.

Other data support the hypothesis that peptides participate in an inflammation–healing–regeneration continuum. Obviously, many peptides interact in pro- and anti-inflammatory actions with the final or clinical result being the sum of the various effects. Sporn and co-workers, in wound-healing studies, found inflammatory cells which are known to be involved in physiological wound healing within wound chambers[25]. Substance P is reported to stimulate regeneration in the amphibian, *N. viridescens*[26].

Table 9.2 Footpad swelling (0.01 mm) in EFA-deficient rats after injections of monosodium urate (MSU), β-endorphin (ED) and MSU, prostaglandin (PGE_2) and MSU, and END + PGE_2 + MSU

Time (h)	*Control* (saline)	*END* (1.5 ng)	PGE_2 (50 ng)	*END* (1.5 ng) + PGE_2 (50 ng)
1	43 ± 20	25 ± 12	75 ± 23	56 ± 20
2	69 ± 31	51 ± 17	119 ± 11	54 ± 16
3	112 ± 22	85 ± 29	150 ± 22	83 ± 24
Number	7	8	7	8
Column*	1	2	3	4

* Statistical comparison of treatment effects:
Col. 1 *cf* col. 2: $p = 0.02$ at 1 h, 0.08 at 2 h, 0.03 at 3 h
Col. 1 *cf* col. 3: $p < 0.01$ at 1, 2, 3 h
Col. 1 *cf* col. 4: p = not significant at 1, 2 h; $p < 0.02$ at 3 h
Col. 3 *cf* col. 4: p = not significant at 1 h; $p < 0.01$ at 2, 3 h

Substance P, a pro-inflammogen, and β-endorphin, an anti-inflammatory agent, both stimulate cartilage metabolism as measured by ^{35}S-incorporation[23] (Tables 9.3 and 9.4).

SUMMARY

Peptides play an important role in the inflammation–healing–regeneration continuum, beginning with response to the noxious environmental factor, its control, and repair of damaged tissue.

Table 9.3 Incorporation of ^{35}S by cartilage explants in semisynthetic media with added β-endorphin

		β-Endorphin per ml	
	Control (saline)	*(25 pg)*	*(12.5 pg)*
cpm/mg	438 ± 184	607 ± 106	494 ± 110
Number	15	15	14
2P*	—	0.005	NS

* Significance of comparison to control mean ± SD
NS = not significant

Table 9.4 Incorporation of ^{35}S by cartilage explants in semisynthetic media with added substance P

		Substance P	
	Control (saline)	*(500 ng)*	*(50 ng)*
cpm/mg	294 ± 80	492 ± 82	313 ± 140
Number	7	6	6
2P*	—	0.002	NS

* Significance of comparison to control mean ± SD
NS = not significant

References

1. Koj, A. (1989). The role of interleukin-6 as the hepatocyte stimulating factor in the network of inflammatory cytokines. *Ann. N.Y. Acad. Sci.*, **557**, 1–8
2. Gauldie, J., Richards, C., Northemann, W., Fey, G. and Baumann, H. (1989). IFN-β_1/BSF2/IL-6 is the monocyte-derived HSF that regulates receptor-specific acute phase gene regulation in hepatocytes. *Ann. N.Y. Acad. Sci.*, **557**, 46–59
3. Schreiber, G., Tsykin, A., Aldred, A. R., Thomas, T., Fung, W.-P., Dickson, P. W., Cole, T., Birch, H., DeJong, F. A. and Milland, J. (1989). The acute phase response in the rodent. *Ann. N.Y. Acad. Sci.*, **557**, 61–86
4. Denko, C. W. and Gabriel, P. (1979). Serum proteins – transferrin, ceruloplasmin, albumin, α_1-acid glycoprotein, α_1-antitrypsin – in rheumatic disorders. *J. Rheumatol.*, **6**, 117–23
5. Denko, C. W., Aponte, J., Gabriel, P. and Petricevic, M. (1982). Serum beta-endorphins in rheumatic disorders. *J. Rheumatol.*, **9**, 827–33
6. Pitt, E. and Lewis, D. A. (1979). Anti-inflammatory properties of alpha-1-antitrypsin. *Int. J. Tissue Reactions*, **1**, 21–32
7. Denko, C. W. (1979). Protective role of ceruloplasmin in inflammation. *Agents Actions*, **9**, 333–6

8. Denko, C. W. and Wanek, K. (1984). Anti-inflammatory action of alpha-1-acidglycoprotein in urate crystal inflammation. *Agents Actions*, **15**, 539–40
9. Denko, C. W. (1980). Phlogistic properties of the serum proteins, albumin and transferrin. *Inflammation*, **4**, 165–8
10. Denko, C. W., Aponte, J., Gabriel, P. and Petricevic, M. (1986). Beta-endorphin, immunological and biochemical changes in synovial fluid in rheumatic disorders. *Clin. Rheumatol.*, **5**, 25–32
11. Denko, C. W. and Gabriel, P. (1985). Effects of peptide hormones in urate crystal inflammation. *J. Rheumatol.*, **12**, 971–5
12. Reinhardt, W. O. and Li, C. H. (1953). Experimental production of arthritis in rats by hypophyseal growth hormone. *Science*, **117**, 295–7
13. Bobalik, G. R., Aldred, J. P., Klesynski, R. R. *et al.* (1974). Effects of calcitonin and combination drug therapy on rat adjuvant arthritis. *Agents Actions*, **4**, 364–9
14. Berczi, L., Nagy, E., Asas, L. and Kovacs, K. (1984). The influence of pituitary hormones on adjuvant arthritis. *Arthritis Rheum.*, **27**, 682–8
15. Levine, J. D., Clark, R., Devor, M. *et al.* (1984). Intraneuronal substance P contributes to the severity of experimental arthritis. *Science*, **226**, 547–9
16. Layton, M. W., Fudman, E. J., Barkan, A., Braunstein, E. M. and Fox, I. H. (1985). Acromegalic arthropathy. *Arthritis Rheum.*, **31**, 1022–7
17. Podgorski, M., Robinson, B., Weissberger, A., Stiel, J., Wang, S. and Brooks, P. M. (1988). Articular manifestations of acromegaly. *Aust. N.Z. J. Med.*, **18**, 28–35
18. Denko, C. W., Moskowitz, R. W. and Heinrich, G. (1972). Interrelated pharmacologic effects of prostaglandin and bradykinin. *Pharmacology*, **3**, 229–42
19. Denko, C. W. (1974). A phlogistic function of prostaglandin E in urate crystal inflammation. *J. Rheumatol.*, **1**, 222–30
20. Denko, C. W. (1974). Effect of prostaglandins in urate crystal inflammation. *Pharmacology*, **12**, 331–9
21. Van Dorp, D. A. (1971). Recent developments in the biosynthesis and the analyses of prostaglandins. *Ann. N. Y. Acad. Sci.*, **180**, 181–99
22. Burr, G. O. and Burr, M. M. (1929). A new deficiency disease produced by the rigid exclusion of fat from the diet. *J. Biol. Chem.*, **82**, 345–67
23. Denko, C. W. (1985). Regeneration, repair and their control by pharmacological agents. In Bonta, I. L., Bray, M. A. and Parnham, M. J. (eds.) *Regeneration and Inflammation: Handbook of Inflammation*, Vol. 5, Ch. 10. (Amsterdam: Elsevier)
24. Lotz, M., Vaughan, J. H. and Carson, D. A. (1988). Effects of neuropeptides on production of inflammatory cytokines by human monocytes. *Science*, **241**, 1218–21
25. Sporn, M. B., Roberts, A. B., Shull, J. H., Smith, J. M., Ward, J. M. and Sodek, J. (1983). Polypeptide transforming growth factors isolated from bovine sources and used for wound healing in vivo. *Science*, **279**, 1329–331
26. Globus, M., Vethamany-Globus, S., Kesick, A. and Milton, G. (1983). Roles of neural peptide substance and calcium in blastoma cell proliferation in the newt *Notophthalmus viridescens*. In Fallon, J. F. and Caplan, A. (eds) *Limb Development and Regeneration*, Part A, pp. 513–535. (New York: Liss)

10
Interleukin 1 as an inflammatory mediator

J. A. SYMONS, J. A. EASTGATE and G. W. DUFF

INTRODUCTION

Interleukin 1 (IL 1) is a polypeptide hormone produced during infection, trauma and antigenic challenge. The original designation of IL 1 derived from the Second International Lymphokine Workshop held in Switzerland in 1979. However, the many biological activities of IL 1 had been previously studied for many years under different acronyms.

Early characterization began with the demonstration of a protein factor in the blood stream of rabbits made febrile after the injection of bacteria, endotoxins or viruses[1]. This circulating pyrogen, termed endogenous pyrogen (EP), was later found to be associated with all other known exogenous pyrogens and was thought to be a common mediator of fever. A few years later a phagocyte product termed leukocytic endogenous mediator (LEM) was proposed to mediate many of the features of the acute phase response[2]. It soon became clear that EP and LEM were either identical molecules or closely related. Initial characterization of EP/LEM revealed considerable size and charge heterogeneity with molecular weights of 38 kD and 15 kD and both neutral and acidic isoelectric points. While work on EP/LEM was in progress immunologists working on lymphocyte function discovered a factor that augmented thymocyte proliferation in response to plant lectins. This factor was termed lymphocyte activating factor (LAF)[3] and further characterization revealed many similarities to EP/LEM. Other immunologists were also discovering the importance of soluble factors produced by activated mononuclear cells on *in vitro* cell culture systems. A factor that directly activated plasma cells, called B cell-activating factor (BAF)[4], was demonstrated to have identical activities to LAF, as were other soluble factors such as thymocyte proliferation factor (TPF) and helper peak-1 (HP-1). Other activities that have since been ascribed to IL 1 include osteoclast activating factor[5], mononuclear cell factor (MCF) that causes prostaglandin and collagenase production from fibroblasts[6] and catabolin, a factor that induces cartilage breakdown[7]. Resolution of the debate of how many biological activities attributed to IL-1 were due to the action of a single molecule were largely resolved with the cloning of murine and human cDNAs coding for IL 1 and their expression as proteins. Many of the important biological activities attributed to IL 1 are shown in Table 10.1.

Table 10.1 Biological activities of IL-1

Cell type	*In vitro*	*In vivo*
Immune system		
T cells	Cytokine induction (IL 2, IL 4) IL 2 receptor expression Radioprotection	
B cells	Proliferative response Augment antibody production Chemotactic	
Monocytes	Prostaglandin production IL 1 induction Cytotoxic Chemotactic	
NK cells	Synergise with IL2 in cytotoxic activity	
Basophils	Degranulation and histamine release	
Neutrophils	Chemotactic Adhesion to endothelial cells Degranulation, thromboxane synthesis, reactive oxygen production	Release from bone marow
Central nervous system		
Astrocytes	Proliferation	
Hypothalamic cells	Prostaglandin production	Fever induction
Liver		
Hepatocytes	Decreased albumin synthesis Increased synthesis of some acute phase proteins	Acute phase protein production Altered plasma metal levels Decreased cytochrome P-450 levels
Musculoskeletal system		
Bone	Resorption Osteoclast activation Osteoblast mitogenesis	Bone marrow radioprotection Cytokine production in bone marrow
Cartilage	Resorption Decreased proteoglycan and collagen synthesis Proteoglycan release	Articular proteoglycan degradation
Fibroblasts	Proliferation Prostaglandin and collagenase production CSF induction	
Synoviocytes	Prostaglandin and collagenase production	
Muscle	Proteolysis	Proteolysis

Table 10.1 (*Contd*)

Cell type	*In vitro*	*In vivo*
Vascular tissue		
Endothelial cells	Proliferation Prostaglandin production Procoagulant activity CSF induction	
Vascular smooth muscle	IL 1 production in response to IL 1	
Other effects		
Cytotoxic/cytostatic	To pancreatic beta islet and some transformed cells Eosinophil degranulation Keratinocyte proliferation	Increased insulin production Induces slow-wave sleep Causes hyoptension Increases steroid levels Increases survival in immune suppressed mice Suppresses appetite Increases sodium excretion Increases cardiac output Hypercalcaemia

IL 1 GENES AND GENE REGULATION

In 1984 the nucleotide sequence for a murine IL 1 cDNA was reported[8]. This clone encoded a 270 amino acid polypeptide precursor lacking a signal peptide with a predicted molecular weight of 31 kD. This protein was processed to form a 17 kD acidic (pI 5.0) mature peptide. This was followed by the cloning of a human monocytic cDNA clone[9] that encoded a 269 amino acid (30.7 kD) precursor also lacking a signal sequence. Cleavage of this propeptide resulted in the formation of a biologically active 17 kD neutral (pI 7.0 peptide). The two nucleotide sequences revealed a 20% homology at the peptide level and 45% at the nucleotide level. A second human IL 1 gene was then cloned[10]; this cDNA encoded a 271 amino acid (30.6 kD) propeptide which was proteolytically cleaved to give a 17.5 kD mature acidic (pI 5.0) molecule. This molecule was found to have a 62% homology to the mouse pI 5.0 IL 1, and was therefore given the name IL 1 alpha (IL 1α), the neutral form was called IL 1β (Table 10.2).

IL 1α and beta have now been characterized at the gene level, and both genes are localized on the long arm of chromosome 2 in the same

Table 10.2 Molecular characteristics of human IL 1

	IL 1α	*IL 1β*
Gene location	Chromosome 2 q13	Chromosome 2 q13–q21
Gene structure	12 kb, 7 exons	9.7 kb, 7 exons
mRNA	2.2 kb	1.6 kb
Propeptide	271aa, 30.6 kD	269aa, 30.7 kD
Mature peptide	159aa, 17.5 kD	153aa, 17.3 kD

chromosomal region (q13–q21)[11,12]. The two genes have a similar overall structure with seven exons and six introns. The human IL 1α gene is 12 kb long[13] and has a similar structural organization to the murine IL 1β gene[14]. The human IL 1β gene[15] spans a 7.5 kb region. Analysis of the two human genes shows that both have comparable exon length and splice site locations; it has therefore been proposed that the IL 1β gene arose by duplication (retrotransposition) of the IL 1α gene[15]. Analysis of the IL 1 genomic sequences identifies many potential regulatory regions; in addition, the conservation of intron structure between the two genes suggests that these may be involved in gene control. Interestingly, in the case of the IL 1α gene the typical TATA box and CAAT box have not been found in the region immediately upstream from the transcription initiation site, but TATA-like sequences can be found further upstream[13]. A 16 bp sequence homologous to the adenovirus 2 major late promoter transcription factor (MLTF) binding site has been identified in the 5′ region of the IL 1α gene; however, the significance of this homology is poorly understood. Other potential regulatory regions include a tandem repeat of a 46 bp sequence in the 6th intron of IL 1α. This repeat contains a glucocorticoid receptor binding site and the binding site of the transcription factor SPI, an enhancer element also found in the immunoglobulin tissue-specific enhancer. Interestingly, this region has been shown to be polymorphic[16], and this may underlie the cause of variable IL-1 production reported among human monocyte cultures[17].

In contrast, the human IL 1β gene has a well-defined TATA box at position −31 and CAAT boxes at positions −75 and −126, which may explain why IL 1β is transcribed more efficiently than IL 1α. Other potential regulatory regions contained within the IL 1β gene include several viral enhancer-like core sequences, a glucocorticoid regulatory element and a binding site for SPI-like transcription factors[15]. Comparison of the two published IL 1β genomic sequences reveals that they differ at eight separate sites in the 5′ regulatory region[15,18], and work performed in our laboratory[28] indicates that these sites show independent variability within the population. Other studies have shown abnormal IL 1β gene regulation associated with chromosomal rearrangements[19].

Pro IL 1β cytoplasmic mRNA is rapidly induced in human peripheral blood monocytes or monocytic cell lines such as THP-1 when stimulated with lipopolysaccharide or phorbol esters, e.g. PMA. Message levels peak at 2–3 h, after which message rapidly falls to a low level[20]. This decrease results from a specific transcriptional repression of the gene 2 h after stimulation, probably mediated by a newly synthesized protein as cycloheximide results in superinduction and stabilization of message levels. In addition to being transcriptionally regulated IL 1 gene expression is also controlled at a post-transcriptional level. Pro IL 1β mRNA is stabilized when cells are stimulated with PMA, whereas the message has a much shorter half-life when induced by LPS[21]. In peripheral blood mononuclear cells IL 1β gene transcription occurs at a greater rate than IL 1α[22]; however, this is not true for all cell types, as in keratinocytes IL 1α transcription predominates[23]. Additionally, the high levels of IL 1β message seen in monocytic cells are probably also due to the greater stability of the mRNA[22] that may be conferred by small differences in the highly conserved AU-rich sequence common to the 3′ untranslated region of cytokine genes[24].

In vivo, IL 1 gene transcription is probably regulated by complex feedback. IL 1 stimulates adrenocorticotrophic hormone (ACTH) production either by a direct action on the anterior pituitary or by stimulating the release of corticotrophin releasing factor from the hypothalamus. IL 1 can enhance the expression of pro-opiomelanocortin, the precursor of both ACTH and the neuropeptide alpha-melanocyte stimulating hormone (α-MSH). Corticosteroids prevent IL 1 gene transcription when added to cells prior to stimulation; however, after transcription has taken place most of the down-regulatory effect of steroids occurs at the level of translation[25,26]. Prostaglandins and prostacyclins seem to have no effect on IL 1 gene transcription, but do block translation[27]. The role of arachidonate derivatives *in vivo* is poorly understood as *in vitro* PGE metabolites accumulate while *in vivo* efficient mechanisms exist to remove them. PGE-induced suppression of IL 1 translation is mediated via the induction of cAMP, which acts by an unknown mechanism.

IL1 BIOCHEMISTRY

The structures of the IL 1 proteins have been analysed by a number of groups. The initial crystal structure determination of the mature IL-1β[29] revealed a molecule composed of 12 β-strands interacting via a complex network of hydrogen bonds to form a barrel-like structure. The overall shape was described as a distorted tetrahedron, each face being triangular with hydrophobic side-chains filling the interior. A refinement of the model[30] from studies at higher resolution confirmed the original structure and also described a high degree of conservation of amino acids located at the interior. There was little clustering of invariant surface amino acids and so the definition of the area involved in receptor recognition was not possible. Other groups[31] showed a similar structural model with predominant β-strands and no α-helix. To account for the high affinity of IL 1 for its receptor it is proposed that a region of large surface area, containing several peptide segments, is necessary for receptor interaction.

The IL 1α crystal structure has also been reported[32] and shows a capped barrel-shaped molecule with similar topology to IL 1β. The N-terminal regions, however, are positioned differently, possibly explaining why the additional propeptide residues in the IL 1β precursor interfere with receptor binding. IL 1β propeptide has been examined using circular dichroism spectra[33]; the data suggest that both mature and precursor forms have similar secondary structure, the latter, though, having some alpha helical regions. The IL 1β propeptide may also have a more open tertiary structure, possibly accounting for its increased protease susceptibility in comparison to the mature form.

Considerable effort has gone into defining the functional domains within the IL-1 molecules. By introducing point mutations, various groups have shown that isolated amino acid changes may result in alterations in local protein structure, but in most cases overall folding and biological activity remain unchanged[34,35]. The histidine at position 30 of IL 1β[36] is important in stabilizing part of the protein structure, while a mutation of Arg 127 to a glycine significantly reduces IL 1β bioactivity with a lesser disruption in receptor binding[37].

Muteins with enhanced activity have been produced[38], these may be due to altered stability or differences in interactions with the receptor molecule. Other mutations that disrupt activity are probably due to disruption of tertiary structure[30]. Truncated IL 1 molecules tested for biological activity mostly show that the loss of a few N or C terminal amino acids considerably reduces the function of both IL 1α and IL 1β[39–41] and this may be due to disruption of the barrel-like structure of the folded molecule[31], as antibodies to the C terminal do not affect receptor binding[42]. Other studies show that monoclonal antibodies binding to regions 133–148 and 351–269 inhibit IL 1β-mediated thymocyte proliferation and fibroblast prostaglandin production[43].

PRODUCTION AND PROCESSING OF IL 1

IL 1α and IL 1β are both produced as 31 kD molecular weight precursors that are cleaved at specific sites to produce the mature molecules. Incorrect processing, leaving or deleting extra amino acids, results in reduced bioactivity[44]. Most work has focused on the cleavage of IL 1β, as the propeptide has little biological or receptor binding activity[45]. The pro IL 1β molecule has 269 amino acids and is processed to the 153 amino acid mature form at the Asp 116–Ala 117[46]. Near the proteolytic site a short sequence of polybasic residues comparable to known processing sites on other prohormones is present. The bond cleaved in the IL 1β precursor is an uncommon substrate for many proteolytic enzymes, being preceded by valine, histidine and aspartate[44]. As mature 17 kD IL 1β is rarely found intracellularly it has been suggested that a cell surface or secreted enzyme is responsible for proteolytic cleavage. However, attempts to isolate the processing enzyme have identified proteolytic activity in both membrane and cytosolic preparations[47,44]. The cytosolic processing activity results in the correct cleavage product as determined by N-terminal sequencing, and increases the bioactivity of the pro IL 1β preparation. In inflammatory disease, enzymes present in exudate fluids may cleave pro IL 1β to a biologically active form[48]. The specificity of this processing activity was not determined, but enzymes such as elastase, collagenase and cathepsin G were all able to increase the level of processed IL 1β.

IL 1 intracellular bioactivity generally exceeds extracellular activity following LPS stimulation[49]. Studies concerning kinetics of IL 1 protein production and release demonstrate that IL 1α is predominantly cell-associated, 95% being retained within the cell, 18 h after stimulation. IL 1β, however, accumulates within the cell during the first 2 h of culture and is then released, resulting in high extracellular levels[50]. Considerable cellular accumulation of IL 1β immunoreactivity is often seen even when substantial secretion occurs; much of this may be the biologically inactive 31 kD propeptide[51]. The presence of unprocessed 31 kD IL 1 in culture supernatants has strengthened the notion that an enzyme responsible for cleavage is either located at the cell surface or is secreted by the cell[44].

Little is known about the mechanisms involved in the secretion of IL 1 from the cell, as neither IL 1 molecule has a recognizable hydrophobic signal sequence[10]. It has been suggested that a 17-residue N-terminal hydrophobic region may substitute for this function[52]. Various studies show that IL 1 molecules are not present in the ER, Golgi or secretory vesicles[53], whereas fusion of a characteristic leader sequence onto the IL 1β molecule results in high levels of secreted, correctly processed IL 1β[54]. Other workers, however, have been unable to achieve secretion from *E. coli* even when a signal region was fused to the IL 1β molecule[55].

A number of secretory pathways for IL 1 have been proposed. The presence of membrane IL 1 has resulted in the theory that a membrane-linked intermediate may play a role in the release of IL 1α[56]; the mechanism of membrane association may involve a lectin-like interaction[57]. However, the existence of membrane IL 1 is controversial and may be due to leakage of IL 1 precursor molecules from the cell following insufficient paraformaldehyde fixation in these experiments[58]. Protein modification may play a role in IL 1 secretion, and it has been shown that the IL 1 propeptides may be covalently linked to myristic acid[59]. Myristylation is thought to occur co-translationally, and directs proteins to the plasma membrane. Phosphorylation may also provide localization signals since LPS stimulation of macrophages results in increased phosphorylation of a number of proteins. IL 1 propeptide phosphorylation has been identified on residue Ser 90 in IL 1α which was phosphorylated to a 10-fold higher level than IL 1β[60]. Phosphate-labelled IL 1α may localize to the lysosomes and be cleaved and secreted from these organelles. The observed association of pro IL-1β with tubulin has led to the proposal that direct transport to the cell surface may be mediated by the microtubular network[61]. Evidence for a novel pathway for IL 1 secretion has been suggested[62], proposing that IL 1 is selectively located within intracellular vesicles that are part of the endocytic pathway. These fuse with the plasma membrane in a temperature- and calcium-dependent manner and propeptide molecules are cleaved upon release. A transporter mechanism that might direct IL 1β to this secretory pathway has yet to be defined. An involvement of calcium in IL 1 secretion has also been suggested[63] after the finding that calcium ionophores enhance release and processing.

CELLULAR SOURCES AND INDUCERS OF IL 1

Many cell types have been shown to produce IL 1, the most studied being the peripheral blood monocyte. However, a wide range of more specialized cell types such as T and B lymphocytes, smooth muscle, endothelial and various brain cells are capable of synthesizing IL 1. The cellular sources and stimulants of IL 1 production are summarized in Tables 10.3 and 10.4.

Interestingly, the amount of IL 1α and IL 1β varies between different cell types. In blood monocytes stimulated with LPS, IL 1β mRNA is found to be 10–50 times more abundant than IL 1α mRNA[10]. However, total IL 1α

Table 10.3 Cellular sources of IL 1

Mononuclear phagocytes	*Skin cells*
Blood monocytes	Langerhans cells
Lung and peritoneal macrophages	Keratinocytes
Synovial cells	
Kupffer's cells	*Brain cells*
Bone marrow macrophages	Astrocytes
Myelomonocytic leukemia cells	Microglia
Lymphocytes	*Other sources*
CD4 positive memory T cells	Corneal epithelial cells
B cells	Gingival exudate cells
Natural killer cells	Renal mesangial cells
Acute T cell leukaemia cells	Fibroblasts
	Neutrophils
Vascular cells	Chondrocytes
Endothelial cells	Dendritic cells
Smooth muscle cells	Noradrenergic neural cells

Table 10.4 Inducers of IL 1 production

Microbial	*Plant lectins*
Viruses	Concanavalin A
Bacteria	Phytohaemagglutinin
Spirochetes	
Yeasts	*Cytokines*
Endotoxins (Gram-negative bacteria)	IL 1
Exotoxins (staphylococci, streptococci)	GM-CSF
Peptidoglycans	TGF-β
	TNF-α
Non-infectious agents	IFN-α, IFN-β
Urate crystals	
Silica	
Asbestos	
Bile salts	

protein often exceeds that of IL 1β[64,50], and this presumably reflects differential translational efficiency or protein stability. Acute T cell leukaemia (ATL) cell lines have also been shown to produce IL 1[65,66]; however, the biological activity produced was only neutralized with anti-IL 1α, and IL 1β mRNA was undetectable. In keratinocytes, cells that make up 95% of the human epidermis, both IL 1α and IL 1β are produced after appropriate stimulation[23,67]; however, unlike blood monocytes, IL 1α mRNA predominates and the protein is effectively translocated into the extracellular medium.

IL 1 RECEPTORS

The 80 kD IL 1 receptor

The IL 1 receptor (IL 1R) was first characterized on a murine T lymphoma[68]. The studies revealed an 80 kD protein with a ligand affinity of 2×10^{-10} mol/L. Receptor number was estimated to be approximately 500 per cell, although higher receptor levels were found on cells of the fibroblast lineage. Further work revealed that the molecule bound both 17 kD IL 1α and IL 1β with a similar affinity[69,70], explaining the almost identical biological activities of the two molecules. Biochemical analysis of the receptor revealed the presence of considerable *N*-linked sugar residues, with *N*-glycanase treatment reducing the molecular weight to 62 kD[71]. Interestingly, the 80 kD IL 1R binds the IL 1α propeptide but not the IL 1β propeptide[72], explaining why the IL 1β precursor has no biological activity. Subsequently the murine 80 kD IL 1R was cloned by direct expression from a murine T cell thymoma cDNA library[73]. The cDNA encodes a protein with a molecular weight of 64.6 kD, a similar size to that estimated following *N*-glycanase treatment. The N-terminal, extracellular domain is composed of 319 amino acids and has seven potential *N*-linked glycosylation sites and contains three immunoglobulin-like domains. The transmembrane region consists of 21 hydrophobic amino acids, while the cytoplasmic domain has 217 residues including a potential protein kinase C phosphorylation site. Purification of the IL 1 receptor protein and microsequencing of proteolytically generated fragments, confirmed the identity of the cloned molecule[73]. Transfection of the IL 1R cDNA into Chinese hamster ovary cells resulted in expression of IL 1R that conferred functional responsiveness to IL 1. Additionally, deletion of the cytoplasmic domain led to expression of high-affinity binding sites for IL 1 but little biological activity[74]. Expression of a cDNA clone encoding only the extracellular region of the receptor resulted in the production of a soluble IL 1R that retained binding activity indistinguishable from the full-length IL 1R[75]. The murine IL 1R cDNA was subsequently used to clone the human T cell IL 1R[76]. The human and mouse receptors show a high degree of sequence conservation with the mature molecules possessing a 69% amino acid homology and 75% nucleotide homology. In addition the IL 1R expressed in human fibroblasts was found to be identical to that expressed in T cells confirming the original finding of similarity between the two molecules[77].

THE 60 kD IL 1 RECEPTOR

A lower molecule weight IL 1R was first described in a human Epstein–Barr virus (EBV) transformed B cell line[78]. The molecular weight was estimated to be 60 kD and although the receptor bound both IL 1α and IL 1β, the affinity for IL 1α was significantly lower. Further reports have shown that this receptor may preferentially bind IL 1β; however, other reports show both high- and low-affinity receptors for IL 1α and B cells[80]. In general the 60 kD receptor appears to have a lower affinity for IL 1 than the 80 kD receptor; this is probably due to a lower association and higher dissociation rate[81].

The 60 kD IL 1R is a distinct gene product from the 80 kD molecule as antibodies specific for the 80 kD receptor do not recognize the smaller molecule and the mRNA for the 80 kD receptor is not found in B cells either by Northern analysis or S1 nuclease protection assay[82,83]. Therefore, the

80 kD IL 1R has been designated type I IL 1R, and the 60 kD IL 1R is known as type II IL 1R. Type I IL 1R are predominantly found on T cells and fibroblasts, whereas type II IL 1R are found on B cells and monocytes, although some cells possess both receptor forms[84].

The two receptors not only differ in their kinetics of binding but also exhibit differences in the internalization and intracellular processing of IL 1[85]. Cells possessing type II IL 1R internalize little of the bound IL 1 (~15%) and a large percentage of the internalized IL 1 is subsequently degraded. In contrast, type I receptor-bearing cells internalize much more of the bound IL 1 which remains intact[85]. The degradation of IL 1 in type II receptor-bearing cells is inhibited in the presence of the lysomotropic agent, chloroquine. Therefore, the pathways for internalization, intracellular trafficking and processing of internalized IL 1 are different for the two receptors. This could obviously have consequences for subsequent IL 1 action and regulation of receptor levels on the cell surface.

SOLUBLE IL 1R

Many cell surface cytokine receptors are known to exist in soluble form and release from the cell surface occurs by two distinct mechanisms. Alternative splicing of the primary RNA transcript can result in protein isoforms that lack transmembrane domains and are therefore secreted, e.g. IL 4R[86]. Proteolytic cleavage of the transmembrane molecule at the cell surface, e.g. IL 2R (p55)[87], may also lead to receptor shedding. Other cytokine receptors that exist in soluble form include those for IL 2 (p75), IL 5, IL 6, IL 7, IFN, TNF (p55 and p75), epidermal growth factor (EGF) and M-CSF.

We have recently described a soluble binding protein specific for IL 1β present in normal human plasma[88], serum, synovial inflammatory exudate, activated blood mononuclear cell supernatants[89] and supernatants of the human B cell line, Raji, a cell that possesses type II IL 1R[90]. Release of this protein is increased by treatment of B cells with dexamethyasone, an agent that stimulates cell surface IL 1R expression and by cholorquine which causes increased IL 1R expression by preventing internalization. Conversely, culture of B cells with the serine protease inhibitor aprotinin, prevents release of the soluble binding protein and, at the same time, increases the level of cell surface IL 1R expression.

Together our data indicate that the soluble IL 1β binding protein is probably a proteolytically cleaved form of a surface IL 1R.

Interestingly, not all cell lines possessing type II IL 1R produce a soluble IL 1 binding protein. Cells possessing type II IL 1R proteins that bind IL 1α and IL 1β with equal affinity, e.g. the macrophage cell lines U937 and P388D_1 and the B cell line 70Z/3, do not release a sIL 1R, whereas cells possessing a type II IL 1R that discriminates between IL 1α and IL 1β, e.g. Raji and COS-7 (a monkey kidney fibroblast), release a 47 kD soluble receptor. This suggests that type II IL 1R may show some form of heterogeneity, or that a third type of IL-1R exists.

IL 1 SIGNAL TRANSDUCTION

Despite the cloning of the type I IL 1R, the mechanism whereby IL 1 transduces a signal to the nucleus of responsive cells has remained poorly defined. A growing number of reports indicate that various second messengers can be induced by IL 1. Some type I IL 1R-bound IL 1 appears to be translocated to the nucleus[91], and IL 1 receptors have been found on nuclear membranes[92]. These receptors show similar binding kinetics to those of the plasma membrane receptor. Therefore internalization and nuclear localization of IL 1 may play a role in the regulation of target gene transcription. However, the cellular response to IL 1 occurs within minutes of cell surface ligand receptor interaction. It would therefore seem likely that second messengers are involved. In a murine T lymphoma line, IL 1 does not cause translocation of protein kinase C or elevation of intracellular calcium[93]. In a human T cell line, IL 1 causes a rapid increase in diacylglycerol and phosphorylcholine levels, but no increase in inositol triphosphate[94]. In contrast IL 1 increases levels of diacylglycerol and phosphoryl ethanolamine rapidly in glomerular mesangial cells, but has no effect on levels of intracellular calcium, phosphorylcholine or inositol triphosphate[95]. Other groups have shown that IL 1 stimulates serine phosphorylation of a cytosolic 65 kD protein[96]. Saklatvala and co-workers[97,98] have shown that IL 1 stimulates progressive serine/threonine phosphorylation of a triad of 27 kD cytosolic heat shock proteins and the epidermal growth factor receptor, independently of protein kinase C. Recent studies of the type I IL 1R reveal that phosphorylation of the receptor occurs within 1 min of ligand binding via the activation of a protein serine/threonine kinase[99]. Shirakawa *et al.*[100] have shown that cAMP accumulates in several cell types in response to IL 1, and this accumulation may be mediated by a G-protein[101]. Similar results have been obtained with human fibroblasts[102].

Type II IL 1R have also been shown to be functional, as IL 1 mediates activation of kappa gene transcription and hence surface IgM expression in the pre-B cell line 70Z/3[103]. IL 1-induced kappa expression is associated with stimulation of Na^+/H^+ exchange and activation of protein kinase C; however, these events are insufficient to trigger kappa expression and transient increases in cAMP may also play an important role[104]. Recently, the mechanism whereby IL 1 activates IL 2 gene transcription has been elucidated. This appears to involve induction of C.Jun with a subsequent cjun/cfos complex binding to an Ap-1-like binding site in 5′ flanking DNA of the IL 2 gene[105]. Activation of NFkB-like factor by IL 1 has also been implicated in the IL 1 induction of acute phase protein target gene such as serum amyloid A[106].

ROLE OF IL 1 AS AN INFLAMMATORY MEDIATOR

Fever and the acute phase response

Fever is most commonly associated with infection; however, non-infectious causes such as inflammation, neoplasia and immune-mediated disease may also result in fever. Pyrogens, the substances that cause fever, may be derived from external sources, i.e. microbial products, toxins or intact microorganisms, or may be endogenous. IL 1 is now recognized as the likely major component of 'endogenous pyrogen' (EP). However, other cytokines such as the interferons, tumour necrosis factors and IL 6 also show pyrogenic activity[107]. Pyrogenic cytokines are thought to cause fever by their ability to alter the function of the hypothalamic thermoregulatory centre, of which the synthesis of PGE_2 has been proposed as important. In this model the antipyretic effect of aspirin would derive from its ability to inhibit the synthesis of cytokine-induced prostaglandins in the hypothalamus. The interaction of IL 1 with the hypothalamus is poorly understood, but it is likely that the production of PGE_2 is derived from the vascular endothelium in the capillaries surrounding the hypothalmus. In addition to PGE_2 production IL 1 induces many other changes in endothelial cells, including expression of adhesion molecules such as ICAM-1 and ELAM-1 and secretion of soluble factors including colony-stimulating factors, platelet activating factor and factors inhibiting fibrinolysis. Systemic injection of IL 1 leads to changes similar to those seen on injection of microbial toxins. Intravenous administration of human recombinant IL 1 results in a decrease in circulating neutrophils after 5 min; 10 min after injection core body temperature begins to rise, reaching a peak between 45 and 55 min after injection[108]. Increases in slow-wave sleep parallel the fever course, but this is independent of the increase in body temperature. Four to six hours after injection, temperature and sleep patterns return to normal; however, an increase in circulating neutrophils is observed. When large amounts of IL-1 (2 μg/kg) are administered a decrease in systemic arterial pressure, systemic vascular resistance and central venous pressure can be observed within 10 min[109].

With the advent of immunoassays for pyrogenic cytokines it has been possible to measure the levels of these factors in the plasma of febrile patients. In human volunteers injected with endotoxin, peak fever occurs after 4 h. Plasma IL 1β concentrations rise slowly, reaching their peak at 3 h[110]. In septic patients or patients receiving high-dose IL 2 therapy peak plasma IL 1 levels also do not correlate with peak fever. These differences may reflect some of the technical difficulties that still exist in the measurement of plasma IL 1. IL 1 may bind to plasma proteins such as $alpha_2$ macroglobulin[111] or the soluble IL 1R[88] and these may mask immunoreactive epitopes. Also circulating IL 1 appears to be rapidly cleared from the circulation, either by cell surface receptors or by excretion in the urine.

IL 1 and the acute phase response

Factors leading to fever elicit a host response referred to as the 'acute phase response'. The most characteristic feature of this response is the change in hepatic protein synthesis which includes the clotting factors, complement components and fibrinogen. In addition, synthesis of a number of proteins not normally found in the healthy state occurs. Two such proteins, serum amyloid A (SAA) protein and C-reactive protein, are classical 'acute phase reactants'. In addition, hepatic synthesis of albumin and transferrin decreases, and these are called negative acute phase reactants. Whereas fever is a very obvious sign of the acute phase response, these other components may be present without clinical manifestations.

The evolutionary conservation of the acute phase response argues that, like fever, it plays a crucial role in survival. The acute phase proteins themselves are a heterogeneous group of inflammatory mediators, protease inhibitors and immunoregulatory molecules. The role of most acute phase proteins is unclear; however, C-reactive protein may opsonize pneumococci or bind serum lipids, whereas SAA is thought to be immunosuppressive. Others, such as ceruloplasmin, may scavenge oxygen free-radicals.

Injection of IL 1 into mice results in the rapid increase in levels of SAA[112]. Maximal SAA levels occur after 4–12 h, suggesting that IL 1 acts by direct interaction with hepatocytes. IL 1 has also been shown to increase the expression of C3, factor B and alpha-acid glycoprotein in hepatocytes[113]. IL 1 also suppresses the synthesis of albumin in cultured hepatocytes. However, it would appear that IL 1 only induces a limited number of acute phase reactants and can even suppress the synthesis of acute phase proteins such as fibrinogen and alpha$_2$-macroglobulin[114]. Recent work has revealed that IL 1 is probably not the major regulator of acute phase protein synthesis. A factor previously known as interferon β_2, hybridoma growth factor, 26 kD protein and B cell-stimulating factor 2 and now known as IL 6[115], appears to be the major acute phase protein inducer. Additionally, IL 1 and IL 6 synergize in the induction of several acute phase reactants and, importantly, IL 1 is one of the most potent inducers of IL 6 production[116].

THE ROLE OF IL 1 IN CHRONIC INFLAMMATION

Rheumatoid arthritis

IL 1 has been implicated as an important mediator in a number of inflammatory diseases; however, particular attention has been directed at the role of IL 1 in inflammatory joint diseases such as rheumatoid arthritis. Rheumatoid arthritis (RA) can be defined as a chronic synovitis affecting predominantly non-axial joints. The disease has a prolonged course with intermittent acute exacerbations and remissions, accompanied by a general systemic inflammatory response. RA is characterized by swelling of the synovial membrane and periarticular soft tissues, subchondral osteoporosis, erosion of articular cartilage and bone, and wasting of associated muscles. There is a higher incidence in women and onset occurs from early childhood onwards. The presence of abnormal immunoglobulins in many patients – autoantibodies (usually IgM) that bind IgG and form inflammatory immune complexes – has led to the idea that RA may be associated with an inappropriate response to exogenous or endogenous antigens. In addition a family history of the disease is often seen and well-documented association with the HLA-DR4 haplotype, indicating that a genetic component plays an important role in the disease. As yet no infectious agent has been consistently demonstrated in RA, although there is growing circumstantial evidence that a microbial agent may be responsible for initiating the disease. The treatment of RA is predominantly symptomatic; non-steroidal anti-inflammatory agents which suppress prostaglandin production being most commonly used. However, these agents fail to correct the underlying abnormality, and more potent non-specific, suppressive agents such as steroids, immunosuppressives, gold salts and antimalarials are often used.

IL 1 and bone

IL 1 is one of the most potent bone-resorbing agents, with much-documented activity on both neonatal murine calavarial and fetal rat long bones[117]. Bone-resorbing agents initially cause osteoclast precursor cells to fuse, forming activated mature osteoclasts. These then form resorption pits on the bone surface. It is thought that IL 1 may stimulate osteoblasts to produce a soluble factor that is responsible for osteoclast activation[118]. Osteoclasts degrade the bone by generating a low pH environment containing lysosomal proteinases. IL 1-induced prostaglandins may also play a role in bone resorption[119]; however, inhibition of prostaglandin synthesis only causes partial inhibition of IL-induced bone resorption[117], and it is likely that prostaglandins enhance bone resorption via actions on osteoblasts rather than osteoclasts.

IL 1 and cartilage

Cartilage consists of a single cell type (chondrocytes) embedded in a matrix of proteoglycans, collagen and water. By retaining water, proteoglycans exert a swelling pressure that enables the tissue to resist compression. The actions of IL 1 have been investigated predominantly in organ cultures where IL 1 causes a dose-dependent release of proteoglycan that is dependent on the presence of live chondrocytes[120]. IL 1 also inhibits the production of new cartilage proteoglycan via inhibition of protein synthesis. The mechanism of IL 1-induced proteoglycan breakdown is still uncertain; however, proteolytic enzymes are implicated, especially the secreted metalloproteinase stromelysin whose production is stimulated by IL 1[120]. Tumour necrosis factor is the only other cytokine able to stimulate proteoglycan breakdown; however, it is about 10-fold less potent than IL 1.

IL 1 and fibrosis

In contrast to its catabolic activities described above, IL 1 increases fibroblast proliferation[77] and collagen synthesis. IL 1 effects on cellular proliferation are influenced by prostaglandin production and large amounts of PGE_2 produced by some fibroblasts may inhibit proliferation. Indeed IL 1-induced fibroblast and smooth muscle cell proliferation is often unobservable unless cyclooxygenase inhibitors are present[121]. The characterization of IL 1 as a factor stimulating PGE_2 production from synovial fibroblasts was first described by Dayer and co-workers[122,123]. The PGE_2 produced by fibroblasts may have an important role in local joint inflammation observed in RA, causing local vasolidatation and enhancing the effect of pain mediators such as bradykinin and substance P.

IL 1 also stimulates the synthesis of metalloproteinases such as collagenase, stromelysin and gelatinase from synovial fibroblasts. These enzymes are secreted as proenzymes that can be subsequently activated by proteinases such as trypsin. Besides causing increased secretion of metalloproteinases, IL 1 augments production of tissue inhibitor of metalloproteinases in the synovial joint and is associated with the extracellular degradation of matrix polymers such as proteoglycans and collagen. Collagen degradation may also be mediated by lysosomal proteinases but the relative contribution of each pathway in inflammation is poorly understood.

Local effects of IL 1 in the joint

The availability of highly purified recombinant IL 1 has allowed the evaluation of IL 1 as a mediator of inflammation *in vivo*. Human IL 1α and IL 1β induced polymorphonuclear leukocyte (PMN) accumulation when injected into the rabbit knee joint[124], and neutrophil accumulation is a common finding in RA synovial fluid. After a single injection of IL 1 into the joint cavity both PMN and monocytes accumulate, with the peak occurring 6 h after injection. Infiltration of the synovial membrane by monocytes also occurs. Although TNF was a weak stimulator of leukocyte infiltration, when co-administered with IL 1 a marked synergy was observed. Single injections of IL 1 result only in acute synovitis; however, repeated injections, especially in animals pretreated with streptococcal peptidoglycan–polysaccharide fragments, leads to pannus formation (chronic synovial proliferation) in 50% of animals[125]. The mechanism of IL 1-induced PMN accumulation appears not to involve changes in vascular permeability as rabbit knee joints injected with IL 1 exhibit no evidence of swelling or histological evidence of oedema. IL 1 probably causes leukocyte infiltration by its action on the endothelium inducing the expression of adhesion proteins and by induction of chemotactic peptides, of which IL 8 is a likely candidate, having been detected at high levels in some RA effusions[126].

Prostaglandins are considered important mediators of pain (hyperalgesia) in the joint since they potentiate the pain-producing effects of histamine and bradykinin. Obviously, IL 1, with its potent effects on PGE_2 production, probably contributes to this; however, it has been demonstrated that IL 1β is also a potent PGE_2-independent hyperalgesic agent when injected into the rat paw[127]. IL 1α was also active but was 3000 times less potent. The IL 1-induced hyperalgesia was only partially inhibited by cyclooxygenase inhibitors, and other studies have demonstrated no role for PGE_2 in IL 1-induced hyperalgesia[128].

Intra-articular injection of IL 1 also causes proteoglycan degradation in rabbits[124]. This cartilage damage occurred independently of leukocyte infiltration as proteoglycan degradation also occurred in leukopenic animals.

Cartilage explants from these animals produced large quantities of both collagenase and stromolysin. Infusions of IL 1α also have been shown to induce osteoclast activation and bone resorption in the rat[129].

IL 1 IN RHEUMATOID ARTHRITIS

Correlation of IL 1 concentration and inflammation

Given the *in-vivo* and *in-vitro* activities of IL 1 it is not surprising that IL 1 was implicated as a possible pathogenic mediator in RA. Initial reports of IL 1 bioactivity in synovial fluid appeared in the early 1980s; however, previously, in 1968, Bodel and Hollingsworth[130] had detected EP activity in inflammatory synovial exudates, some of which would have been due to IL 1. The early demonstrations of IL 1 in joint fluid required fractionation before the sample yielded reliable measurements[131]. It was, however, possible to demonstrate that mononuclear cells isolated either from the synovial fluid[132] or synovial membrane[133] produced biologically active IL 1 *in vitro*. The bioassays were unable to distinguish between IL 1α and IL 1β, and were often inhibited by biological fluids, so it was not until the development of specific immunoassays that the measurement of *ex-vivo* IL 1 became possible. However, technical problems still occurred and it apears that IL 1 is carried in the circulation bound to a number of soluble binding proteins. These may mask the epitopes recognized by the antibodies used in the immunoassays. As noted previously, two proteins known to bind IL 1β in the plasma are α_2-macroglobulin[111] and the soluble IL 1R[88]. Due to the presence of these and other interfering substances a number of extraction procedures have been developed that probably exposed antibody recognition sites. Cannon *et al.*[134] have developed a chloroform extraction procedure that results in the appearance of both bioactive and immunoreactive IL 1α and IL 1β with a molecular weight below 30 kD.

We used the Cannon extraction protocol on plasma samples, collected into EDTA with protease inhibitors, from patients with RA and from controls. The extracted samples were subsequently tested for IL 1α and IL 1β using specific immunoassays. The mean plasma level of IL 1β was significantly higher in patients with RA than in healthy controls of similar age. Using standard clinical and laboratory measurements of disease activity, significant cross-sectional correlations were found between plasma IL 1β and pain score, joint tenderness, erythrocyte sedimentation rate and haemoglobin concentration[135]. No such correlations were found cross-sectionally in a group of RA patients tested for plasma IL 1α[136]. There were, however, significant correlations between the indices of inflammation and both forms of IL 1 within individual patients with active disease who were tested at regular intervals over a 4–5-week period[136]. Both forms of IL 1 have been identified in the synovial fluid (SF) of patients with rheumatic diseases[137,138] using immunoassay, but significant correlations with disease activity were not found[138]. To overcome this problem, SF from patients with symmetrical and asymmetrical knee joint inflammation were studied[139]. In patients with symmetrical joint involvement almost identical levels of IL 1β were detected in the right and left knee joints. In contrast, in patients exhibiting asymmetrical knee joint involvement, IL 1β levels in the inflamed joints were significantly higher than in the contralateral joints, indicating that inflammation in an individual joint is related to the local concentration of IL 1β.

IL 1 mRNA in the rheumatoid joint

To understand the pathogenic mechanisms of IL 1 in RA it is important to define the cellular source(s) of IL 1 within the joint. The absence of IL 1 mRNA in resting blood monocytes suggests that the gene is not constitutively expressed. However, following stimulation with endotoxin, IL 1 mRNA accumulates rapidly and IL 1 protein can be detected after 45 min[140]. Confirmation that IL 1 is produced locally within rheumatoid joint tissue has come from mRNA studies using Northern blotting and *in situ* hybridization.

Analysis of synovial tissue mRNA reveals a single 1.6 kb band that hybridizes an IL 1β probe and a 2.2 kb band hybridizing with an IL 1α probe[141] (Wood, Dickens, Symons and Duff, submitted for publication), demonstrating that each gene expresses a single transcript within RA synovial tissues. Although IL 1β is usually the predominant form in RA synovia, the ratio of β- to α-mRNA is reduced and sometimes reversed in some RA synovial extracts[141]. By using the techniques of *in situ* hybridization we have found that IL 1β mRNA-containing cells were more numerous than those expressing IL 1α in most RA synovial tissue sections[142]. Recently, using a concurrent *in situ* hybridization and cellular immunophenotyping technique we have demonstrated that the predominant cell type producing IL 1β mRNA in RA synovium is the CD14-positive macrophage. Cells expressing the IL 1β gene were especially frequent in the 'transitional' areas of the synovial membrane that contain macrophages, lymphocytes and plasma cells. Macrophages within the lining area also contained IL 1β mRNA. Other workers have used *in situ* hybridization techniques on enzymatically dispersed synovial tissue, synovial fluid mononuclear cells[143] and cultured primary synoviocytes[144]. The results revealed that IL 1β probe hybridized with cells located in stromal areas remote from lymphocyte-rich follicles. In dispersed synovial tissue approximately 10% of cells expressed detectable message for IL 1β, whereas IL 1β probe did not significantly hybridize with synovial fluid mononuclear cells. Fractionation of synovial tissue cells confirmed that the majority of IL 1β gene expressing cells were macrophages[143].

IL 1 and immune responses in the rheumatoid joint

In vitro experiments reveal that IL 1 plays an important role during the immune response. IL 1 augments the maturation and proliferation of both B and T cells and their differentiation into antibody-producing B cells or into lymphokine-producing T cells. IL 1 does not act as a direct growth factor for T cells, but enhances the production of the major T cell growth factor (IL 2) as well as the expression of the IL 2 receptors[145]. Interestingly, studies of both IL 2 and IL 1 using immunoassays to measure levels in RA synovial fluid demonstrated a significant correlation ($n = 31, r = 0.82, p < 0.001$) between IL 1$\beta$ and IL 2[137].

Human IL 2R are composed of two different polypeptide chains (p55 and p75) each capable of binding IL 2 with different affinity[146]. The p55 chain, also known as the Tac protein (CD25) can be shed from the cell membrane and can be detected in sera, SF and culture supernatants by ELISA[147]. Shedding of the soluble receptor occurs in proportion to its cell surface expression (i.e. immune cell activation) and therefore soluble IL 2 receptor (sIL 2R) concentration can be thought of as a measure of immune activation *in vivo*. In RA and many other inflammatory or immune-mediated diseases serum sIL 2R levels are raised compared to healthy controls[148]. Additionally SF levels of sIL 2R in RA correlate significantly ($n = 30$, $r = 0.62$, $p < 0.001$) with SF ILβ concentrations. The association of IL 2R and IL 1β is also found within the RA synovium. *In situ* localization of IL 1β and IL 2R (p55) using monoclonal antibodies on RA synovia demonstrates that both are expressed in the same cellular aggregates[149]. Taken together the evidence would suggest that IL 1, and particularly IL 1β, may play a role in the potentiation of IL 2 and IL 2R production within the synovium, and thus lead to increased immune-mediated inflammation.

IL 1 inhibitors and anti-inflammatory agents

Manipulation of IL 1 can be achieved at three distinct levels: induction, synthesis and secretion, and receptor binding/signal transduction. As yet the signals inducing IL 1 gene transcription and mRNA translation are poorly understood, and therefore it has been impossible to design a rational approach to specific inhibition of IL 1 gene transcription. However, inhibition of IL 1β protein production can be specifically inhibited by the use of antisense oligonucleotides[150]. Using antisense phosphorothioate oligonucleotides complementary to the 5′ untranslated and exon 6 regions of the IL 1β gene, IL 1β protein production was inhibited by 98% without any reduction in overall protein synthesis. Levels of IL 1α and TNF alpha production were also reduced in the cells to which IL 1β antisense oligonucleotides had been added, this may be related to IL 1β inhibition. This approach could have therapeutic potential assuming that correct delivery and stability of the antisense reagents can be achieved or, alternatively, they could be used to model bioavailable synthetic agents.

Processing of IL 1β activates it from an inactive precursor, and this takes place at the same time or shortly after secretion. Inhibition of this may therefore lead to down regulation of IL 1 activity. The proteolytic enzymes responsible for IL 1β processing are currently being characterized[44]. A number of non-specific protease inhibitors have been shown to inhibit the *in vitro* processing of precursor IL 1β[151]; however, these are unlikely to be of therapeutic use. In our laboratory we have used synthetic peptides (spanning the cleavage site) as competitors for the processing enzyme(s). However, although secreted processing activity was inhibited by the synthetic peptide, membrane-associated processing activity was unaffected and it is possible that the peptide does not share the epitopes required for binding of the membrane enzyme. Synthetic peptides have previously been used successfully to inhibit the processing activity of the HIV 1 protease[152].

Much of the work directed towards specific IL 1 inhibition has focused on the interaction of IL 1 with its cell surface receptor, as this offers a specific target for pharmacological intervention. As yet there are no synthetic agents described that interfere with specific IL 1 binding. However, a number of natural products have been found that inhibit IL 1 receptor interaction.

Inhibitory activity towards IL 1 was originally identified in supernatants from mononuclear cells[153] and the urine of patients with monocytic leukemia and juvenile RA[154,155]. The mechanism of action was shown to be competitive antagonism of the IL 1R[156]. Subsequently, the IL 1 receptor antagonist (IL 1 ra) was purified to homogeneity[157], sequenced and cloned[158]. The gene encodes a 152 amino acid peptide that is glycosylated. The IL 1 ra exhibits 26% homology to IL 1β and 19% homology to IL 1α. The IL 1 ra has similar affinity for type 1 IL 1R as IL 1α and IL 1β, but it has no bioactivity and is therefore a pure receptor antagonist. The IL 1 ra does not appear to interact with type II IL 1R, and therefore only antagonizes IL 1 activities mediated via type I IL 1R found on T cells and fibroblasts. As well as antagonizing the *in vitro* activity of IL 1, for example, IL 1-induced bone resorption[159], the IL 1 ra reduces the lethality of both IL 1 and endotoxin-induced shock in rabbits[160]. As yet no human studies with the IL 1 ra have been reported, although they are in progress.

Another potential mechanism for IL 1 inhibition is the use of soluble IL 1 receptors that lack transmembrane and cytoplasmic domains. A soluble form of type I IL 1R has been constructed from a cDNA clone encoding the extracellular domain of type I IL 1R[75]. The soluble type I IL 1R (sIL 1R I) retains the binding properties of the full-length IL 1R. *In vitro* studies demonstrated that sIL 1R I can inhibit IL 1-induced B cell proliferation[161], while *in vivo* administration of sIL 1R I inhibited the rejection of heterotopic heart allografts, with survival being prolonged from 12 days in controls to 17 days in mice treated with sIL 1R I[162]. Inhibition was overcome by simultaneous administration of IL 1, indicating that the sIL 1R I acts by neutralizing IL 1.

Given the high affinity of the naturally occurring soluble IL 1R (sIL 1R II) for IL 1β, the molecule may function as a specific inhibitor of IL 1β *in vivo*. To test this we performed binding studies using EL-4 NOB.1, a T cell clone with a type I IL 1R and Raji cells that possess a type II IL 1R. The results showed that the sIL 1R II inhibited IL 1β binding to both cell lines in a dose-dependent fashion; however, IL 1α binding to EL-4 NOB.1 was not inhibited[163]. Similar results have been reported by other authors[164]; therefore, the natural sIL 1R may be useful in modulating the actions of IL 1β *in vivo*, especially where immunopathogenesis is associated specifically with IL 1β as seems to be the case, for example, with insulin secretion from pacreatic beta islets[165].

THE FUTURE

Though much information is now available on the basic biochemistry and biology of IL 1 this has not, as yet, shed much light on its role in normal homeostasis or in the mediation of chronic inflammatory diseases. Such questions may be resolved in the future with the development of transgenic animal models including those with disrupted IL 1 genes. Current work on polymorphic sequences in regulatory areas of IL 1 genes may well elucidate genetically determined aspects of the inflammatory response and important mechanisms in viral patheogenesis. Future developments in IL 1 biology, though perhaps not so prolific as in the past, should be much more informative in terms of its physiological and pathological significance.

References

1. Atkins, E. (1960). Pathogenesis of fever. *Physiol. Rev.*, **40**, 580–646
2. Kampschmidt, R. F. (1981). Leukocyte endogenous mediator/endogenous pyrogen. In Powanda, M. C. and Canonico, P. G. (eds), *The Physiologic and Metabolic Responses of the Host*, pp. 55–73 (Amsterdam: Elsevier)
3. Gery, I. and Waksman, B. H. (1972). Potentiation of the T lymphocyte response to mitogens II the celullar source of potentiating mediator(s). *J. Exp. Med.*, **136**, 143–55
4. Wood, D. D. and Cameron, P. M. (1976). Stimulation of the release of a B cell-activating factor from human monocytes. *Cell. Immunol.*, **21**, 88–96
5. Dewhirst, F. E., Stashenko, P. P., Mole, J. E. and Tsurumachi, T. (1985). Purification and partial sequence of human osteoclast activating factor: identity with interleukin 1 beta. *J. Immunol.*, **135**, 2562–8
6. Mizel, S. B., Dayer, J.-M., Krane, S. M. and Mergenhagen, S. E. (1981). Stimulation of rheumatoid synovial cell collagenase and prostaglandin production by partially purified lymphocyte-activating factor/interleukin-1). *Proc. Natl. Acad. Sci. USA*, **78**, 2474–7
7. Saklatvala, J. (1981). Characterisation of catabolin, the major product of pig synovial tissue that induces resorption of cartilage proteoglycan *in vitro*. *Biochem. J.*, **199**, 705–14
8. Lomedico, P. T., Gubler, U., Hellmann, C. P., Dukovich, M., Giri, J. G., Pan, Y.-C. E., Collier, K., Semionow, R., Chua, A. O. and Mizel, S. B. (1984). Cloning and expression of murine interleukin-1 cDNA in *E. coli*. *Nature*, **312**, 458–61
9. Auron, P. E., Webb, A. C., Rosenwasser, L. J., Mucci, S. F., Rich, A., Wolff, S. M. and Dinarello, C. A. (1984). Nucleotide sequence of human monocytic interleukin 1 precursor cDNA. *Proc. Natl. Acad. Sci. USA*, **82**, 7907–11
10. March, C. J., Moseley, B,., Larsen, A., Cerretti, D. P., Braedt, G., Price, V., Gillis, S., Henney, C. S., Kronheim, S. R., Grabstein, K., Conlon, P. J., Hopp, T. P. and Cosman, D. (1985). Cloning, sequence and expression of two distinct human interleukin-1 complementory DNAs. *Nature*, **315**, 641–7
11. Modi, W. S., Masuda, A., Yamada, M., Oppenheim, J. J., Matsushima, K. and O'Brien, S. J. (1988). Chromosomal localization of the human interleukin 1 alpha (IL-1 alpha) gene. *Genomics*, **2**, 310–14
12. Webb, A. C., Collins, K. L., Auron, P. E., Eddy, R. L., Nakai, H., Byers, M. G., Haley, L. L., Henry, W. M. and Shows, T. B. (1986), Interleukin 1 (IL-1) assigned to long arm of human chromosome 2. *Lymphokine Res.*, **5**, 77–85
13. Furutani, Y., Notake, M., Fukui, T., Ohue, M., Nomura, H., Yamada, M. and Nakamura, S. (1986). Complete nucleotide sequence of the gene for human interleukin 1 alpha. *Nucl. Acids Res.*, **14**, 3167–79
14. Telford, J. L., Macchia, G., Massone, A., Carina, V., Palla, E. and Melli, M. (1986). The murine interleukin 1 beta gene: structure and evolution. *Nucl. Acids Res.*, **14**, 9955–63
15. Clark, B. D., Collins, K. L., Gandy, M. S., Webb, A. C. and Auron, P. E. (1986). Genomic sequence for human prointerleukin 1 beta: possible evolution from a reverse transcribed prointerleukin 1 alpha gene. *Nucl. Acids Res.*, **14**, 7897–914

16. Hangen, A., Mann, D., Murray, C., Weston, A. and Willey, J. C. (1989). Interleukin 1 alpha gene intron containing variable repeat region coding for the SP1 Transcription Factor Recognition Sequence is polymorphic. *Mol. Carcinogen.*, **2**, 68–71
17. Molvig, J., Baek, L., Christensen, P., Manogue, R., Viassara, H., Platz, P., Nielsen, L. S., Svejgaard, A. and Nerup, J. (1988). Endotoxin-stimulated human monocyte secretion of interleukin I, tumor necrosis factor alpha and prostaglandin E_2 shows stable interindividual differences. *Scand. J. Immunol.*, **27**, 705–16
18. Bensi, G., Raugei, G., Palla, E., Carinci, V., Buonamassa, D. T. and Melli, M. (1987). Human interleukin-1 beta gene. *Gene*, **52**, 95–101
19. Silver, A., Boultwood, J., Breckon, G., Masson, W., Adam, J., Shaw, A. R., and Cox, R. (1989). Interleukin 1 beta deregulation associated with chromosomal rearrangement: a candidate initiating event for murine radiation-myeloid leukemogenesis? *Mol. Carcinog.*, **2**, 226
20. Fenton, M. J., Clark, B. D., Collins, K. L., Webb, A. C., Rich, A. and Auron, P. E. (1987). Transcriptional regulation of the human prointerleukin 1 beta gene. *J. Immunol.*, **138**, 3972–9
21. Fenton, M. J., Vermeulen, M. W., Clark, B. D., Webb, A. C. and Auron, P. E. (1988). Human pro-IL-1 beta gene expression in monocytic cells is regulated by two distinct pathways. *J. Immunol.*, **140**, 2267–73
22. Turner, M., Chantry, D., Buchan, G., Barrett, K. and Feldmann, M. (1989). Regulation of expression of human IL-1 alpha and IL-1 beta genes. *J. Immunol.*, **143**, 3556–61
23. Kupper, T. S., Ballard, D. W., Chua, A. O., McGuire, J. A., Flood, P. M., Horowitz, M. C., Langdon, R., Lightfoot, L. and Gubler, U. (1986). Human keratinocytes contain mRNA indistinguishable from monocyte interleukin 1 alpha and beta mRNA: keratinocytes epidermal cell-derived thymocyte activating factor is identical to interleukin 1. *J. Exp. Med.*, **164**, 2095–100
24. Shaw, G. and Kamen, R. (1986). A conserved AU sequence from the 3′ untranslated region of GM-CSF mRNA mediates selective mRNA degradation. *Cell*, **46**, 659–67
25. Knudsen, P. J., Dinarello, C. A. and Strom, T. B. (1987). Glucocorticoids inhibit transcriptional and post-transcriptional expression of interleukin 1 in U937 cells. *J. Immunol.*, **139**, 4129–34
26. Kern, J. A., Lamb, R. J., Reed, J. C., Daniels, R. P. and Nowell, P. C. (1988). Dexamethasone inhibition of interleukin 1 beta production by human monocytes: post-transcriptional mechanisms. *J. Clin. Invest.*, **81**, 237–44
27. Knudsen, P. J., Dinarello, C. A. and Strom, T. B. (1986). Prostaglandins post-transcriptionally inhibit monocyte expression of interleukin 1 activity by increasing intracellular cyclic adenosine monophosphate. *J. Immunol.*, **137**, 3189–94
28. Di Giovine, F. S., Takhsh, E., Sim, E., McDowell, T. L., Symons, J. A. and Duff, G. W. (1990). Genetic variation of interleukin 1 beta in RA. *Br. J. Rheumatol.*, **29**, 90A
29. Priestle, J. P., Schar, H.-P. and Grutter, M. G. (1988). Crystal structure of the cytokine interleukin-1 beta. *EMBO J.*, **7**, 339–43
30. Priestle, J. P., Schar, H.-P. and Grutter, M. G. (1989). Crystallographic refinement of interleukin 1 beta at 2.0 A resolution. *Proc. Natl. Acad. Sci.*, **86**, 9667–71
31. Frizel, B. C., Clancy, L. L., Holland, D. R., Muchmore, S. W., Watenpaugh, K. D. and Einspahr, H. M. (1989). Crystal structure of recombinant human interleukin 1 beta at 2.0 A resolution. *J. Mol. Biol.*, **209**, 779–91
32. Graves, B. J., Hatada, M. H., Hendrickson, W. A., Miller, J. K., Madison, V. S. and Satow, Y. (1990). Structure of interleukin 1 alpha at 2.7 A resolution. *Biochemistry*, **29**, 2679–84
33. Hazuda, D., Webb, R. L., Simon, P. and Young, P. (1989). Purification and characterisation of human recombinant precursor interleukin 1 beta. *J. Biol. Chem.*, **264**, 1689–93
34. Driscoll, P. C., Clore, G. M., Marion, D., Wingfield, P. T. and Gronenbom, A. M. (1990). Complete resonance assignment for the polypeptide backbone of interleukin 1 beta using three-dimensional heteronuclear NMR spectroscopy. *Biochemistry*, **29**, 3542–56
35. Gronenborn, A. M., Clore, G. M., Schmeissner, V. and Wingfield, P. (1986). A 'H-NMR study of human interleukin-1 beta: sequence-specific assignment of aromatic residues using site-directed mutant proteins. *Eur. J. Biochem.*, **161**, 37–43
36. MacDonald, H. R., Wingfield, P., Schmeissner, U., Shaw, A., Clore, G. M. and Gronenbom, A. M. (1986). Point mutations of human interleukin 1 with decreased receptor binding affinity. *FEBS Lett.*, **209**, 295–8

37. Gehrke, L., Jobling, S. A., Paik, L. S. K., McDonald, B., Rossenwasser, L. J. and Auron, P. E. (1990). A point mutation uncouples human interleukin-1 beta biological activity and receptor binding. *J. Biol. Chem.*, **265**, 5922–5
38. Huang, J. J., Newton, R. C., Horuk, R., Matthew, J. B., Covington, M., Pezzella, K. and Lim, Y. (1987). Muteins of human interleukin-1 show enhanced bioactivities. *FEBS Lett.*, **223**, 294–8
39. Dechiara, T. M., Young, D. and Semionow, R. (1986). Structure–function analysis of murine interleukin 1: biologically active polypeptides are at least 127 amino acids long and are derived from the carboxyl terminus of a 270 amino acid precursor. *Proc. Natl. Acad. Sci.*, **83**, 8303–7
40. Mosely, B., Dower, S. K., Gillis, S. and Cosman, D. (1987). Determination of the minimum polypeptide lengths of the functionally active sites of human interleukins 1 alpha and beta. *Proc. Natl. Acad. Sci.*, **84**, 4572–6
41. Zurawski, S. M., Pope, K., Cherwinski, H. and Zurawski, G. (1986). Expression in *E. coli* of synthetic human interleukin 1 alpha genes encoding the processed active protein, mutant proteins and beta-galactosidase fusion proteins. *Gene*, **49**, 61–8
42. Lillquist, J. S., Simon, P. L., Summers, M., Jonak, Z. and Young, P. R. (1988). Structure-activity studies of human IL-1 beta with mature and truncated proteins expressed in *E. coli*. *J. Immunol.*, **141**, 1975–81
43. Massone, A., Baldari, C., Censini, S., Bertalini, M., Nucci, D., Boraschi, D. and Telford, J. L. (1988). Mapping of biologically relevant sites on human IL-1 beta using monoclonal antibodies. *J. Immunol.*, **140**, 3812–16
44. Black, R. A., Kronheim, S. R., Cantrell, M., Deeley, M. C., March, C. J., Prickett, K. S., Wignall, J., Conlon, P. J., Cosman, D., Hopp, T. A. and Mochizuki, D. Y. (1988). Generation of biologically active interleukin 1 beta by proteolytic cleavage of the inactive precursor. *J. Biol. Chem.*, **263**, 9437–42
45. Mosely, B., Urdal, D. L., Prickett, K. S., Larsen, A., Cosman, D., Conlon, P. J., Gillis, S. and Dower, S. K. (1987). The interleukin-1 receptor binds the human interleukin-1 alpha precursor but not the interleukin 1 beta precursor. *J. Biol. Chem.*, **262**, 2941–4
46. Cameron, P., Limjuco, G., Rodkey, J., Bernett, C. and Schmidt, J. A. (1985). Amino acid sequence analysis of human interleukin 1 (IL-1): Evidence for biochemically distinct forms of IL-1. *J. Exp. Med.*, **162**, 790–801
47. Black, R. A., Kronheim, S. R., Merriam, J. E., March, C. J. and Hopp, T. P. (1989). A pre-aspartate-specific protease from human leukocytes that cleaves pro-interleukin-1 beta. *J. Biol. Chem.*, **264**, 5323–6
48. Hazuda, D. J., Strickler, J., Kueppers, F., Simon, P. L. and Young, P. R. (1990). Processing of precursor interleukin-1 beta and inflammatory disease. *J. Biol. Chem.*, **265**, 6318–22
49. Gery, I. and Lepe-Zuniga, J. L. (1984). Interleukin 1: uniqueness of its production and spectrum of activities. In: Pick, E. and Landy, M. (eds), *Lymphokines*, pp. 109–125 (New York: Academic Press).
50. Di Giovine, F. S., Symons, J. A. and Duff, G. W. (1991). Kinetics of IL-1 beta mRNA and protein accumulation in human mononuclear cells. *Immunol. Lett.*, **29**, 211–18
51. Auron, P. E., Warner, S. J. C., Webb, A. C., Cannon, J. G., Bernheim, H. A., McAdam, K. J. P. W., Rosenwasser, L. J., LoPreste, G., Mucci, S. F. and Dinarello, C. A. (1987). Studies on the molecular nature of human interleukin 1. *J. Immunol.*, **138**, 1447–56
52. Auron, P. E., Rosenwasser, L. J., Matsushima, K., Copeland, T., Dinarello, C. A., Oppenheim, J. J. and Webb, A. C. (1985). Human and murine interleukin 1 possess sequence and structural similarities. *J. Mol. Cell. Immunol.*, **2**, 169–77
53. Singer, I. I., Scott, S., Hall, G. L., Limjuco, G., Chin, J. and Schmidt, J. A. (1988). Interleukin 1 beta is localised in the cytoplasmic ground substance but is largely absent from the golgi apparatus and plasma membranes of stimulated human monocytes. *J. Exp. Med.*, **167**, 389–407
54. Baldari, C., Murray, J. A. H., Ghiara, P., Cesareni, G. and Galeotti, C. L. (1987). A novel leader peptide which allows efficient secretion of a fragment of human interleukin 1 beta in *Saccharomyces cerevisiae*. *EMBO J.*, **66**, 229–34
55. Denefle, P., Kovarick, S., Ciora, T., Gosselet, N., Benichon, J.-C., Latta, M., Guinet, F., Ryder, A. and Mayaux, J.-F. (1989). Heterologous protein export in *E. coli*: influence of bacterial signal peptides on the export of human interleukin 1 beta. *Gene*, **85**, 499–510
56. Bakouche, O., Brown, D. C. and Lachman, L. B. (1987). Subcellular localisation of human

monocyte interleukin 1: evidence for an inactive precursor molecule and a possible mechanism for IL-1 release. *J. Immunol.*, **138**, 4249–55
57. Brody, D. T. and Durum, S. K. (1989). Membrane IL-1: IL-1 alpha precursor binds to the plasma membrane via a lectin-like interaction. *J. Immunol.*, **143**, 1183–7
58. Suttles, J., Carruth, L. M. and Mizel, S. B. (1990). Detection of IL-1 alpha and IL-1 beta in the supernatants of paraformaldehyde-treated human monocytes. *J. Immunol.*, **144**, 170–4
59. Burnstein, S. L., Locksley, R. M., Ryan, J. L. and Lovett, D. H. (1988). Acylation of monocyte and glomerular mesangial cell proteins: myristyl acylation of the interleukin 1 precursors. *J. Clin. Invest.*, **82**, 1479–88
60. Beuscher, H. V., Nickells, M. W. and Colten, H. R. (1988). The precursor of interleukin 1 alpha is phosphorylated at residue serine 90. *J. Biol. Chem.*, **263**, 4023–8
61. Baldari, C. T. and Telford, J. L. (1989). The intracellular precursor of IL1 beta is associated with microtubules in activated U937 cells. *J. Immunol.*, **142**, 785–91
62. Rubartelli, A., Cozzolino, F., Talio, M. and Sitia, R. (1990). A novel secretory pathway for interleukin-1 beta, a protein lacking a signal sequence. *EMBO J.*, **9**, 1503–10
63. Suttles, J., Giri, J. G. and Mizel, S. B. (1990). IL-1 secretion by macrophages enhancement of IL-1 secretion and processing by calcium ionophores. *J. Immunol.*, **144**, 175–82
64. Endres, S., Cannon, J. G., Ghorbani, R., Dempsey, R. A., Sisson, S. D., Lonnemann, G., van der Meer, J. W. M., Wolff, S. M. and Dinarello, C. A. (1989). In vitro production of IL-1 beta, IL-1 alpha, TNF and IL-2 in healthy subjects: Distribution, effect of cycloxygenase inhibition and evidence of independent gene regulation. *Eur. J. Immunol.*, **19**, 2327–33
65. Yamashita, U., Shirakawa, F. and Nakamura, H. (1987). Production of interleukin 1 by adult T cell leukemia (ATL) cell lines. *J. Immunol.*, **138**, 3284–9
66. Cerdan, C., Martin, Y., Brailly, H., Courcoul, M., Flavetta, S., Costello, R., Mawas, C., Birg, F. and Olive, D. (1991). IL-1 alpha is produced by T lymphocytes activated via the CD2 plus CD28 pathways. *J. Immunol.*, **146**, 550–9
67. McKenzie, R. C., Arsenault, T. V., Sauder, D. N. and Harley, C. B. (1990). Expression of interleukin 1 beta in a human keratinocyte cell line. *Lymphokine Res.*, **9**, 391–403
68. Dower, S. K., Kronheim, S. R., March, C. J., Conlon, P. J., Hopp, T. P., Gillis, S. and Urdal, D. L. (1985). Detection and characterization of high affinity plasma membrane receptors for human interleukin 1. *J. Exp. Med.*, **162**, 501–15
69. Dower, S. K., Kronheim, S. R., Hopp, T. P., Cantrell, M., Deeley, M., Gillis, S., Henney, C. S. and Urdal, D. L. (1986). The cell surface receptors for interleukin 1 alpha and interleukin 1 beta are identical. *Nature*, **324**, 266–8
70. Bird, T. A. and Saklatvala, J. (1986). Identification of a common class of high affinity receptors for both types of porcine interleukin-1 on connective tissue cells. *Nature*, **324**, 263–6
71. Urdal, D. L., Call, S. M., Jackson, J. L. and Dower, S. K. (1988). Affinity purification and chemical analysis of the interleukin 1 receptor. *J. Biol. Chem.*, **261**, 2870–7
72. Mosely, B., Urdal, D. L., Prickett, K. S., Larsen, A., Cosman, D., Conlon, P. J., Gillis, S. and Dower, S. K. (1987). The interleukin 1 receptor binds the human interleukin 1 alpha precursor but not the interleukin 1 beta precursor. *J. Biol. Chem.*, **262**, 2941–4
73. Sims, J. E., March, C. J., Cosman, D., Widmer, M. B., MacDonald, H. R., McMahan, C. J., Grubin, C. E., Wignal, J. M., Jackson, J. L., Call, S. M., Friend, D., Alpert, A. R., Gillis, S., Urdal, D. L. and Dower, S. K. (1988). cDNA Expression cloning of the IL-1 receptor, a member of the immunoglobulin superfamily. *Science*, **241**, 585–9
74. Curtis, B. M., Gallis, B., Overell, R. W., McMahan, C. J., DeRoos, P., Ireland, R., Eisenman, J., Dower, S. K., Sims, J. E. (1989). T cell interleukin-1 receptor cDNA expressed in Chinese hamster ovary cells regulates functional responses to interleukin 1. *Proc. Natl. Acad. Sci.*, **86**, 3045–9
75. Dower, S. K., Wignal, J. M., Schodey, K., McMahan, C. J., Jackson, J. L., Prickett, K. S., Lupton, S., Cosman, D. and Sims, J. E. (1989). Retention of ligand binding activity by the extracellular domain of the Il-1 receptor. *J. Immunol.*, **142**, 4314–20
76. Sims, J. E., Acres, R. B., Grubin, C. E., McMahan, C. J., Wignall, J. M., March, C. J. and Dower, S. K. (1989). Cloning the interleukin 1 receptor from human T cells. *Proc. Natl. Acad. Sci.*, **86**, 8946–50
77. Dower, S. K., Call, S. M., Gillis, S. and Urdal, D. L. (1986). Similarity between the interleukin 1 receptors on a murine T-lymphoma cell line and on a murine fibroblast cell line. *Proc. Natl. Acad. Sci.*, **83**, 1060–4

78. Matsushima, K., Akahoshi, T., Yamada, M., Furutani, Y. and Oppenheim, J. J. (1986). Properties of a specific interleukin 1 (IL-1) receptor on human Epstein Barr virus-transferred B lymphocytes; identity of the receptor for IL-1 alpha and IL-1 beta. *J. Immunol.*, **136**, 4495–502
79. Scapigliati, G., Ghiara, P., Bartalini, M., Tagliabue, A. and Boraschi, D. (1989). Differential binding of IL-1 alpha and IL-1 beta to receptors on B and T cells. *FEBS Lett.*, **243**, 394–8
80. Benjamin, D., Wormsley, S. and Dower, S. K. (1990). Heterogeneity in interleukin (IL-1) receptors expressed on human B cell lines; differences in the nolecular properties of IL-1 alpha and IL-1 beta binding sites. *J. Biol. Chem.*, **265**, 9943–51
81. Horuk, R. and McCubrey, J. A. (1989). The interleukin-1 receptor in Raji human B-lymphoma cells; molecular characterisation and evidence for receptor-mediated activation of gene expression. *Biochem. J.*, **260**, 657–63
82. Chizzonite, R., Truitt, T., Kilian, P. L., Stern, A. S., Numes, P., Parker, K. P., Kaffka, K. L., Chua, A. O., Lugg, D. K. and Gubler, U. (1989). Two high-affinity interleukin 1 receptors represent separate gene products. *Proc. Natl. Acad. Sci.*, **86**, 8029–33
83. Bomsztyk, K., Sims, J. E., Stanton, T. H., Slack, J., McMahan, C. J., Valentine, M. A. and Dower, S. K. (1989). Evidence for different interleukin-1 receptors in murine B and T cell lines. *Proc. Natl. Acad. Sci.*, **86**, 8034–8
84. Benjamin, D. and Dower, S. K. (1990). Human B cells express two types of interleukin-1 receptors. *Blood*, **10**, 2017–23
85. Horuk, R. (1991). Differences in internalisation and intracellular processing of interleukin-1 associated with the two forms of interleukin-1 receptor found in B cells and T cells. *Biochem. J.*, **273**, 79–83
86. Mosely, B., Beckman, M. P., March, C. J., Idzerda, R. L., Gimpel, S,. D., Bos, T. V., Friend, D., Alpert, A., Anderson, D., Jackson, J., Wignal, J. M., Smith, C., Gallis, G., Sims, J. E., Urdal, D., Widner, M. B., Cosman, D. and Park, L. S. (1989). The murine interleukin 4 receptor; molecular cloning and characterisation of secreted and membrane bound forms. *Cell*, **59**, 335–48
87. Robb, J. R. and Kutny, R. M. (1987). Structure–function relationships for the IL-2 receptor system II Analysis of sequence and ligand binding properties of soluble Tac protein. *J. Immunol.*, **139**, 855–62
88. Eastgate, J. A., Symons, J. A. and Duff, G. W. (1990). Identification of an interleukin 1 beta binding protein in human plasma. *FEBS Lett.*, **260**, 213–16
89. Symons, J. A., Eastgate, J. A. and Duff, G. W. (1990). A soluble binding protein specific for interleukin 1 beta is produced by activated mononuclear cells. *Cytokine*, **2**, 190–8
90. Symons, J. A. and Duff, G. W. (1990). A soluble form of the interleukin-1 receptor produced by a human B cell line. *FEBS Lett.*, **272**, 133–6
91. Curtis, B. M., Widmer, M. B., DeRoos, P. and Qwarnstrom, E. E. (1990). IL-1 and its receptor are translocated to the nucleus. *J. Immunol.*, **144**, 1295–303
92. Grenfell, S., Smithers, N., Miller, K. and Solari, R. (1989). Receptor-mediated endocytosis and nuclear-transport of human interleukin-1 alpha. *Biochem. J.*, **264**, 813–22
93. Abraham, R. T., Ho, S. N., Barna, T. J. and McKean, D. J. (1987). Transmembrane signalling during interleukin-1 dependent T cell activation. *J. Biol. Chem.*, **262**, 2719–28
94. Rossoff, P. M., Savage, N. and Dinarello, C. A. (1988). Interleukin-1 stimulates diacylglycerol production in T lymphocytes by a novel mechanism. *Cell.*, **54**, 73–81
95. Kester, M., Simonsen, M. S., Mene, P. and Desor, J. R. (1989). Interleukin-1 alpha generates transmembrane signals from phospholipids through novel pathways in cultured rat mesangial cells. *J. Clin. Invest.*, **83**, 718–23
96. Matsushima, K., Koyayashi, Y., Copeland, T. D., Akahoshi, T. and Oppenheim, J. J. (1987). Phosphorylation of a cytosolic 65-KDa protein induced by interleukin-1 in glycocorticoid pretreated normal human peripheral blood mononuclear leukocytes. *J. Immunol.*, **139**, 3367–74
97. Kaur, P. and Saklatvala, J. (1988). Interleukin-1 and tumour necrosis factor increase phosphorylation of fibroblast proteins. *FEBS Lett.*, **241**, 6–10
98. Bird, T. A. and Saklatvala, J. (1988). IL-1 and TNF transmodulate epidermal growth factor receptors by a protein kinase C-independent mechanism. *J. Immunol.*, **142**, 126–33
99. Gallis, B., Prickett, K. S., Jackson, J., Slack, J., Schooley, K., Sims, J. E. and Dower, S. K. (1989). IL-1 induces rapid phosphorylation of the IL-1 receptor. *J. Immunol.*, **143**, 3235–40
100. Shirakawa, F., Yamashita, V., Chedid, M. and Mizel, S. B. (1988). Cyclic AMP; an intracellular second messenger for interleukin-1. *Proc. Natl. Acad. Sci.*, **85**, 8201–5

101. Chedid, M., Shirakawa, F., Naylor, P. and Mizel, S. B. (1989). Signal transduction pathways for IL-1; involvement of a pertussis toxin-sensitive GTP-binding protein in the activation of adenylate cyclase. *J. Immunol.*, **142**, 4301–6
102. Zhang, Y., Lin, J. X., Yip, Y. K. and Vilcek, J. (1988). Enhancement of cAMP levels and of protein kinase activity by tumour necrosis factor and interleukin-1 in human fibroblasts; role in the induction of interleukin-6. *Proc. Natl. Acad. Sci.*, **85**, 6802–5
103. Stanton, T. H., Maynard, M. and Bomsztyk, K. (1986). Effect of interleukin-1 on intracellular concentration of sodium, calcium and potassium in 70Z/3 cells. *J. Biol. Chem.*, **261**, 5699–701
104. Bomsztyk, K., Toivota, B., Emery, D. W., Rooney, J. W., Dower, S. K., Rachie, N. A. and Sibley, C. H. (1990). Role of cAMP in interleukin-1-induced k light chain gene expression in murine B cell line. *J. Biol. Chem.*, **265**, 9413–17
105. Muegge, K., Williams, T. M., Kant, J., Karin, M., Chin, R., Schmidt, A., Sieken List, V., Young, H. A. and Durum, S. K. (1989). Interleukin-1 costimulatory activity on the interleukin-2 promoter via AP-1. *Science*, **246**, 249–51
106. Edbrooke, M. R., Burt, D. W., Cheshire, J. K. and Woo, P. (1989). Identification of cis-acting sequences responsible for phorbolester induction of human serum amyloid A gene expression via a nuclear factor kB-like transcription factor. *Mol. Cell. Biol.*, **9**, 1908–16
107. Dinarello, C. A. (1989). Interleukin-1 and its biologically related cytokines. *Adv. Immunol.*, **44**, 153–205
108. Dinarello, C. A., Cannon, J. G., Mier, J., Bernheim, H. A., LoPreste, G., Lynn, D. L., Love, R. N., Webb, A. C., Auron, P. E., Reuken, R. C., Rich, A., Woltt, S. M. and Putney, S. D. (1986). Multiple biological activities human recombinant interleukin-1. *J. Clin. Invest.*, **77**, 1734–9
109. Okusawa, S., Gelfand, J. A., Ikejima, T., Connolly, R. A. and Dinarello, C. A. (1988). Interleukin-1 induces a shock-like state in Rabbits: synergism with tumour necrosis factor and the effect of cyclooxygenase inhibition. *J. Clin. Invest.*, **81**, 1162–72
110. Dinarello, C. A. (1989). Fever. In Bomford, R. and Henderson, B. (eds), *Interleukin-1. Inflammation and Disease*, pp. 175–90 (Oxford: Elsevier)
111. Borth, W. and Lugar, T. A. (1989). Identification of alpha$_2$ macroglobulin as a cytokine binding plasma protein; binding of interleukin-1 beta to 'F' alpha$_2$ macroglobulin. *J. Biol. Chem.*, **264**, 5818–25
112. Sztein, M. B., Vogel, S. N., Sipe, J. D., Murphy, P. A., Mizel, S. B., Oppenheim, J. J. and Rosenstreich, D. L. (1981). The role of macrophytes in the acute phase response; SAA inducer is closely related to lymphocyte activating factor and endogenous pyrogen. *Cell Immunol.*, **63**, 164–76
113. Perlmutter, D. H., Goldberger, G., Dinarello, C. A., Mizel, S. B. and Cotten, H. R. (1986). Regulation of class III major histocompatibility complex gene products by interleukin-1. *Science*, **232**, 850–2
114. Whicher, J. T., Gauldie, J., Baumann, H. and Westacott, C. (1989). Acute phase proteins. In Bomford, R. and Henderson, B. (eds), *Interleukin-1, Inflammation and Disease*, pp. 191–216 (Oxford: Elsevier)
115. Hirano, T., Yasukawa, K., Harada, H., Taga, T., Watanake, Y., Matsuda, T., Kashiwamura, S., Sakiyama, F., Matsui, H., Takahara, Y., Taniguchi, T. and Kishimoto, T. (1986). Complementary DNA for a novel human interleukin (BSF-2) that induces B lymphocytes to produce immunoglobulin. *Nature*, **324**, 73–6
116. Content, J., DeWit, L., Ponpart, P., Opdenakker, G., Van Damme, J. and Billiau, A. (1985). Induction of a 26-KDa-protein mRNA in human cells treated with an interleukin-1-related leukocyte-derived factor. *Eur. J. Biochem.*, **152**, 253–7
117. Gowan, M., Wood, D. D., Ihrie, E. J., McGuire, M. K. B. and Russell, R. G. G. (1983). An interleukin-1-like factor stimulates bone resorption *in vitro*. *Nature*, **306**, 378–80
118. Thompson, B. M., Saklatvala, J. and Chambers, T. J. (1986). Osteoblasts mediate interleukin-1 stimulation of bone resorption by rat osteoblasts. *J. Exp. Med.*, **164**, 104–12
119. Sato, K., Fujii, Y., Kasono, K., Safi, M., Tsushima, T. and Shizume, K. (1986). Stimulation of prostaglandin E_2 and bone resorption by recombinant human interleukin-1 of cartilage breakdown and production of collagenase and proteoglucanase by human chondrocytes but not by human osteoblasts *in vitro*. *Biochim. Biophys. Acta*, **797**, 186–93
120. Gowan, M., Wood, D. D., Ihrie, E. J., Meats, J. E. and Russell, R. G. G. (1984). Stimulation by human interleukin 1 of cartilage breakdown and production of collagenase and

proteoglycanase by human chondrocytes but not by human osteoblasts *in vitro*. *Biochim. Biophys. Acta*, **797**, 186–93

121. Korn, J. H., Halushka, P. V. and Le Roy, E. C. (1980). Mononuclear cell modulation of connective tissue function; suppression of fibroblast growth by endogenous prostaglandin production. *J. Clin. Invest.*, **65**, 543–54
122. Mizel, S. B., Dayer, J. M., Krane, S. M. and Mergenhagen, S. E. (1981). Stimulation of rheumatoid synovial cell collagenase and prostaglandin production by partially purified lymphocyte activating factor (interleukin-1). *Proc. Natl. Acad. Sci.*, **78**, 2474–7
123. Daer, J. M., Rochemonteix, B. de, Burrus, B., Demczuk, S. and Dinarello, C. A. (1986). Human recombinant interleukin-1 stimulates collagenase and prostaglandin E_2 production by human synovial cells. *J. Clin. Invest.*, **77**, 645–8
124. Pettipher, E. R., Higgs, G. A. and Henderson, B. (1986). Interleukin-1 induces leukocyte infiltration and cartilage proteoglycan degradation in the synovial joint. *Proc. Natl. Acad. Sci.*, **83**, 8749–53
125. Stimpson, S. A., Dalldorf, F. G., Otterness, I. G. and Schwab, J. H. (1988). Exacerbation of arthritis by IL-1 in rat joints previously injured by peptidoglycan-polysaccharide. *J. Immunol.*, **140**, 2964–9
126. Brennan, F. M., Zacharie, C. O. C., Chantry, D., Larsen, C. G., Turner, M., Maini, R. N., Matsushima, K. and Feldmann, M. (1990). Detection of interleukin-8 biological activity in synovial fluids from patients with rheumatoid arthritis and production of interleukin-8 mRNA by isolated synovial cells. *Eur. J. Immunol.*, **20**, 2141–4
127. Ferreira, S. M., Lorenzetti, B. B., Bristow, A. F. and Poole, S. (1988). Interleukin-1 beta as a potent hyperalgesic agent antagonised by a tripeptide analogue. *Nature*, **334**, 698–700
128. Follenfant, R. L., Nakamura-Craig, M., Henderson, B. and Higgs, G. A. (1989). Inhibition by neuropeptides of interleukin-1 beta-induced prostaglandin-independent hyperalgesia. *Br. J. Pharmacol.*, **98**, 41–3
129. Sabatini, M., Boyce, B., Aufolemorte, T., Bonewald, L. and Mundy, G. R. (1988). Infusions of recombinant human interleukin-1 alpha and beta cause hypercalcemia in normal mice. *Proc. Natl. Acad. Sci.*, **85**, 5235–9
130. Bodel, P. and Hollingsworth, J. W. (1969). Pyrogen release from human synovial exudate cells. *Br. J. Exp. Pathol.*, **49**, 11–19
131. Wood, D. D., Ihrie, E. J., Dinarello, C. A. and Cohen, P. L. (1983). Isolation of an interleukin-1-like factor from human joint effusions. *Arthritis Rheum.*, **26**, 975–83
132. Di Giovine, F. S., Malawista, S. E., Nuki, G. and Duff, G. W. (1987). Interleukin (IL-1) as a mediator of crystal arthritis; stimulation of T cell and synovial fibroblast mitogenesis by urate crystal-induced IL-1. *J. Immunol.*, **138**, 3213–18
133. Wood, D. D., Ihrie, E. J. and Hammerman, D. (1985). Release of interleukin-1 from human synovial tissue *in vitro*. *Arthritis Rheum.*, **28**, 853–61
134. Cannon, J. G., Van der Meer, J. W. M., Kwiatowski, D., Endres, S., Lonnemann, G., Birke, J. F. and Dinarello, C. A. (1988). Interleukin-1 beta in human plasma; optimisation of blood collection, plasma extraction and radioimmunoassay methods. *Lymphokine Res.*, **7**, 457–67
135. Eastgate, J. A., Symons, J. A., Wood, N. C., Grinlinton, F. M., Di Giovine, F. S. and Duff, G. W. (1988). Correlation of plasma interleukin-1 levels with disease activity in rheumatoid arthritis. *Lancet*, **2**, 706–9
136. Eastgate, J. A., Symons, J. A., Wood, N. C., Capper, S. J. and Duff, G. W. (1991). Plasma levels of interleukin-1 alpha in rheumatoid arthritis. *Br. J. Rheumatol.*, **30**. 295–7
137. Symons, J. A., McDowell, T. L., DiGiovine, F. S., Wood, N. C., Capper, S. J. and Duff, G. W. (1989). Interleukin-1 in rheumatoid arthritis; potentiation of immune responses within the joint. *Lymphokine Res.*, **8**, 365–72
138. DiGiovine, F. S., Poole, S., Situnayake, R. D., Wadhwa, M. and Duff, G. W. (1990). Absence of correlations between indices of systematic inflammation and synovial fluid interleukin-1 (alpha and beta) in rheumatic diseases. *Rheumatol. Int.*, **9**, 259–64
139. Rooney, M., Symons, J. A. and Duff, G. W. (1990). Interleukin-1 beta in synovial fluid is related to local disease activity in rheumatoid arthritis. *Rheumatol. Int.*, **10**, 217–19
140. Di Giovine, F. S., Symons, J. A. and Duff, G. W. (1991). Kinetics of IL-1 beta mRNA and protein accumulation in human mononuclear cells. *Immunol. Lett.*, **29**, 211–18
141. Buchan, G., Barrett, K., Turner, M., Chantry, D., Maini, R. N. and Feldmann, M. (1988).

Interleukin-1 and tumour necrosis factor mRNA expression in rheumatoid arthritis; prolonged production of IL-1 alpha. *Clin. Exp. Immunol.*, **73**, 449–55

142. Duff, G. W., Dickens, E., Wood, N., Manson, J., Symons, J. A., Poole, S. and diGiovine, F. S. (1988). Immunoassay, bioassay and *in situ* hybridisation of monokines in human arthritis. In Oppenheim, J. J., Dimarello, C. A. and Kluger, M. (eds.), *Monokines and Other Non-lymphatic Cytokines*, pp. 387–92 (New York: Alan R. Liss)
143. Firestein, G. S., Alvaro-Garcia, J. M. and Maki, R. (1990). Quantitative analysis of cytokine gene expression in rheumatoid arthritis. *J. Immunol.*, **144**, 3347–53
144. Macnaul, K. L., Hutchinson, N. I., Parsons, J. N., Bayne, E. K. and Tocci, M. J. (1990). Analysis of IL-1 and TNF alpha gene expression in human rheumatoid synoviocytes and normal monocytes by in situ hybridisation. *J. Immunol.*, **145**, 4154–66
145. Durum, S. K., Schmidt, J. A. and Oppenheim, J. J. (1985). Interleukin-1; an immunological perspective. *Ann. Rev. Immunol.*, **3**, 263–87
146. Wang, H. M. and Smith, K. A. (1987). The interleukin-2 receptor; functional consequences of its bimolecular structure. *J. Exp. Med.*, **166**, 1055–69
147. Rubin, L. A., Kurman, C. C., Fritz, M. E., Biddison, W. E., Boutin, B., Yarchoan, R. and Nelson, D. L. (1985). Soluble interleukin-2 receptors are released from activated human lymphoid cells *in vitro*. *J. Immunol.*, **135**, 3172–7
148. Symons, J. A., Wood, N. C., diGiovine, F. S. and Duff, G. W. (1988). Soluble IL-2 receptor in rheumatoid arthritis; correlation with disease activity, IL-1 and IL-2 inhibition. *J. Immunol.*, **141**, 2612–18
149. Duff, G. W. (1989). Interleukin-1 inflammatory joint disease. In Bomford, R. and Henderson, B. (eds), *Interleukin-1. Inflammation and Disease*, pp. 243–55 (Oxford: Elsevier)
150. Manson, J., Brown, T. and Duff, G. W. (1990). Modulation of interleukin-1 beta gene expression using antisense phosphorothioate oligonucleotides. *Lymphokine Res.*, **9**, 35–42
151. Black, R. A., Kronheim, S. R. and Sleath, P. R. (1989). Activation of interleukin-1 beta by a co-induced protease. *FEBS Lett.*, **247**, 386–90
152. Meek, T. D., Lambert, D. M., Dreyer, G. B., Carr, T. J., Tomaszek, T. A., Moore, M. L., Strickler, J. E., Debonck, C., Hyland, L. J., Matthews, T. J., Metcalf, B. W. and Petteway, S. R. (1990). Inhibition of HIV-1 protease in infected T lymphocytes by synthetic peptide analogues. *Nature*, **343**, 90–2
153. Arend, W. P., Joslin, F. G. and Massoni, R. J. (1985). Effects of immune complexes on production by human monocytes of interleukin-1 or an interleukin-1 inhibitor. *J. Immunol.*, **134**, 3868–75
154. Balavoine, J. F., de Rochemonteix, B., Williamson, K., Seckinger, P., Cruchand, A. and Dayer, J. M. (1986). Prostaglandin E_2 and collagenase production by fibroblasts and synovial cells is regulated by urine derived human interleukin-1 and inhibitor(s). *J. Clin. Invest.*, **78**, 1120–4
155. Prier, A. M., Kaufman, M. T., Griscelli, C. and Dayer, J. M. (1987). Specific interleukin-1 inhibitor in serum and urine of children with systematic juvenile chronic arthritis. *Lancet*, **2**, 1240–2
156. Seckinger, P., Lowenthal, J. W., Williamson, K., Dayer, J. M. and MacDonald, H. R. (1987). A urine inhibitor of interleukin-1 activity that blocks ligand binding. *J. Immunol.*, **139**, 1546–9
157. Hannum, C. H., Wilcox, C. J., Arend, W. P., Joslin, F. G., Dripps, D. J., Heindal, P. L., Armes, L. G., Sommer, A., Eisenberg, S. P. and Thompson, R. C. (1990). Interleukin-1 receptor antagonist activity of a human interleukin-1 inhibitor. *Nature*, **343**, 336–40
158. Eisenberg, S. P., Evans, R. J., Arend, W. P., Verderker, E., Brewer, M. T., Hannum, C. H. and Thompson, R. C. (1990). Primary structure and functional expression from complementary DNA of a human interleukin-1 receptor antagonist. *Nature*, **343**, 341–6
159. Seckinger, P., Klein-Nulend, J., Alander, C., Thompson, R. C., Dayer, J. M. and Raisz, L. G. (1990). Natural and recombinant human IL-1 receptor antagonists block the effects of IL-1 on bone resorption and prostaglandin production. *J. Immunol.*, **145**, 4181–4
160. Ohlsson, K., Bjork, P., Bergenfeldt, M., Hageman, R. and Thompson, R. C. (1990). Interleukin-1 receptor antagonist reduces mortality from endotoxin shock. *Nature*, **348**, 550–2
161. Maliszewski, C. R., Sato, T. A., Vanden Bos, T., Waugh, S., Dower, S. K., Slack, J., Beckmann, M. P. and Grabstein, K. H. (1990). Cytokine receptors and B cell functions I Recombinant soluble receptors specifically inhibit IL-1 and IL-4 induced B cell activities

in vitro. *J. Immunol.*, **144**, 3028–33

162. Fanslow, W. C., Sims, J. E., Sassenfeld, H., Morrissey, P. J., Gillis, S., Dower, S. K. and Widmer, M. B. (1990). Regulation of alloreactivity *in vivo* by a soluble form of the interleukin-1 receptor. *Science*, **248**, 739–42
163. Symons, J. A., Eastgate, J. A. and Duff, G. W. (1991). Purification and characterisation of a novel soluble receptor for interleukin-1. *J. Exp. Med.*, **174**
164. Giri, J. G., Newton, R. C. and Horuk, R. (1990). Identification of soluble interleukin-1 binding protein in cell-free supernatants; evidence for soluble interleukin-1 receptor. *J. Biol. Chem.*, **265**, 17416–19
165. Bendtzen, K., Mandrup-Poulson, T., Nerup, J., Nielson, J. H., Dinarello, C. A. and Svenson, M. (1986). Cytotoxicity of human pI 7 interleukin-1 for pancreatic islets of Langerhans. *Science*, **232**, 1545–7

11
Tumour necrosis factor (TNF) and inflammation

P. J. McLAUGHLIN

INTRODUCTION

Adequate biological defences against infection by foreign organisms are essential to the survival of the host. A phylogenetically relatively primitive, but nevertheless essential, aspect of these defences is the inflammatory response. In contrast to the immune responses involving antibodies and effector T lymphocytes, inflammation is relatively non-specific, but it does provide a quick and usually effective anti-invasive response. The inflammatory response is mediated by host cells and their soluble products, the cytokines, and in general is beneficial to the host, limiting potentially lethal infections. However, inflammation may also be accompanied by local pathological effects leading to host tissue damage or to systemic deleterious effects such as shock and catabolic states. These inflammatory changes are orchestrated and mediated by cytokines. Tumour necrosis factor (TNF) is one of these soluble mediators and it appears to have a central role in the initiation, development and augmentation of inflammation, as well as in the tissue remodelling and healing events occurring after the response.

TNF was originally identified as an endotoxin-induced serum factor causing necrosis of tumours *in vivo* and tumour cell cytotoxicity *in vitro*[1]. The protein responsible for this tumour necrotic effect was later shown to be the same molecule as cachectin, a factor producing wasting in trypanosome-infected rabbits[2,3]. The major source of TNF is the macrophage[4], although other cell types may be induced to produce significant amounts of the TNF under mitogenic, cytokine or other stimuli[5-7]. TNF usually occurs as a soluble product, but a macrophage membrane-bound form has been described[8] which may provide one of the killing mechanisms of activated macrophages[9]. It is a protein of molecular weight about 17 kD[10], but its biologically most active form is probably a trimer[11]. The molecule is highly conserved between species[12], but although its biological effects usually cross species barriers, it is often most effective in homologous systems[6,13].

TNF exerts its cellular effects through a receptor[14], and most cells and tissues including liver, kidney, muscle, placenta, adipocytes, endothelial cells, epithelial cells, monocytes, polymorphs, lymphocytes and haematopoietic cells express surface TNF receptor[10,15–20] and are thus potential targets for TNF-mediated effects. The cytotoxic signals and mechanisms following binding of TNF to its receptor appear to involve a GTP-binding protein, phospholipase A2 and products of arachidonic acid metabolism[21,22]. However, other effects such as cell stimulation may involve different pathways including up-regulation of cellular oncogenes[23] and growth factor receptors[24]. TNF may have very specific effects on certain sensitive cell types. The wasting diathesis seen in conditions associated with systemic release of TNF[2] may be due to its post-receptor-binding effects on adipocytes, inhibiting lipoprotein lipase activity[10] and so preventing access of free fatty acids into the circulation. The nature of these post-receptor-binding events may in some cases depend on the structure of the TNF receptor, and a 138 kD polypeptide has been described which appears to be associated with sensitivity to TNF-mediated cytotoxicity[25]. A related cytokine, lymphotoxin, also termed tumour necrosis factor-beta (TNFβ) (under this nomenclature tumour necrosis factor/cachectin is termed tumour necrosis factor-alpha, TNFα) may act through the same receptor[26], although post-receptor binding events may be different for this cytokine[27].

The most potent stimulus for TNF production seems to be endotoxin[1]. However, many invasive stimuli including bacterial[28], viral[29], and parasitic[30] infections are known to induce TNF. In addition, other types of immune response may also be associated with TNF secretion, including autoimmunity[31], graft versus host disease[32], graft rejection[33], inflammatory joint disease[34] and cancer[35]. TNF may act directly on a wide range of cell types, having diverse actions including cellular cytostasis and cytotoxicity or, in contrast, cell activation and proliferation. Recruitment of inflammatory cells may be brought about by TNF through its chemotactic action, and these cells may then be induced to produce other cytokines and soluble mediators which themselves have inflammatory actions, or may act to enhance the actions of TNF. Alternatively, TNF may act on the potential cellular targets of the inflammatory response, inducing cell surface interaction molecules to increase their accessibility to inflammatory cells. It is therefore clear that the net effect of TNF on a cell will depend on other co-factors which may affect the signal transduction pathways following TNF binding and thus act to modulate the intensity and diversity of the cellular actions of TNF (Table 11.1).

CYTOTOXIC VERSUS PROLIFERATIVE ACTIONS OF TNF

The definitive property of TNF is its cytotoxicity for tumour cells[36], and this is greatly enhanced by interferon gamma (IFNγ)[37]. This effect has been

Table 11.1 Cellular actions of TNF

Cell	*Action*	*Involvement of other cytokines*
Tumour	Cytotoxicity/cytostasis	IFNγ
	Increased expression of MHC class I antigens	
	Increased expression of other cell interaction molecules	IFNγ
Endothelial	Cytotoxicity/cytostasis	IFNγ
	Increased expression of cell interaction molecules	
	Induction of procoagulant activity	
	Release of IL 1 and GM-CSF	
Phagocyte	Proliferation	M-CSF
	Activation	IFNγ, IL 1
	Chemotaxis	IL 1
	Increased expression of MHC class II antigens	
	Increased expression of other cell interaction molecules	
	Release of IL 1, TNF, CSF and prostaglandins	
Fibroblast	Proliferation	
	Cytotoxicity/cytostasis	IFNγ, IL 1
	Release of IL 6 and GM-CSF	
Hypothamic neuron	Release of prostaglandins and IL 1	
Adipocyte	Inhibition of lipoprotein lipase activity	
Hepatocyte	Release of acute reactants	
Virus-infected	Cytotoxicity	

IFNγ = interferon gamma, IL 1 = interleukin 1, IL 6 = interleukin 6, GM-CSF = granulocyte/macrophage colony stimulating factor, M-CSF = macrophage colony stimulating factor, TNF = tumour necrosis factor, MHC = major histocompatibility complex.

observed repeatedly, more recently, using cells taken from fresh biopsy specimens of malignant neoplasms[38] where picomolar concentrations of TNF were cytotoxic for tumour cells, IFNγ providing a strong synergistic stimulus. Other, non-transformed, cell types may be susceptible to TNF-induced cytotoxicity or cytostatic activity, particularly in the presence of IFNγ, and these include normal epithelial[39] and endothelial cells[40]. This clearly has implications in inflammatory processes involving skin and vasculature. TNF has a cytotoxic effect on virus-infected cells which is augmented by IFNγ[41]. This contrasts with its antiviral effect, protecting cells from viral cytopathic effects, possibly mediated by TNF induction of cytokines of the IFN group[42]. Thus, the balance between TNF-mediated cytotoxicity and proliferation seems to be dependent on the presence of other cytokines. These may be produced by cells attracted to the vicinity of the inflammatory response or by the target cells themselves. There is evidence that potential target cells may protect themselves from TNF-mediated cytolysis by elaborating protective proteins[43] which may act by altering pathways of signal transduction following binding of TNF to its receptor. The interaction of TNF with other factors is therefore clearly an important consideration in interpreting experimental effects of TNF. For example, pure recombinant TNF inhibits *in vitro* angiogenesis, probably due to cytostatic and cytotoxic actions on vascular endothelium[40]. In contrast, peritoneal macrophage products, containing similar concentrations of TNF, together with unknown other factors, stimulate angiogenesis both *in vivo* and *in vitro*[44]. Presumably, in this environment TNF is acting in cooperation with growth-stimulating factors. Recently many other observations of cytokines modulating the effects of TNF have been documented. For example, on its own, TNF is a mitogen for fibroblasts[45,46]; however, it strongly synergizes with IFNγ and interleukin 1 (IL 1) to inhibit proliferation of normal fibroblasts, even though IL 1 itself is slightly stimulatory[46]. Similarly, in the presence of IFNγ, TNF suppresses haematopoiesis[47,48] and reverses granulocyte/macrophage colony stimulating factor (GM-CSF)-driven proliferation of precursor cells[49]. In contrast, in the absence of IFNγ, TNF synergizes with macrophage colony stimulating factor (M-CSF) to enhance proliferation of macrophage precursors[50]. This proliferative effect of TNF may also be mediated through other cytokines. For example, administration of TNF to patients leads to release of IL 6 into the circulation[51]. It is possible that fibroblasts may be the source of these TNF-induced IL 6 phosphoglycoproteins which may then act in an autocrine manner stimulating fibroblast proliferation[52]. Endothelial cells may also be a source of growth stimulatory factors induced by TNF[53], and interaction of TNF and growth factors may have an important homeostatic role leading to the controlled cell proliferation of tissue repair, following inflammatory damage. TNF may also have proliferative effects on lymphocytes, acting as a growth factor for T cells in the thymus[54] and in *in vitro* culture[13,55]. This appears to be a direct effect, not mediated by other cytokines, and the observations that TNF may regulate the mixed lymphocyte reaction[56] and the generation of cytolytic T cells[57] further indicates a central role of TNF in the development of T cell-mediated immune responses. An involvement of TNF-mediated proliferation/cytostatic control in clinical inflammatory disease is indicated by its action on bone and cartilage-derived cells. TNF induces osteoblast-like cells to proliferate[58], and also stimulates DNA synthesis in cultured chondrocytes[59]. However, it may inhibit synthesis and stimulate resorption of proteoglycan in cartilage[53,60], induce prostaglandin synthesis in osteoblasts[58], and produce bone resorption in mice[61], suggesting an involvement in inflammatory disease of joints. Supporting this, TNF has been detected in synovial fluid taken from patients with rheumatoid arthritis[62].

It would therefore seem that the ultimate effect on TNF on cell growth depends on the presence of other cytokines in the vicinity. In particular, IFNγ appears to lead to a cytostatic or cytotoxic response to TNF. In contrast, on its own, or in the presence of growth factors, TNF usually stimulates cell proliferation. These contrasting effects of TNF may be important during the course of the inflammatory response when, early on, there may be IFN production related to invasive stimuli, while later TNF may aid tissue repair after the infection/invasion has been effectively dealt with, and when many of the host cells at the site of the inflammatory lesion may be capable of producing growth factors, especially in the presence of TNF. Even in the absence of an inflammatory lesion, it has been suggested that TNF may have natural role in turnover of senescent tissue proteins[63].

CHEMOTACTIC ACTIONS OF TNF

Sites of inflammation are often associated with an apparent influx of phagocytic cells. This may be due to release of chemotactic factors attracting cells to, or preventing their migration away from, the inflammatory focus, effectively leading to a build-up of their numbers. It has been observed that TNF is chemotactic *in vivo*, causing an influx of polymorphonuclear neutrophils (PMN) when injected into the mouse peritoneal cavity[64]. In this action TNF appears to require accessory cells or cytokines to express chemotactic activity as it is not chemotactic for PMN or monocytes when used alone in an *in vitro* system[65]. It may act through endothelial cells, which produce a chemotactic factor on stimulation with TNF or IL 1[66], but optimal chemotactic effects may also require the presence of cytokines such as IL 1[67]. It is likely that, in the initiation of an inflammatory response, TNF acts in synergy with other cells and their products, producing positive feedback and so expanding the infiltration of phagocytes. This is illustrated by its interactions with other chemotactic factors such as transforming growth factor beta (TGFβ) which is chemotactic for macrophages and may induce them to produce TNF[68]. This in turn is chemotactic in the presence of other macrophage products such as IL 1, causing an influx of PMN[67].

ACTIVATION OF CELLS BY TNF

The major cellular targets of TNF-mediated activation appear to be the phagocytic cells for which it is chemotactic. Once these cells have been sequestered in the inflammatory site they may be activated for optimal phagocytosis and killing of invasive organisms; in this respect TNF increases neutrophil phagocytic activity for opsonised particles[69], and enhances cytotoxicity for *Candida albicans*[70]. The increased phagocytic activity of TNF-treated neutrophils may be a result of increased expression of receptors for complement components C3b and C3bi[71], enhancing neutrophil interaction with invasive stimuli which have activated the complement cascade. The enhanced killing of organisms subsequent to phagocytosis may be associated with TNF-induced superoxide anion[72] and lysozyme[73] release. In these effects TNF does not appear to act alone, but in concert with other activation signals either provided by cytokines such as IFNγ and IL 1[74] or by other signals such as those provided by cell adhesion[72], or treatment with phorbol ester or chemotactic peptide[73].

The ability of TNF to recruit, and then activate, phagocytic cells in an inflammatory site suggests a role for this factor in initiation and augmentation of the initial non-specific cellular response to invasion. Other factors such as activation of the complement cascade and production of cytokines by inflammatory cells may also be required for optimizing these TNF-mediated effects.

INDUCTION OF SOLUBLE MEDIATORS BY TNF

TNF may act on a variety of cell types stimulating production of soluble mediators which may have inflammatory actions of their own, or which interact with TNF to modulate inflammatory responses. Administration of TNF *in vivo* gives rise to circulating detectable growth factors and cytokines including M-CSF, GM-CSF, IL 1[75] and IL 6[51]. The cellular source of these factors has been suggested by studies showing TNF may cause release of IL 1 from endothelial[76] and mononuclear cells[77] and release of CSF and IL 6 from fibroblasts[52,78], endothelial cells[79] and monocytes[80]. The direct action of TNF in recruitment and activation of phagocytes may be further augmented by TNF-mediated enhancement of leukotriene production by these cells[81], which in turn may amplify the cellular or inflammatory response by their chemotactic action on phagocytes[82]. Prostaglandin formation may be stimulated by TNF in cell populations found in joints[58] and in kidney[83], suggesting an involvement of TNF in inflammatory diseases of these organs and in renal graft rejection, where involvement of TNF is further implicated by the finding of circulating cytokine in association with rejection episodes[34]. TNF may also be involved in initiating the acute phase reaction by its action on liver cells enhancing serum amyloid A protein mRNA and factor B gene expression, and increasing C3 and caeruloplasmin biosynthesis[84]. These effects are also mediated by IL 6, which in turn may be induced by TNF[78].

INDUCTION OF SURFACE MOLECULES BY TNF

TNF is a potent inducer of cell surface membrane molecules which facilitate immune and inflammatory interactions between cells. It can act at both the target cell and immune effector cell level, increasing their mutual interaction. Some of the best-studied of these surface molecules are the major histocompatibility complex (MHC) antigens. The group termed MHC class I act as targets for attack by cytotoxic effector cells. TNF increases expression of MHC class I antigens on vascular endothelial cells[85,86] and on tumour cells taken from fresh human malignant tissue[87], and this TNF-induced expression of MHC class I increases target cell susceptibility to cytotoxic cell attack[87]. This may be a factor in the antitumour effects of TNF *in vivo*. TNF also acts to increase MHC class II expression on macrophage-like cells[88] which may augment the immune response by enhancing cell cooperation and antigen presentation.

Another group of cell surface molecules which facilitate interaction between target and effector cells are the cell-adhesion related molecules. These may also be modulated by TNF, which induces expression of the cell adhesion molecule ICAM-1 on endothelial[89] and tumour cells[90]. These molecules may participate in adhesion of lymphocytes to TNF-treated endothelial cells[91]. Treatment of phagocytes or vascular endothelial cells with TNF increases their mutual adherence, associated with increased expression of the CD18 leukocyte cell surface glycoproteins[92,93]. The action of TNF in increasing expression of cell interaction molecules clearly has an important role in influencing direct effector–target cell interactions. However, its action in bringing together cells in close proximity also enhances the paracrine effects of other soluble mediators secreted by these cells. These actions of TNF allow for multiple sensitive and specific areas for interaction by cells or cytokines for the initiation, augmentation and resolution of the inflammatory response.

INFLUENCE OF TNF ON COAGULATION

Vascular endothelial cells appear to be the mediators through which TNF induces changes in local haemostatic activity. Exposure of endothelial cells to TNF induces procoagulant activity, enhances tissue factor-like coagulant activity and suppresses antithrombotic mechanisms[94]. TNF also decreases expression of thrombomodulin, by increasing internalization and degradation of the molecule[95] and plasminogen activator inhibitor[97,98]. These changes in vascular endothelial procoagulant activity may contribute to the antitumour effects of TNF *in vivo* by causing endothelial deposition of fibrin and the formation of occlusive thrombi in the tumour vasculature[99]. This leads to ischaemic damage and ultimate necrosis of tumour tissue. These effects are not limited to tumours, and there may be a role for TNF in the induction of procoagulant activity in many immune and inflammatory conditions associated with microvascular injury. For example, it is likely that the thrombohaemorrhagic component of the Schwartzmann reaction may be initiated by the synergistic actions of TNF and IL 1 produced by endotoxin-activated macrophages[100]. Also, in this context, the thrombotic effects in rejecting renal grafts may be exacerbated by cyclosporin A, which acts to enhance TNF-induced thromboplastic activity in renal grafts[101]. The action of TNF on endothelial cells, altering haemostatic and cell surface properties, may be an early event in producing the vascular responses associated with inflammation, including intravascular coagulation, adherence of blood cells to endothelium and increased vascular permeability leading to leakage of macromolecules into the tissue space.

PYROGENIC ACTIVITY OF TNF

The acute toxicity events following TNF administration to patients include rigors, chills and fever[102–103]. This pyrogenic response may result from a direct effect of TNF on the thermoregulatory centre, stimulating prostaglandin release from the hypothalamic neurons[104,105]. The mechanisms of the TNF and IL 1-mediated pyrogenic effect are different, TNF having a direct central action, whereas IL 1 depends on release of other thermogenic factors[106]. TNF has recently been implicated in producing the fever associated with antithymocyte globulin administration in renal allograft patients[107], and in the pyrogenic effect of IL 2 administration in cancer patients[108]. These reports indicate that TNF may act as an endogenous pyrogen for a variety of fever-producing stimuli.

TNF: A PERSPECTIVE

TNF provides an early non-specific mechanism for host protection against invasive stimuli. Its diverse actions on cells seem to depend on the cell type and also on the presence of other cytokines or growth factors (Table 10.1). Its cytotoxic action against target cells/organisms is usually greatly enhanced by other cytokines, particularly IFNγ, which may also be released at the inflammatory site. Host phagocytic cells are recruited and activated in the inflammatory site, effector–target cell interactions are favoured and target cells sensitized by the various local actions of TNF. Systemic actions include pyrogenicity, which may inhibit the proliferation of many invading organisms, and mobilization of adipocyte energy reserves, which may serve to meet the metabolic demands of fever and inflammation. In the longer term when IFNγ levels have fallen, TNF may stimulate the proliferation of fibroblasts, particularly in the presence of other growth factors. This may be important in tissue repair and remodelling after the acute inflammatory response has subsided.

Thus, under normal circumstances, TNF is an essential mediator of the acute response to infection, but later on may have a role in wound healing. However, under circumstances resulting in rapid release of large amounts of TNF, or chronic long-term release of the cytokine, profound pathological effects may be encountered such as shock or chronic wasting conditions. TNF is clearly a powerful endogenous factor in host protection which is also capable of profound deleterious effects on the host. There is currently interest in investigating the multiple actions of TNF, so that its impressive array of actions may be better understood and ultimately manipulated to the benefit of patients.

References

1. Carswell, E. A., Old, L. J., Kassel, R. L., Green, S., Fiore, N. and Williamson, B. (1975). An endotoxin-induced serum factor that causes necrosis of tumors. *Proc. Natl. Acad. Sci. USA*, **72**, 3666–70
2. Rouzer, C. and Cerami, A. (1980). Hypertriglyceridemia associated with *Trypanosoma brucei* infection in rabbits; role of defective triglyceride removal. *Mol. Biochem. Parasitol.*, **2**, 31–8
3. Caput, D., Beutler, B., Hartog, K., Brown-Shimer, S. and Cerami, A. (1986). Identification of a common muclotide sequence in the 3′ untranslated region of mRNA molecules specifying inflammatory mediators. *Proc. Natl. Acad. Sci. USA*, **83**, 1670–4
4. Mannel, D. N., Moore, R. N. and Mergenhagen, S. E. (1980). Macrophages as a source of tumoricidal activity (tumor-necrotizing factor). *Infect. Immun.*, **30**, 523–30
5. Sung, S. S., Jung, L. K., Walters, J. A., Chen, W., Wang, C. Y. and Fu, S. M. (1988). Production of tumor necrosis factor/cachectin by human B cell lines and tonsillar B cells. *J. Exp. Med.*, **168**, 1539–51
6. Ranges, G. E., Zlotnik, A., Espevik, T., Dinarello, C. A., Cerami, A. and Palladino, M. A. Jr (1988). Tumor necrosis factor/cachetin is a growth factor for thymocytes. Synergistic interctions with other cytokines. *J. Exp. Med.*, **167**, 1472–8
7. Turner, M., Londei, M. and Feldmann, M. (1987). Human T cells from autoimmune and normal individuals can produce tumor necrosis factor. *Eur. J. Immunol.*, **17**, 1807–14
8. Kreigler, M., Perez, C., De Fay, K., Albert, I. and Lu, S. D. (1988). A novel form of human TNF/cachectin is a cell surface cytotoxic transmembrane protein: ramifications for the complex physiology of TNF. *Cell*, **53**, 45–53

9. Decker, T., Lohmann-Matthes, M.-L. and Gifford, G. E. (1987). Cell-associated tumor necrosis factor (TNF) as a killing mechanism of activated cytotoxic macrophages. *J. Immunol.*, **138**, 957–62
10. Beutler, B., Mahoney, J., Le Trang, N., Pekala, P. and Cerami, A. (1985). Purification of cachectin, a lipoprotein lipase suppressing hormone secreted by endotoxin-induced RAW 264.7 cells. *J. Exp. Med.*, **161**, 984–95
11. Smith, R. A. and Baglioni, C. (1987). The active form of tumor necrosis factor is a trimer. *J. Biol. Chem.*, **262**, 6951–4
12. Marmenout, A., Fransen, L., Tavernier, J., Van Der Heyden, J., Tizard, R., Ruysschaert, M. R., van Vliet, A. and Fiers, W. (1985). Molecular cloning and expression of human tumor necrosis factor. *Eur. J. Biochem.*, **152**, 512–22
13. Ranges, G. E., Bombara, M. P., Aiyer, R. A., Rice, G. G. and Palladino, M. A. Jr (1989). Tumor necrosis factor alpha as a proliferative signal an IL-2-dependent T cell line: strict species specificity of action. *J. Immunol.*, **142**, 1203–8
14. Kull, F. C. Jr, Jacobs, S. and Cuatrecasas (1985). Cellular receptor for ^{125}I-labelled tumor necrosis factor: specific binding, affinity labelling and relationship to sensitivity. *Proc. Natl. Acad. Sci. USA*, **82**, 5756–60
15. Nawroth, P. P., Bank, I., Handley, D., Cassimeris, J., Chess, L. and Stern, D. (1986). Tumor necrosis factor/cachectin interacts with endothelial cell receptors to induce release of interleukin 1. *J. Exp. Med.*, **163**, 1363–75
16. Munker, R., Di Persio, J. and Koeffler, H. P. (1987). Tumor necrosis factor: receptors on hematopoietic cells. *Blood*, **70**, 1730–4
17. Pichyangkul, S., Schick, D., Jia, F. L., Berent, S., Bollon, A. and Kahn, A. (1987). Binding of tumor necrosis factor alpha (TNF-alpha) to high affinity receptors on polymorphonuclear cells. *Exp. Hematol.*, **15**, 1055–9
18. Eades, D. K., Cornelius, P. and Pekala, P. H. (1988). Characterization of the tumour necrosis factor receptor in human placenta. *Placenta*, **9**, 247–51
19. Imamura, K., Spriggs, D. and Kufe, D. (1987). Expression of tumor necrosis factor receptor on human monocytes and internalization of receptor bound ligand. *J. Immunol.*, **139**, 2989–92
20. Scheurich, P., Maxeiner, B., Ucer, U. and Pfizenmaier, K. (1987). Interferon gamma production by activated human T lymphocytes is stimulated by tumor necrosis factor alpha. *J. Interferon Res.*, Suppl (1), **6**, 112 (abstract 43)
21. Suffys, P., Beyaert, R., Van Roy, F. and Fiers, W. (1987). Reduced tumour necrosis factor-induced cytotoxicity by inhibitors of the arachidonic acid metabolism. *Biochem. Biophys. Res. Commun.*, **149**, 735–43
22. Hepburn, A., Boeynaems, J. M., Fiers, W. and Dumont, J. E. (1987). Modulation of tumor necrosis factor alpha cytotoxicity in L929 cells by bacterial toxins, hydrocortisone and inhibitors of arachidonic acid metabolism. *Biochem. Biophys. Res. Commun.*, **149**, 815–22
23. Lin, J.-X. and Vilcek, J. (1987). Tumor necrosis factor and interleukin-1 cause a rapid and transient stimulation of c-fos and c-myc mRNA levels in human fibroblasts. *J. Biol. Chem.*, **262**, 11908–11
24. Palombella, V. J., Yamashiro, D. J., Maxfield, F. R., Decker, S. J. and Vilcek, J. (1987). Tumor necrosis factor increases the number of epidermal growth factor receptors on human fibroblasts. *J. Biol. Chem.*, **262**, 11908–11
25. Creasey, A. A., Yamamoto, R. and Vitt, C. R. (1987). A high molecular weight component of the human tumor necrosis factor receptor is associated with cytotoxicity. *Proc. Natl. Acad. Sci. USA*, **84**, 3293–7
26. Aggarwal, B. B., Eessalu, T. E. and Hass, P. E. (1985). Characterisation of receptors for human tumour necrosis factor and their regulation by gamma-interferon. *Nature*, **318**, 665–7
27. Broudy, V. C., Harlan, J. M. and Adamson, J. W. (1987). Disparate effects of tumour necrosis factor alpha/cachectin and tumour necrosis factor-beta/lymphotoxin on hematopoietic growth factor production and neutrophil adhesion molecule expression by cultured human endothelial cells. *J. Immunol.*, **138**, 4298–302
28. Waage, A., Halstensen, A. and Espevik, T. (1987). Association between tumor necrosis factor in serum and fatal outcome in patients with meningococcal disease. *Lancet*, **1**, 355–7
29. Aderka, D., Holtmann, H., Toker, L., Hahn, T. and Wallach, D. (1986). Tumor necrosis induction by Sendai virus. *J. Immunol.*, **136**, 2938–42
30. Scuderi, P., Sterling, K. E., Lam, K. S., Finley, P. R., Ryan, K. J., Ray, C. G., Petersen, E.,

Slymen, D. S. and Salomon, S. E. (1986). Raised serum levels of tumour necrosis factor in parasitic infections. *Lancet*, **2**, 1364–5

31. Jacob, C. O. and McDevitt, H. O. (1988). Tumour necrosis factor-alpha in murine autoimmune 'lupus' nephritis. *Nature*, **331**, 356–8
32. Piguet, P.-F., Grau, G. E., Allet, B. and Vassalli, P. (1987). Tumor necrosis factor/cachectin is an effector of the skin and gut lesions of the acute phase of graft-vs.-host disease. *J. Exp. Med.*, **166**, 1280–9
33. Maury, C. P. J. and Teppo, A.-M. (1987). Raised serum levels of cachectin/tumor necrosis factor alpha in renal allograft rejection. *J. Exp. Med.*, **166**, 1132–7
34. Bertolini, D. R., Nedwin, G. E., Bringman, T. S., Smith, D. D. and Mundy, G. R. (1986). Stimulation of bone resorption and inhibition of bone formation *in vitro* by human tumor necrosis factors. *Nature*, **319**, 516–88
35. Balkwill, F., Burke, F., Talbot, D., Tavernier, J., Osborne, S., Naylor, H., Durbin, H. and Fiers, W. (1987). Evidence for tumour necrosis factor/cachectin production in cancer. *Lancet*, **2**, 1229–32
36. Old, L. J. (1985). Tumour necrosis factor (TNF). *Science*, **230**, 630–2
37. Sugarman, B. J., Aggarwal, B. B., Hass, P. E., Figari, I. S., Palladino, M. A. Jr and Shepard, H. M. (1985). Recombinant human tumor necrosis factor-alpha: effects on proliferation of normal and transformed cells in vitro. *Science*, **230**, 943–5
38. Salmon, S. E., Young, L., Scuderi, P. and Clark, B. (1987). Antineoplastic effects of tumor necrosis factor alone and in combination with gamma-interferon on tumor biopsies in clonogenic assay. *J. Clin. Oncol.*, **5**, 1816–21
39. Taverne, J., Rayner, D. C., van der Meide, P. H., Lydyard, P. M., Bidey, S. P. and Cooke, A. (1987). Cytotoxicity of tumor necrosis factor for mitogenic action in fibroblasts. *J. Cell. Physiol.*, Suppl. **5**, 57–61
40. Sato, N., Fukuda, K., Nariuchi, H. and Sagara, N. (1987). Tumor necrosis factor inhibiting angiogenesis *in vitro*. *J. Natl. Cancer Inst.*, **79**, 1383–91
41. Wong, G. H. W., Krowka, J. F., Stites, D. P. and Goeddel, D. V. (1988). *In vitro* anti-human immunodeficiency virus activities of tumor necrosis factor-alpha and interferon-gamma. *J. Immunol.*, **140**, 120–4
42. Ito, M. and O'Malley, J. A. (1987). Antiviral effects of recombinant human tumor necrosis factor. *Lymphokine Res.*, **6**, 309–18
43. Matthews, N. and Watkins, J. F. (1978). Tumor necrosis factor from the rabbit. I. Mode of action, specificity and physicochemical properties. *Br. J. Cancer*, **38**, 302–9
44. Leibovich, S. J., Polverini, P. J., Shepard, H. M., Wiseman, D. M., Shively, V. and Nuseir, N. (1987). Macrophage-induced angiogenesis is mediated by tumour necrosis factor-alpha. *Nature*, **329**, 630–2
45. Vilcek, J., Tsujimoto, M., Palombella, V. J., Kohase, M. and Jumming, L. E. (1987). Tumor necrosis factor: receptor binding and mitogenic action in fibroblasts. *J. Cell. Physiol.*, Suppl. **5**, 57–61
46. Elias, J. A. (1988). Tumor necrosis factor interacts with interleukin-1 and interferon to inhibit fibroblast proliferation via fibroblast prostaglandin-dependent and -independent mechanisms. *Am. Rev. Respir. Dis.*, **138**, 652–8
47. Broxmeyer, H. E., Williams, D. E., Lu, L., Cooper, S., Anderson, S. L., Beyer, G. S., Hoffman, R. and Rubin, B. Y. (1986). The suppressive influences of human tumor necrosis factors on bone marrow hematopoietic progenitor cells from normal donors and patients with leukemia: synergism of tumor necrosis factor and gamma-interferon. *J. Immunol.*, **136**, 4487–95
48. Herrman, F., Bambach, T., Bonifer, R., Lindemann, A., Riedel, D., Oster, W. and Mertelsmann, R. (1988). The suppressive effects of recombinant tumor necrosis factor alpha on normal and malignant myelopoiesis: synergism with interferon-gamma. *Int. J. Cell. Cloning*, **6**, 241–61
49. Murphy, M., Perussia, B. and Trinchieri, G. (1988). Effects of recombinant tumor necrosis factor, lymphotoxin and immune interferon on proliferation and differentiation of enriched hematopoietic precursor cells. *Exp. Hematol.*, **16**, 131–8
50. Branch, D. R., Turner, A. R. and Guilbert, L. J. (1989). Synergistic stimulation of macrophage proliferation by the monokines tumor necrosis factor-alpha and colony-stimulating factor 1. *Blood*, **73**, 307–11
51. Jablons, D. M., Mule, J. J., McIntosh, J. K., Seghal, P. B., May, L. T., Huang, C. M.,

Rosenberg, S. A. and Lotze, M. T. (1989). Il-6/IFN-beta-2 as a circulating hormone. Induction by cytokine administration in humans. *J. Immunol.*, **142**, 1542–7
52. Kohase, M., Henriksen-De Stefano, D., May, L. T., Vilcek, J. and Sehgal, P. B. (1986). Induction of beta-2 interferon by tumor necrosis factor: a homeostatic mechanism in the control of cell proliferation. *Cell*, **45**, 659–66
53. Hajjar, K. A., Hajjar, D. P., Silverstein, R. L. and Nachman, R. L. (1987). Tumor necrosis factor-mediated release of platelet-derived growth factor from cultured endothelial cells. *J. Exp. Med.*, **166**, 235–45
54. Ranges, G. E., Zlotnik, A., Espevik, T., Dinarello, C. A., Cerami, A. and Palladino, M. A. Jr (1988). Tumour necrosis factor alpha/cachectin is a growth factor for thymocytes. Synergistic interactions with other cytokines. *J. Exp. Med.*, **167**, 1472–8
55. Hackett, R. J., Davis, L. S. and Lipsky, P. E. (1988). Comparative effects of tumor necrosis factor-alpha and IL-1 beta on mitogen-induced T cell activation. *J. Immunol.*, **140**, 2639–44
56. Shalaby, M. R., Espevik, T., Rice, G. C., Figari, I. S., Ammann, A. J., Ranges, G. E. and Palladino, M. A. Jr (1988). The involvement of human tumour necrosis factors alpha and beta in the mixed lymphocyte reaction. *J. Immunol.*, **141**, 499–503
57. Ranges, G. E., Figari, T., Espevik, T. and Palladino, M. A. Jr (1987). Inhibition of cytotoxic T cell development by transforming growth factor-beta and reversal by recombinant tumor necrosis factor-alpha. *J. Exp. Med.*, **166**, 991–8
58. Gowen, M., MacDonald, B. R. and Russel, R. G. (1988). Actions of recombinant human gamma-interferon and tumor necrosis factor alpha on the proliferation and osteoblastic characteristics of human trabecular bone cells in vitro. *Arthritis Rheum.*, **31**, 1500–7
59. Ikebe, T., Hirata, M. and Koga, T. (1988). Effects of human recombinant tumor necrosis factor alpha and interleukin-1 on the synthesis of glycosaminoglycan and DNA in cultured rat costal chondrocytes. *J. Immunol.*, **140**, 827–31
60. Saklatvala, J. (1986). Tumour necrosis factor alpha stimulates resorption and inhibits synthesis of proteoglycan in cartilage. *Nature*, **322**, 547–9.
61. Johnson, R. A., Boyce, B. F., Mundy, G. R. and Roodman, G. D. (1989). Tumors producing human tumor necrosis factor induced hypercalcemia and osteoclastic bone resorption in nude mice. *Endocrinology*, **124**, 1424–7
62. Hopkins, S. J. and Meager, A. (1988). Cytokines in synovial fluid. II. The presence of tumor necrosis factor and interferon. *Clin. Exp. Immunol.*, **73**, 88–92
63. Vlassara, H., Brownlee, M., Manogue, K. R., Dinarello, C. A. and Pasagian, A. (1988). Cachectin/TNF and IL-1 induced by glucose-modified proteins: role in normal tissue remodelling. *Science*, **240**, 1546–8
64. Sayers, T. J., Wiltrout, T. A., Bull, C. A., Denn, A. C. 3rd, Pilaro, A. M. and Lokesh, B. (1988). Effect of cytokines on polymorphonuclear infiltration in the mouse. Prostaglandin and leukotriene-independent induction of infiltration by IL-1 and tumor necrosis factor. *J. Immunol.*, **141**, 1670–7
65. Mrowietz, U., Schroder, J. M. and Christophers, E. (1988). Recombinant human tumor necrosis factor alpha lacks chemotactic activity for human peripheral blood neutrophils and monocytes. *Biochem. Biophys. Res. Commun.*, **153**, 1223–8
66. Strieter, R. M., Kunkel, S. L., Showell, H. J. and Marks, R. M. (1988). Monokine-induced gene expression of a human endothelial cell-derived neutrophil chemotactic factor. *Biochem. Biophys. Res. Commun.*, **156**, 1340–5
67. Wankowicz, Z., Megyeri, P. and Issekutz, A. (1988). Synergy between tumour necrosis factor alpha and interleukin-1 in the induction of polymorphonuclear leukocyte migration during inflammation. *J. Leukocyte Biol.*, **43**, 349–56
68. Wiseman, D. M., Polverini, P. J., Kamp, D. W. and Leibovich, S. J. (1988). Transforming growth factor beta (TGF beta) is chemotactic for human monocytes and induces their expression of angiogenic activity. *Biochem. Biophys. Res. Commun.*, **157**, 793–800
69. Ozaki, Y., Ohashi, T., Niwa, Y. and Kume, S. (1988). Effects of recombinant DNA-produced tumor necrosis factor on various parameters of neutrophil function. *Inflammation*, **12**, 297–309
70. Djeu, J. Y., Blanchard, D. K., Halkias, D. and Friedman, H. (1986). Growth inhibition of *Candida albicans* by human polymorphonuclear neutrophils: activation by interferon-gamma and tumor necrosis factor. *J. Immunol.*, **137**, 2980–4
71. Berger, M., Wetzler, E. M. and Wallis, R. S. (1988). Tumor necrosis factor is the major monocyte product that increases complement receptor expression on mature human

neutrophils. *Blood*, **71**, 151–8
72. Kownatzki, E., Kapp, A. and Uhrich, S. (1988). Modulation of human neutrophilic granulocyte functions by recombinant human tumor necrosis factor and recombinant human lymphotoxin. Promotion of adherence, inhibition of chemotactic migration and superoxide anion release from adherent cells. *Clin. Exp. Immunol.*, **74**, 143–8
73. Berkow, R. L., Wang, D., Larrick, J. W., Dodson, R. W. and Howard, T. H. (1987). Enhancement of neutrophil superoxide production by preincubation with recombinant human tumor necrosis factor. *J. Immunol.*, **139**, 3783–91
74. Philip, R. and Epstein, L. B. (1986). Tumour necrosis factor as immunomodulator and mediator of monocyte cytotoxicity induced by itself, gamma-interferon and interleukin-1. *Nature*, **323**, 86–9
75. Kaushansky, K., Broudy, V. C., Harlan, J. M. and Adamson, J. W. (1988). Tumor necrosis factor-alpha and tumor necrosis factor-beta stimulate the production of granulocyte-macrophage colony-stimulating factor, macrophage colony-stimulating factor and IL-1 *in vivo*. *J. Immunol.*, **141**, 3410–15
76. Nawroth, P. P., Bank, I., Handley, D., Cassimeris, J., Chess, L. and Stern, D. (1986). Tumor necrosis factor/cachectin interacts with endothelial cell receptors to induce release of IL-1. *J. Exp. Med.*, **163**, 1363–75
77. Dinarello, C. A., Cannon, J. G., Wolff, S. M., Bernheim, H. A., Beutler, B., Cerami, A., Figari, I. S., Palladino, M. A. Jr and O'Connor, J. V. (1986). Tumor necrosis factor (cachectin) is an endogenous pyrogen and induces production of interleukin 1. *J. Exp. Med.*, **163**, 1433–50
78. Munker, R., Gasson, J., Ogawa, M. and Koeffler, H. P. (1986). Recombinant human TNF induces production of granulocyte/monocyte colony stimulating factor. *Nature*, **323**, 79–82
79. Broudy, V. C., Kaushansky, K., Segal, G. M., Harlan, J. M. and Adamson, J. W. (1986). Tumor necrosis factor type alpha stimulates human endothelial cells to produce granulocyte/macrophage colony-stimulating factor. *Proc. Natl. Acad. Sci. USA*, **83**, 7467–71
80. Oster, W., Lindemann, A., Horne, S., Mertelsmann, R. and Herrmaun, F. (1987). Tumor necrosis factor TNF-alpha but not TNF-beta induces the secretion of colony stimulating factor for macrophages (CSF-1) by human monocytes. *Blood*, **70**, 1700–3
81. Roubin, R., Elsas, P. P., Fiers, W. and Dessein, A. J. (1987). Recombinant human tumour necrosis factor (rTNF) enhances leukotriene biosynthesis in neutrophils and eosinophils stimulated with the Ca^{2+} ionophore A23187. *Clin. Exp. Immunol.*, **70**, 484–90
82. Ford-Hutchinson, A. W., Bray, A. W., Doig, M. V., Shipley, M. E. and Smith, M. J. H. (1980). Leukotriene B: a potent chemokinetic and aggregating substance released from polymorphonuclear leukocytes. *Nature*, **286**, 264–5
83. Baud, L., Perez, J., Friedlander, G. and Ardaillou, R. (1988). Tumor necrosis factor stimulates prostaglandin production and cyclic AMP levels in rat cultured mesangial cells. *FEBS Lett.*, **239**, 50–4
84. Ramadori, G., van Damme, J., Rieder, H. and Meyer-zum-Buschenfelde, K. H. (1988). Interleukin-6, the third mediator of acute phase reaction, modulates hepatic protein synthesis in human and mouse. Comparison with interleukin 1 beta and tumor necrosis factor alpha. *Eur. J. Immunol.*, **18**, 1259–64
85. Pober, J. S. (1987). Effects of tumour necrosis factor and related cytokines on vascular endothelial cells. *Ciba Found. Symp.*, **131**, 170–84
86. Wedgwood, J. F., Hatam, L. and Bonagura, V. R. (1988). Effect of interferon-gamma and tumor necrosis factor on the expression of Class I and Class II major histocompatibility molecules by cultured human umbilical vein endothelial cells. *Cell. Immunol.*, **111**, 1–9
87. Vanky, F., Stuber, G., Rotstein, S. and Klein, E. (1989). Autotumor recognition following *in vitro* induction of MHC antigen expression on solid human tumors: stimulation of lympahocytes and generation of cytotoxicity against the original MHC-antigen-negative tumor cells. *Cancer Immunol. Immunother.*, **28**, 17–21
88. Portillo, G., Turner, M., Chantry, D. and Feldman, M. (1989). Effect of cytokines on HLA-DR and IL-1 production by a monocytic tumour THP-1. *Immunology*, **66**, 170–5
89. Pober, J. S., Gimbrone, M. A. Jr, Lapierre, C. A., Mendrick, D. L., Fiers, W., Rothlein, R. and Springer, T. A. (1986). Overlapping patterns of activation of human endothelial cells by interleukin 1, tumor necrosis factor, and immune interferon. *J. Immunol.*, **137**, 1893–6
90. Rothlein, R., Czajkowski, M., O'Neill, M. M., Marlin, S. D., Mainolfi, E. and Merluzzi, V. J. (1988). Induction of intercellular adhesion molecule 1 on primary and continuous

cell lines by pro-inflammatory cytokines. Regulation by pharmacologic agents and neutralizing antibodies. *J. Immunol.*, **141**, 1665–9
91. Cavender, D. E., Haskard, D. O., Maliakkal, D. and Ziff, M. (1988). Separation and characterization of human T lymphocytes with varying adhesiveness for endothelial cells. *Cell. Immunol.*, **117**, 111–26
92. Pohlman, T. H., Stanness, K. A., Beatty, P. G., Ochs, H. D. and Haslan, J. M. (1986). An endothelial cell surface factor(s) induced *in vitro* by lipopolysaccharide, interleukin 1, and tumor necrosis factor-alpha increases neutrophil adherence by a CDw 18-dependent mechanism. *J. Immunol.*, **136**, 4548–53
93. Lamas, A. M., Mulroney, C. M. and Schleimer, R. P. (1988). Studies on the adhesive interaction between purified human eosinophils and cultured vascular endothelial cells. *J. Immunol.*, **140**, 1500–5
94. Stern, D. M. and Nawroth, P. P. (1986). Modulation of endothelial hemostatic properties by tumor necrosis factor. *J. Exp. Med.*, **163**, 740–5
95. Moore, K. L., Esman, C. T. and Esman, N. L. (1989). Tumor necrosis factor leads to internalization and degradation of thrombomodulin from the surface of bovine aortic endothelial cells in culture. *Blood*, **73**, 159–65
96. Camussi, G., Bussolino, F., Salvidio, G. and Baglioni, C. (1987). Tumor necrosis factor/cachectin stimulates peritoneal macrophages, polymorphonuclear neutrophils, and vascular endothelial cells to synthesize and release platelet-activating factor. *J. Exp. Med.*, **166**, 1390–404
97. Dosne, A. M., Dubor, F., Lutcher, F., Parant, M. and Chedid, L. (1988). Tumor necrosis factor (TNF) stimulates plasminogen activator inhibitor (PAI) production and decreases blood fibrinolytic activity in the rat. *Thromb. Res. Suppl.*, **8**, 115–22
98. Medcalf, R. L., Kruithof, E. K. and Schleuning, W. D. (1988). Plasminogen inhibitor 1 and 2 are tumor necrosis factor/cachectin-responsive genes. *J. Exp. Med.*, **168**, 751–9
99. Nawroth, P., Handley, D., Matsueda, G., De-Waal, R., Gerlach, H., Blohm, D. and Stern, D. (1988). Tumor necrosis factor/cachectin-induced intravascular fibrin formation in meth A fibrosarcomas. *J. Exp. Med.*, **168**, 637–47
100. Movat, H. Z., Burows, C. E., Cybulsky, M. I. and Dinarello, C. A. (1987). Acute inflammation and a Schwartzman-like reaction induced by interleukin-1 and tumor necrosis factor. Synergistic action of the cytokines in the induction of inflammation and microvascular injury. *Am. J. Pathol.*, **129**, 463–76
101. Carlsen, E., Flatmark, A. and Prydz, H. (1988). Cytokine-induced procoagulant activity in monocytes and endothelial cells, further enhancement by cyclosporine. *Transplantation*, **46**, 575–80
102. Creaven, P. J., Plager, J. E., Dupere, C., Huben, R. P., Takita, H., Mittelman, A. and Proefrock, A. (1987). Phase I clinical trial of recombinant human tumor necrosis factor. *Cancer Chemother. Pharmacol.*, **20**, 137–44
103. Selby, P., Hobbs, S., Viner, C., Jackson, E., Jones, A., Newell, D., Calvert, A. H., McElwain, T., Fearon, K., Humphreys, J. and Shiga, T. (1987). Tumor necrosis factor in man: clinical and biological observations. *Br. J. Cancer*, **56**, 803–8
104. Dinarello, C. A., Cannon, J. G., Wolff, S. M., Bernheim, H. A., Beutler, B., Cerami, A., Figari, I. S., Palladine, M. A. Jr and O'Connor, J. V. (1986). Tumour necrosis factor (cachectin) is an endogenous pyrogen and induces production of interleukin 1. *J. Exp. Med.*, **163**, 1433–50
105. Nakamura, H., Seto, Y., Motoyoshi, S., Kadokawa, T. and Sunahara, N. (1988). Recombinant human tumor necrosis factor causes long-lasting and prostaglandin-mediated fever, with little tolerance in rabbits. *J. Pharmacol. Exp. Ther.*, **245**, 336–41
106. Rothwell, N. J. (1988). Central effectsof TNF alpha on thermogenesis and fever in the rat. *Biosci. Rep.*, **8**, 845–52
107. Debets, J. M., Leunissen, K. M., van-Hooff, H. J., van-den-Linden, C. J. and Buurman, W. A. (1989). Evidence of involvement of tumor necrosis factor in adverse reactions during treatment of kidney allograft rejection with antithymocyte globulin. *Transplantation*, **47**, 487–92
108. Mier, J. W., Vachino, G., van-der-Meer, J. W., Numerof, R. P., Adams, S., Cannon, J. G., Bernheim, H. A., Atkins, M. B., Parkinson, D. R. and Dinarello, C. A. (1988). Induction of circulating tumor necrosis factor (TNF alpha) as the mechanism for the febrile response to interleukin-2 (IL-2) in cancer patients. *J. Clin. Immunol.*, **8**, 426–36

12
Interleukin 6: a consequence of inflammation

S. W. EVANS

INTRODUCTION

Interleukin 6 (IL 6) is a polypeptide mediator with many different biological activities. The pleiotropic nature of this cytokine is reflected by its identification in a number of different guises: hepatocyte stimulating factor, hybridoma/plasmacytoma growth factor, interferon β_2, 26 kD protein and B cell stimulatory factor 2. The molecular cloning of genes encoding proteins with these activities has established that the molecules responsible are identical[1–5]. It is now clear that IL 6 is a cytokine with important roles in a wide variety of systems including regulation of the immune response, the acute phase reaction and haematopoiesis.

BIOCHEMICAL AND MOLECULAR PROPERTIES OF IL 6

Structure of IL 6

Human IL 6 is a glycoprotein with an apparent molecular weight of between 21 and 28 kD as determined by SDS-PAGE. The molecule consists of 212 amino acids which includes a 28 residue hydrophobic signal sequence, two potential N-linked and several potential O-linked glycosylation sites. The observed heterogeneity of natural IL 6 has been attributed to different glycosylation, phosphorylation and acylation states of the molecule and to heterogeneity in signal peptide cleavage[6,7].

The gene for IL 6 has been located on chromosome 7 in humans and 5 in the mouse, occupying approximately 5 and 7 kb respectively[10,11]. Both genes consist of five exons and four introns, and closely resemble each other and those of growth hormone, prolactin, erythropoietin and G CSF[8,12,13] (Figure 12.1). Further investigation of the human IL 6 gene has located the gene to 7p21 and established that there are at least three polymorphic forms. MspI, BgiI and BstNI restriction sites reveal three, two and four allele polymorphism respectively (Table 12.1)[14]. The MspI and BgiI polymorphism appear to be due to base pair substitutions, MspI in the vicinity of the fifth exon and BgiI in the 5′ flanking region. The BstNI polymorphism appears to be due to an insertion/deletion event 3′ of the fifth exon.

IL 6 gene regulation

Many different cell types are able to synthesize IL 6 in response to a variety of different stimuli. Some of the major cellular sources of IL 6 include: B

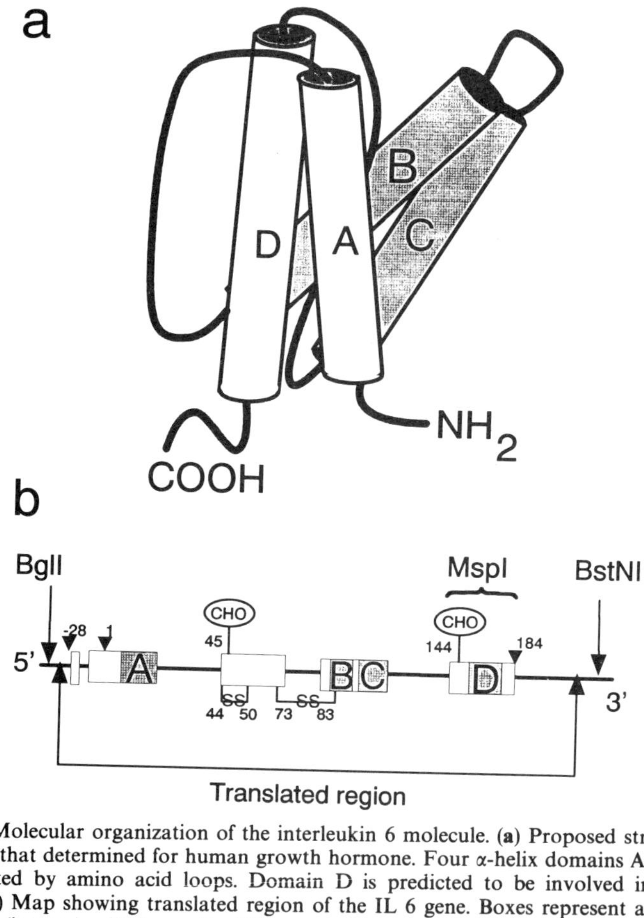

Figure 12.1 Molecular organization of the interleukin 6 molecule. (**a**) Proposed structure for IL 6 based on that determined for human growth hormone. Four α-helix domains A, B, C and D are connected by amino acid loops. Domain D is predicted to be involved in receptor recognition. (**b**) Map showing translated region of the IL 6 gene. Boxes represent amino acid coding regions (introns) solid boxes (A–D) correspond to the α-helix domains in (a). Proposed location of polymorphic regions (BglI, MspI and BstNI), disulphide bridge loops (s-s) and potential *N*-linked glycosylation sites (CHO) are marked.

Table 12.1 Interleukin 6 gene polymorphism[14]

Allele	*MspI*			*BglII*		*BstNI*			
RFLP (kb)	8	7.5	4.0	7.6	5.7	1.6	1.5	1.44	1.37
f (Caucasian)	0.0	0.55	0.45	0.04	0.96	0.05	0	0.11	0.84

Table 12.2 Some major cellular sources of interleukin 6

Cell type	*Secretagogue*	*Refs*
Monocyte/macrophage	Lipopolysaccharide Interleukin 1α/β HIV virus	15–17
Fibroblasts	Interleukin 1α/β poly(I). poly(C) Viruses Tumour necrosis factor α	18–20
Endothelial cells	Interleukin 1α/β Tumour necrosis factor α	21
Epidermal cells		22
Chondrocytes		23
Synoviocytes	Interleukin 1α/β Tumour necrosis factor α	24
Endometrial cells	Interleukin 1α	25
Astrocytes	Interleukin 1α/β Tumour necrosis factor α Virus	26
Microglia cells	Virus	26

cells, monocytes and non-lymphoid cells such as endothelial cells, keratinocytes and fibroblasts (Table 12.2).

Relatively little is known about the mechanism of IL 6 gene expression. However, the variety of stimuli able to induce IL 6 synthesis and sequence analysis of the 5′ flanking region of the IL 6 gene suggest that several different signal transduction pathways, including both cAMP-dependent and protein kinase C-activating systems, have the potential to participate[18,27].

Several lines of evidence suggest that a c-fos-like, serum responsive element (SRE) contains important *cis*-acting regulatory elements (CRE) controlling IL 6 gene transcription. A c-fos SRE like sequence has been located 5′ (−173 to −145) to the IL 6 gene CRE[28]. Other regulatory sequences are located either side of the CRE region, 5′–two glucocorticoid response elements and an AP-1 binding sequence and 3′–one NF-kB binding site and one TATA box (Figure 12.2)[29]. Using Hela cells transfected with IL 6 promoter–CAT constructs, phorbol esters, IL 1 and virus were able to induce transcription which was dependent upon the intact c-fos-like SRE. Two overlapping transcription control elements have been identified within the c-fos SRE homology region, NF-IL 6 and the multiple response element (MRE)[29,30]. Several glucocorticoid responsive elements are present in the 5′ flanking region and it has been shown that dexamethasone inhibits IL 6 production[31].

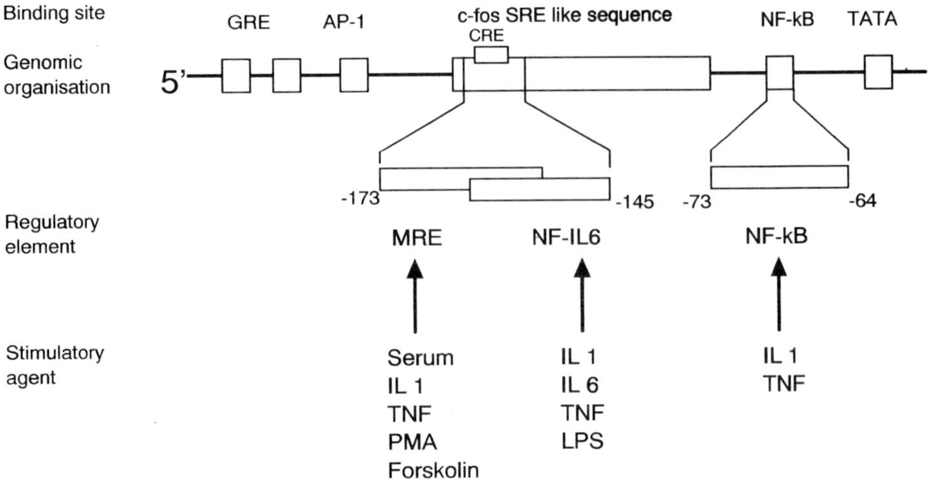

Figure 12.2 Molecular organization of the regulatory region 5′ to the IL 6 coding region[28,29].

IL 6 receptors and signal transduction

Specific receptors for IL 6 have been demonstrated on a variety of normal and transformed cell types (Table 12.3). Analysis by Scatchard plot has revealed high- and low-affinity forms of the IL 6 receptor on a human myeloma cell line[32]. A membrane-associated receptor for IL 6 has been identified and the gene encoding this protein cloned[33]. A single polypeptide chain constitutes the ligand binding site and the transmembrane region of the receptor. This 468 amino acid protein has an apparent molecular weight of 80 kD and has six potential N-linked glycosylation sites[33]. In contrast to IL 6, IL 6 receptor expression is increased by glucocorticoids[34]. At the molecular level the IL 6 receptor resembles the receptors for growth hormone, prolactin, erythropoietin and the p75 chain of the IL 2 receptor[35]. Sequence homology with immunoglobulin light chain, CD4, poly-Ig receptor and α_{1B}-glycoprotein suggest that the IL 6 receptor gene might be a member of

Table 12.3 Cells expressing the interleukin 6 receptor[32–34]

Cells	*Receptors/cell*
Hepatocytes	
Hepatoma cell lines	~2500
Activated B cells	~500
Resting B cells	Non-detected
Myeloma cells (and lines)	100–20 000
Resting T cells	~300
Myeloid cells	
Myeloid cell lines	~2500

the immunoglobulin supergene family[36].

Binding of IL 6 to its receptor is thought to involve association of the receptor with an accessory protein gp130[38]. It is possible that gp130 plays a role in signal transduction, although the nature of that role is not known. It has been reported that extracellular calcium is required for IL 6-stimulated growth of plasmacytoma cells[39]. An important role for calcium is also suggested by the ability of lead and cadmium, competitive inhibitors of calcium-dependent processes, to inhibit IL 6-stimulated proliferation of a hybridoma cell line[40] and IL 6-stimulated synthesis of α_1-antichymotrypsin (S. Evans and J. Whicher, unpublished). Phorbol esters stimulate the accumulation of acute phase protein mRNA in hepatoma cells and protein kinase C 'burn-out' experiments ablate IL 6-stimulated accumulation of acute phase protein mRNA, suggesting but not establishing a role for the calcium-dependent protein kinase C in IL 6 signal transduction[41,42].

PLEIOTROPIC PROPERTIES OF IL 6; ROLE OF IL 6 IN INFLAMMATION

IL 6 has a wide variety of different biological activities *in vitro* (Table 12.4). At least two distinct types of property can be discerned, differentiation and proliferation. The wide variety of cells which can be activated or which differentiate in response to IL 6 suggest an important *in vivo* regulatory role for this cytokine. In the following sections those activities of IL 6 which are most relevant to the inflammatory response are described.

IL 6 as a mediator of acute phase protein synthesis

One of the most apparent consequences of inflammation is the production of acute phase proteins (Chapter 13). A wide variety of molecules have been implicated in regulation of the synthesis of acute phase proteins. Speculation that IL 1 was the hepatocyte stimulating factor (HSF) followed the demonstration that this cytokine induced synthesis of murine serum amyloid A and haptoglobin *in vivo* and *in vitro*[48]. Subsequently it was demonstrated that the major HSF activity and IL 1 could be separated, the HSF activity being

Table 12.4 Some biological activities of interleukin 6

Cell types	*Effect of IL 6*	*Refs*
Acute phase response		
Hepatocyte	Acute phase protein synthesis	42
Adrenal cortex	Corticosterone release	43
Immune response		
B cell	Differentiation	5
Plasma cell	Growth as plasmacytoma	2
T cell	T_C differentiation	44
	IL 2 receptor expression	
Haematopoieses and repair		
Stem cells	Differentiation	45
Megakaryocyte	Differentiation	46
PC12	Neural differentiation	47

attributed to IL 6[1,49]. Using a variety of different cells including primary hepatocytes and hepatoma cell lines, recombinant IL 6 and antibodies specific for IL 6, it has now been clearly established that this cytokine is one of the predominant mediators controlling acute phase protein production[50]. There is growing evidence that, while IL 6 is the main regulator of acute phase protein synthesis, other soluble mediators acting on hepatocytes can influence the pattern of acute phase protein production. In addition to IL 1 and IL 6, three other cytokines, TGFβ, TNFα and IFNγ, have been shown to play a role in regulation of some aspects of acute phase protein production, modulating the IL 6-stimulated synthesis of distinct groups of acute phase proteins[51,52]. More recently a third hepatocyte stimulating factor (HSF III), immunochemically distinct from IL 6 but biologically indistinguishable, has been described[53]. Because of its biological identity with IL 6, this cytokine, also called leukaemia inhibitory factor (LIF), may have an important role in the regulation of acute phase protein synthesis. Two additional regulatory molecules which have attracted some attention are glucocorticoid hormones (dexamethasone) and insulin. It has recently been shown that both of these mediators can modulate some of the effects of IL 6[54]. For instance, dexamethasone will increase synthesis of fibrinogen by IL 6-stimulated HepG2 cells, and insulin will inhibit synthesis of this protein but only in the presence of both dexamethasone and IL 6.

IL 6 as a mediator of fever

Fever is the regulated rise in body temperature which occurs as a response to infection, trauma or malignant disease. It has been recognized for many years that fever is one component of the acute phase response, and as such must be regulated by a mediator circulating in the blood, the endogenous pyrogen. A number of cytokines have been implicated as endogenous pyrogens including IL 1, TNFα, IFNγ, IFNα, IL 8 and IL 6. Several laboratories have shown that these cytokines when injected peripherally will cause fever, with IL 1α and IL 1β being the most potent endogenous pyrogens. Studies of the thermogenic action of cytokines injected directly into the brain suggest an order of potency IL 1β > IL 6, IL 8 > IL 1α > TNFα[55] and inter-cerebroventricular injection of antibodies to IL 1β or IL 6 inhibit fever and thermogenesis[56].

As described below, a number of cytokines can act on the hypothalamic–pituitary–adrenal axis. One action of IL 1β is the stimulation of corticotrophin releasing factor (CRF), a molecule involved in many of the physiological responses to stress, including fever[57]. Pretreatment of animals with antibodies to CRF or with ibuprofen, an antagonist to CRF release, inhibits the thermogenic properties of either IL 1β or IL 6.

Although IL 1β appears to be the most potent centrally acting endogenous pyrogen there is no good evidence that circulating concentrations of IL 1β in infection or trauma patients are sufficient to account for the observed fever. Intra-cerebroventricular injection of IL 1, however, induces high concentrations of circulating IL 6[5], suggesting that IL 1β may act via induction of IL 6. The available evidence then suggests that IL 6 is the best candidate for a circulating physiological mediator of fever[59].

IL 6 interaction with hypothalamic–pituitary–adrenal axis

An intriguing property of cytokines produced by inflammatory cells is their interaction with the hypothalamic–pituitary–adrenal axis. One consequence of this interaction is the induction of corticosteroid release by the adrenal gland. The anti-inflammatory role of corticosteroids is well described in Chapter 4.

It has been shown that several monocyte-derived cytokines can act on the hypothalamic–pituitary–adrenal axis, stimulating adrenal cells to release corticosteroid hormones. Injection of IL 6 into rats results in an increase in concentrations of ACTH in the plasma[60]. This effect can be blocked by a previous injection of antiserum to corticotrophin-releasing factor, suggesting that IL 6 acts at the hypothalamic level or higher to induce ACTH production[60]. IL 1 has been shown to stimulate the release of several hormones, including ACTH, by pituitary cells[61]. More recently it has been shown that IL 1 and IL 6 can also act directly on the adrenal cells to induce corticosteroid release[43,62,63]. In humans, several days after trauma, there is a marked lack of correlation between concentrations of ACTH and cortisol, concentrations of cortisol remaining high in the presence of relatively low ACTH concentrations[64]. It is therefore possible that one important physiological role of IL 6 is to act synergistically with relatively low concentrations of ACTH to increase corticosteroid concentrations. An important consequence of corticosteroid production is suppression of the inflammatory response (Chapter 4).

Action of IL 6 on myeloid and lymphoid production

A major requirement for the provision of efficeint defence systems is the replenishment by haematopoiesis of those cells utilized in the immune and inflammatory responses. Haematopoiesis is a complicated process regulated by a wide variety of cytokines. IL 6 interacts with many of these cytokines to enhance the growth of multipotent progenitor, erythroid, myeloid and megakaryocytic cells.

IL 6 and IL 3 appear to act synergistically to support proliferation of multipotent progenitor cells *in vitro*[45,65] and act synergistically with GM-CSF to support the production of granulocytes[66]. Differentiation of M1 and WEHI 3B myeloid leukaemic cells is induced by IL 6[67] and the IL 6 gene is regulated by a variety of other agents that induce differentiation of myeloid leukemic cells[68]. Maturation of megakaryocytes *in vitro* and increased platelet count *in vivo* have been achieved using recombinant IL 6, suggesting that this cytokine acts as a thrombopoietic factor[46,69,70]. Further evidence that IL 6 is a thrombopoietic factor comes from IL 6 transgenic mice which have increased numbers of megakaryocytes in their bone marrow[71].

IL 6 and the immune response

If the local defence mechanism fails to control an infection then an antigen-specific immune response is normally elicited. Cytokines produced by cells at the site of inflammation appear to play an important role in controlling the developing immune response. In particular IL 6 regulates some aspects of the developing immune response, stimulating differentiation events in both T and B lymphocytes.

Effects on B lymphocytes

IL 6 has been identified as an essential and late-acting factor in mitogen-activated immunoglobulin production, stimulating the synthesis of IgM, IgG and IgA and inhibiting B cell proliferation[72,73]. IL 6 has also been shown to act as a growth factor for plasmacytoma cells, myeloma cells, EBV transformed cells and B cell hybridoma[73–75]. Castleman's disease is a benign hyperplastic lymphadenopathy, characterized by large plasma cell-rich lymph node follicles and hypergammaglobulinaemia. Constitutive IL 6 production by cells in the germinal centre of affected lymph nodes has been reported[78]. Other characteristics of this disease include fever and raised concentrations of acute phase proteins, events attributed to increased concentrations of plasma IL 6.

Effects on T lymphocytes, natural killer cells and lymphokine-activated killer cells; a possible role in the antitumour response

Inflammation often occurs as a consequence of cancer. In particular the process of metastasis has been associated with local tissue damage and inflammation. It would not be surprising then if antitumour defence systems responded to inflammatory mediators. IL 6, which has a well-defined endocrine function in the regulation of acute phase protein synthesis and which has a number of actions on T lymphocytes, natural killer (NK) and lymphokine-activated killer (LAK) cells, is an ideal candidate for such a tumour response mediator.

Cytolytic T cells play a central role in the defence against virus induced tumors. However, there is no convincing evidence that they have any role in protection against 'spontaneous' or chemically induced tumours. The main defence against non virius induced tumours appears to be mediated by LAK cells, NK cells and macrophages. A number of reports suggest that IL 6 plays a role in the generation and activation of each of these cell types (Table 12.5). IL 6 has also been shown to have an antitumour activity when injected in to mice[77]. It has not been demonstrated that IL 6 has an *in vivo* role in the up-regulation of the antitumour response. However, it is an attractive hypothesis that IL 6, a cytokine which is produced at sites of inflammation, can activate cells involved in cell-mediated antitumour responses.

Table 12.5 Interleukin 6 and the immune response to tumours

Cell type	*Action*	*Refs*
Human NK cells	Activated by IL 6 *in vitro*	78
Human LAK cells	Activated by IL 6 *in vitro*	79
Human and murine cytotoxic T cells	Differentiate in response to IL 6 *in vitro*	44, 80, 81
Tumour-associated macrophages and epithelial cells	Produce IL 6	82

Does IL 6 play a role in the regulation of protein glycosylation?

It has been recognized for some time that changes in protein glycosylation occur in inflammation. Changes in the glycosylation patterns of immunoglobulins, acute phase proteins, salivary kallikriens and cell surface glycoproteins have all been described in individuals with inflammatory disease[83–85]. To a large extent the physiological function of, and the mechanisms controlling, such changes in glycosylation are not known.

Changes in protein glycosylation in inflammation

In rheumatoid arthritis, Crohn's disease, tuberculosis and erythema nodosum leprosum (ENL), immunoglobulins appear to have a reduced galactosylation of terminal *N*-acetylglucosamine groups on some oligosaccaride chains[83,86]. This change in immunoglobulin galactosylation is not seen in systemic lupus erythematosus (SLE) (unless accompanied by Sjögren's syndrome), osteoarthritis, sarcoidosis and lepromatous (except ENL) or tubercoloid leprosy. The change appears to be seen only in disease states associated with both an acute phase response and a major T cell involvement[87]. Some reports suggest that the observed change reflects a reduced galactosyltransferase activity in B cells[88]. Increased concentrations of haptoglobins and alpha-1-antichymotrypsin (α_1-ACT) which bind to a fucose-specific lectin have also been reported in individuals with rheumatoid arthritis and cancer[89,90]. It is possible that this increased binding represents altered fucose content of carbohydrate side-chains or else that reduced terminal galactose groups change the affinity of the lectin for side-chain fucose groups.

Concanavalin A (Con A) binding forms of alpha-1-acid glycoprotein (AGP) have been reported to be decreased in individuals with rheumatoid arthritis or ankylosing spondylitis, remain unchanged in SLE and increased in recurrent infection or pregnancy[91,92]. Low pI forms of AGP have been described in cancer and rheumatoid arthritis[91,93]. It seems likely that these changes can be accounted for by increased N-terminal sialic acid groups. Tissue kallikreins in the saliva of individuals with connective tissue disease have also been reported to have a reduced pI, which has been attributed to increased sialation[87]. Similar changes have been observed in kallikreins from individuals with active but not inactive inflammatory bowel disease, suggesting that the change in glycosylation is a consequence of the inflammation[40]. Sialyltransferase activity in the small intestine has been reported to increase following thermal injury to rats, further supporting the idea that changes in glycosylation occur in response to inflammation[94].

The majority of membrane and secreted proteins involved in regulating the activity of cells of the immune and inflammatory systems are glycoproteins. The precise role of the carbohydrate moieties of these molecules is unknown; however, there is some evidence, especially for the membrane proteins, that they can contribute significantly to glycoprotein function. For instance, it has been reported that desialation of spleen cells leads to enhanced accessory cell activity, neuraminidase treatment of macrophages stimulates cytotoxic T cell responses and natural killer cell activity, and that abrogating the negative charge of heavily glycosylated surface molecules increases clustering of T cells around accessory cells[95–97].

Role of IL 6 in the modulation of glycosylation

Changes in the glycosylation of acute phase proteins has been studied *in vitro* using hepatocytes, hepatoma cell lines. In these *in vitro* systems IL 6 stimulates synthesis of acute phase protein and changes in their glycosylation. These changes occur in parallel, and it is not yet clear to what extent regulation of glycosylation is independent of the regulation of protein synthesis and export. Conflicting results have been obtained using different cell lines. In Hep3B, IL 6 stimulated forms of alpha-1-proteinase inhibitor (α_1-PI), caeruloplasm and α-fetoprotein with enhanced Con A binding, while in HepG2 IL 6 stimulated production of proteins with reduced Con A binding. Using primary human hepatocyte cultures IL 6 has been shown to stimulate synthesis of AGP with enhanced Con A binding.

Changes in the glycosylation of serum proteins and cell surface molecules clearly occur in inflammation. These changes have the potential to affect the outcome of an inflammatory response, altering cell–cell interaction and changing the function and/or catabolism of serum proteins[95–99]. It has been clearly shown that IL 6 can modulate glycosylation of acute phase proteins. Whether IL 6 is responsible for the glycosylation changes seen in other serum and cell surface molecules, which occur in inflammation, remains to be established. B cells have functional receptors for IL 6, and IL 6 stimulates immunoglobulin synthesis by activated B cells. It will be interesting to determine how IL 6 effects changes in the glycosylation of immunoglobulins. IL 6 is produced by many cells, but the major source in inflammation is thought to be the activated macrophage. Presumably any role for IL 6 in modulating glycosylation will depend on macrophage production of IL 6. However, it has been suggested that a T cell event is involved in the altered glycosylation of immunoglobulins seen in inflammatory diseases[100]. The role of IL 6 in the regulation of immunoglobulin glycosylation and the nature of the proposed T cell event remain to be established. It is possible that changes in protein glycosylation play an important role in the regulation of inflammation, and that an inability to effect proper changes or 'abnormal' glycosylation is associated with aberrant T cell activity and inflammatory disease.

IL 6 IN INFLAMMATION

Using both bioassay and immunoassay methods, IL 6 has been detected in the serum, plasma and urine of patients with a variety of different inflammatory conditions. IL 6 concentrations have been reported to increase before those of acute phase proteins in individuals suffering from severe burns, surgical trauma, transplant rejection or inflammatory bowel disease[101–105]. In individuals with serious burns or surgical trauma, plasma concentrations of IL 6 have been correlated with C-reactive protein concentrations and the degree of fever. In Crohn's disease, but not ulcerative colitis, IL 6 concentrations correlate well with the type and extent of disease[105]. Endotoxaemia and sepsis are frequent complications of bacterial infection and are associated with an acute phase response. IL 6 concentrations are elevated in both conditions[106,107]. Elevated concentrations of IL 6 have also been reported in the serum and synovial fluid of individuals with inflammatory joint disease, where IL 6 concentrations appear to correlate well with IgG concentrations[108,109]. The conclusion then is that circulating concentrations of IL 6 correlate well with the extent of inflammation observed.

IL 6 REGULATION OF THE INFLAMMATORY RESPONSE

IL 6 is a pleiotropic cytokine which appears to have an important role in the regulation of the inflammatory response. Many of the biological activities of IL 6 can shown to be relevant to the down-regulation of inflammation. Thus in the normal course of events, transiently elevated concentrations of IL 6 might be considered a marker of the successful conclusion of an inflammatory episode (Figure 12.3). On the other hand, sustained periods of raised IL 6 concentrations suggest an underlying chronic inflammatory condition.

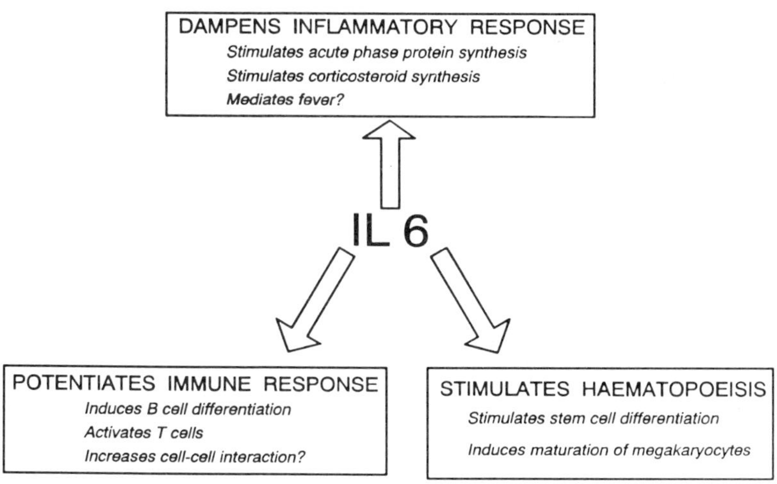

Figure 12.3 Role of interleukin 6 in controlling inflammation and the immune response.

Acknowledgements

I am grateful to J. T. Whicher and D. Thompson for their helpful comments, and to the Yorkshire Cancer Research Campaign for generous financial support.

References

1. Gauldie, J., Richards, C., Harnish, D., Lansdrop, P. and Baumann, H. (1987). Interferon β2/B-cell stimulatory factor type 2 shares identity with monocyte-derived hepatocyte-stimulating factor and regulates the major acute phase protein response in liver cells. *Proc. Natl. Acad. Sci.*, **84**, 7251–5
2. Van-Damme, J., Opdenakker, G., Simpson, R. J., Rubira, M. R., Cayphas, S., Vink, A., Billiau, A. and Van Snick, J. (1987). Identification of the human 26 kD protein, interferon β2 (INFβ2), as a B cell hybridoma/plasmacytoma growth factor induced by interleukin 1 and tumor necrosis factor. *J. Exp. Med.*, **165**, 914–19
3. Zilberstein, A., Ruggier, R., Korn, J. and Revel, M. (1986). Structure and expression of cDNA and genes for human interferon beta 2, a distinct species inducible by growth-stimulatory cytokines. *EMBO J.*, **5**, 2529–37
4. Haegeman, G., Content, J., Volckaert, G., Drynck, R., Tavernier, J. and Friers, W. (1986). Structural analysis of the sequence encoding for an inducible 26 kDa protein in human fibroblasts. *Eur. J. Biochem.*, **159**, 625–32
5. Hirano, T., Yasukawa, K., Harada, H., Taga, T., Watanaba, Y., Matsuda, T., Kashiwamura, S., Nakajima, K., Koyama, K., Iwamatu, A., Tsunaswa, S., Sakiyama, F., Matsui, H., Takahara,. Y., Taniguchi, T. and Kishimoto, T. (1987). Complementary DNA for a novel human interleukin (BSF-2) that induces B lymphocytes to produce immunoglobulin. *Nature*, **324**, 73–6
6. Gross, V., Andus, T., Castell, J., Von-Berg, D., Heinrich, P. C. and Gerok, W. (1989). O- and N-glycosylation lead to different molecular mass forms of human monocyte interleukin-6. *FEBS Lett.*, **247**, 323–6
7. May, L. T., Santhanam, U., Tatter, S. B., Ghrayeb, J. and Sehgal, P. B. (1989). Multiple forms of human interleukin-6. Phosphoglycoproteins secreted by many different tissues. *Ann. N.Y. Acad. Sci.*, **557**, 114–19
8. Bazan, J. F. (1990). Haemopoietic receptors and helical cytokines. *Immunol. Today*, **11**, 350–4
9. Abdel-Meguid, S. S., Shieh, H. S., Smith, W. W., Dayringer, H. E., Violand, B. N. and Bentle, L. A. (1987). Three-dimensional structure of a genetically engineered variant of porcine growth hormone. *Proc. Natl. Acad. Sci. USA*, **84**, 6434–7
10. Bowcock, A. M., Kidd, J. R., Lathrop, G. M., Daneshvar, L., May, L. T., Ray, A., Sehgal, P. B., Kidd, K. K. and Cavalli-Sforza, L. L. (1988). The human 'interferon-beta 2/hepatocyte stimulating factor/interleukin-6' gene: DNA polymorphism studies and localization to chromosome 7p21. *Genomics*, **3**, 8–16
11. Mock, B. A., Nordan, R. P., Justice, M. J., Kozak, C., Jenkins, N. A., Copeland, N. G., Clark, S. C., Wong, G. G. and Rudikoff, S. (1989). The murine IL-6 gene maps to the proximal region of chromosome 5. *J. Immunol.*, **142**, 1372–6
12. Yasukawa, K., Hirano, T., Watanaba, Y., Muratani, K., Yamamura, Y. and Kishimoto, T. (1987). Structure and expression of human B cell stimulatory factor 2 (BSF-2/IL 6) gene. *EMBO J.*, **6**, 2937–45
13. Tanabe, O., Akira, S., Kamiya, T., Wong, G. G., Hirano, T. and Kishimoto, T. (1988). Genomic structure of the murine IL-6 gene; high degree conservation of potential regulatory sequences between mouse and human. *J. Immunol.*, **141**, 3875–81
14. Bowcock, A. M., Ray, A., Erlich, H. A. and Sehgal, P. B. (1989). The molecular genetics of beta-2 interferon/interleukin-6 (IFN beta 2/IL6) alpha. *Ann. N.Y. Acad. Sci.*, **557**, 345–52
15. Bauer, J., Ganter, U., Geiger, T., Jacobshagen, U., Hirano, T., Matsuda, T., Kishimoto, T., Andus, T., Acs, G., Gerok, W. and Ciliberto, G. (1988). Regulation of interleukin 6 expression in cultured human blood monocytes and monocyte-derived macrophages. *Blood*, **72**, 1134–40
16. May, L. T., Ghrayeb, J., Santhanam, U., Tatter, S. B., Stoeger, Z., Helfgott, D. C., Chiorazzi, N., Grieninger, G. and Sehgal, P. B. (1988). Synthesis and secretion of multiple forms of

beta-2-interferon/B-cell differentiation factor 2/hepatocyte stimulating factor by human fibroblasts and monocytes. *J. Biol. Chem.*, **263**, 7760–6
17. Molina, J. M., Schindler, R., Ferriani, R., Sakaguchi, M., Vannier, E., Dinarello, C. A. and Groopman, J. E. (1990). Production of cytokines by peripheral blood monocytes/macrophages infected with human immunodeficiency virus type 1 (HIV-1). *J. Infect. Dis.*, **161**, 888–93
18. Helfgott, D. C., May, L. T., Sthoeger, Z., Tamm, I. and Sehgal, P. B. (1987). Bacterial lipopolysaccharide (endotoxin) enhances expression and secretion of $\beta 2$ interferon by human fibroblasts. *J. Exp. Med.*, **166**, 1300–8
19. Zhang, Y., Lin, J-X. and Vilcek, J. (1988). Synthesis of interleukin 6 (interferon-$\beta 2$/B cell stimulatory factor 2) in human fibroblasts is triggered by an increase in intracellular cyclic AMP. *J. Biol. Chem.*, **263**, 6177–82
20. Van Damme, J., Schaafsma, M. R., Fibbe, W. E., Frederik, J. H., Falkenburg, J. H. F., Opendenkker, G. and Billiau, A. (1989). Simultaneous production of interleukin 6, interferon β and colony stimulating activity by fibroblasts after viral and bacterial infection. *Eur. J. Immunol.*, **19**, 163–8
21. Jirij, F. R., Podor, T. J., Hirano, T., Kishimoto, I., Loskutoff, D. J., Carson, D. A. and Lotz, M. (1989). Bacterial lipopolysaccaride and inflammatory mediators augment IL-6 secretion by human endothelial cells. *J. Immunol.*, **142**, 144–7
22. Kirnbauer, R., Kock, A., Schwartz, T., Urbanski, A., Krutmann, J., Borth, W., Damm, D., Shipley, G., Ansel, J. C. and Luger, T. A. (1989). IFN-$\beta 2$, B cell differentiation factor 2, or hybridoma growth factor (IL 6) is expressed and released by human epidermal cells and epidermoid carcinoma cell lines. *J. Immunol.*, **142**, 1922–8
23. Bunning, R. A., Russell, R. G. and Van-Damme, J. (1990). Independent induction of interleukin 6 and prostaglandin E2 by interleukin 1 in human articular chondrocytes. *Biochem. Biophys. Res. Commun.*, **166**, 1163–70
24. Guerne, P.-A., Zuraw, B. L., Vaughan, J. H., Carson, D. A. and Lotz, M. (1989). Synovium as a source of interleukin 6 in vivo. *J. Clin. Invest.*, **83**, 585–92
25. Tabibzadeh, S. S., Santhanam, U., Sehgal, P. B. and May, L. T. (1989). Cytokine induced production of IFN$\beta 2$/IL-6 by freshly explanted human endometrial cells. *J. Immunol.*, **142**, 3134–9
26. Frei, K., Malipiero, U. V., Leist, T. P., Zinkernagel, R. M., Schab, M. E. and Fontana, A. (1989). On the cellular source and function of interleukin 6 produced in the central nervous system in viral disease. *Eur. J. Immunol.*, **19**, 689–94
27. Sehgal, P. B., Walther, Z. and Tamm, I. (1987). Rapid enhancement of $\beta 2$-interferon/B cell differentiation factor BSF-2 gene expression in human fibroblasts by diacylglycerols and the calcium ionophore A23187. *Proc. Natl. Acad. Sci. USA*, **84**, 3633–67
28. Ray, A., Sassone-Corsi, P. and Sehgal, P. B. (1989). A multiple cytokine and second messenger-responsive element in the enhancer of the human interleukin-6 gene: similarities with c-fos gene regulation. *Mol. Cell. Biol.*, **9**, 5537–47
29. Hirano, T., Akira, S., Taga, T. and Kishimoto, T. (1990). Biological and clinical aspects of interleukin 6. *Immunol. Today*, **11**, 443–9
30. Isshiki, H., Akira, S., Tanabe, O., Nakajima, T., Shimamoto, T., Hirano, T. and Kishimoto, T. (1990). Constitutive and interleukin-1 (IL-1)-inducible factors interact with the IL-1-responsive element in the IL-6 gene. *Mol. Cell. Biol.*, **10**, 2757–64
31. Zander, B., Walz, G., Wieder, K. J. and Strom, T. B. (1990). Evidence that glucocorticoids block expression of the human interleukin 6 gene by accessory cells. *Transplantation*, **49**, 183–5
32. Taga, T., Kawanishi, K., Hardy, R. R., Hirano, T. and Honjo, T. (1987). Receptors for B cell stimulatory factor 2 (BSF-2): quantitation, specificy, distribution and regulation of the expression. *J. Exp. Med.*, **166**, 967–79
33. Yamasaki, K., Taga, T., Hirata, Y., Kawanishi, Y., Seed, B., Taniguchi, T., Hirano, T. and Kishimoto, T. (1988). Cloning and expression of the human interleukin-6 (BSF-2/INFβ) receptor. *Science*, **241**, 825–8
34. Snyers, L., De-Wit, L. and Content, J. (1990). Glucocorticoid up-regulation of high affinity interleukin 6 receptors on human epithelial cells. *Proc. Natl. Acad. Sci. USA*, **87**, 2838–42
35. Bazan, J. F. (1989). A novel family of growth factor receptors: a common binding domain in the growth hormone, prolactin, erythropoietin and IL-6 receptors, and the p75 IL-2 receptor beta-chain. *Biochem. Biophys. Res. Commun.*, **164**, 788–95
36. Hirano, T. and Kishimoto, T. (1990). Interleukin 6. In Spoon, M. B. and Roberts, A. B.

(eds), *Handbook of Experimental Pharmacology*, vol. 95/I: *Peptide Growth Factors and their Receptors, I*, pp. 633–65, (Berlin, Heidelberg: Springer-Verlag)
37. Snyers, L., Fontaine, V. and Content, J. (1989). Modulation of interleukin 6 receptors in human cells. *Ann. N.Y. Acad. Sci.*, **557**, 388–93
38. Hibi, M., Murakami, M., Saito, M., Hirano, T., Taga, T. and Kishimoto, T. (1990). Molecular cloning and expression of an IL 6 signal transducer gp130. *Cell*, **63**, 1149–57
39. Nordan, R. P., Mock, B. A., Neckers, L. M. and Rudikoff, S. (1989). The role of plasmacytoma growth factor in the *in vitro* response of murine plasmacytoma cells. *Ann. N.Y. Acad. Sci.*, **557**, 200 – 5
40. Orupabo, I., Hay, A. W. M. and Evans, S. W. (1991). Effects of metals on interleukin 6 mitogenic stimulation of murine hybridoma cells. *Immunology* (Submitted)
41. Evans, E., Courtois, G., Kilian, P. L., Fuller, G. M. and Crabtree, G. R. (1987). Induction of fibrinogen and a subset of acute phase response genes involves a novel monokine which is mimicked by phorbol esters. *J. Biol. Chem.*, **262**, 10850–4
42. Baumann, H., Isseroff, H., Latimer, J. J. and Jahreis, G. P. (1989). Phorbol ester modulates interleukin 6 and interleukin 1 regulated expression of acute phase plasma proteins in hepatoma cells. *J. Biol. Chem.*, **265**, 17390–6
43. Salas, M. A., Evans, S. W., Levell, M. J. and Whicher, J. T. (1990). Interleukin 6 and ACTH act synergistically to stimulate the release of corticosterone from adrenal gland cells. *Clin. Exp. Immunol.*, **79**, 470–3
44. Smyth, M. J., Ortaldo, J. R., Bere, W., Yagita, H., Okumura, K. and Young, H. A. (1990). IL-2 and IL-6 synergize to augment the pore-forming protein gene expression and cytotoxic potential of human peripheral blood T cells. *J. Immunol.*, **145**, 1159–66
45. Ogawa, M. and Clark, S. C. (1988). Synergistic interaction between interleukin-6 and interleukin-3 in support of stem cell proliferation in culture. *Blood*, **14**, 329–337
46. Bruno, E. and Hoffman, R. (1989). Effect of interleukin 6 on *in vitro* human megakaryocytopoiesis: its interaction with other cytokines. *Exp. Hematol.*, **17**, 1038–43
47. Satoh, T., Nakamura, S., Taga, T., Matsuda, T., Hirano, T., Kishimoto, T. and Kaziro, Y. (1988). Induction of neuronal differentiation in PC12 cells by B-cell stimulatory factor 2/interleukin 6. *Mol. Cell. Biol.*, **8**, 3546–9
48. Koji, A., Gauldie, J., Regoeczi, E., Sauder, D. N. and Sweeney, G. D. (1984). The acute phase response of cultured rat hepatocytes. System characterization and the effect of human cytokines. *Biochem. J.*, **224**, 505–14
49. Andus, T., Geiger, T., Hirano, T., Northoff, H., Ganter, U., Bauer, J., Kishiomoto, T. and Heinrich, P. C. (1987). Recombinant human B cell stimulatory factor 2 (BSF-2/IFNβ2) regulates β-fibrinogen and albumin mRNA levels in Fao-9 cells. *FEBS Lett.*, **221**, 18–22
50. Heinrich, P. C., Castell, J. V. and Andus, T. (1990). Interleukin 6 and the acute phase response. *Biochem. J.*, **265**, 621–36
51. Magielska-Zero, D., Bereta, J., Czuba-Pelech, B., Pajdak, V., Gauldie, J. and Koj, A. (1988). Inhibitory effect of human interferon gamma on synthesis of acute phase proteins in human hepatoma Hep G2 cells stimulated by leukocyte cytokines, TNFα and IFN-β2/BSF-2/IL 6. *Biochem. Int.*, **17**, 17–23
52. Mackiewicz, A., Ganapathi, M. K., Schultz, D., Brabenec, A., Weinstein, J., Kelley, M. F. and Kuschner, I. (1990). Transforming growth factor β1 regulates production of acute phase proteins. *Proc. Natl. Acad. Sci. USA*, **87**, 1491–5
53. Baumann, H., Won, K. A. and Jahreis, G. P. (1989). Human hepatocyte-stimulating factor-III and interleukin-6 are structurally and immunologically distinct but regulate the production of the same acute phase plasma proteins. *J. Biol. Chem.*, **264**, 8046–51
54. Thomson, D., Harrison, S. P., Evans, S. W. and Whicher, J. T. (1991). Effects of insulin and dexamethasone on acute phase protein production in the human hepatoma cell line, Hep G2. *Cytokine* (In press)
55. Rothwell, N. J. (1990). Mechanisms of the pyrogenic actions of cytokines. *Eur. Cytokine Net.*, **1**, 211–13
56. Rothwell, N. J., Busbridge, N. J., Humphray, H. and Hissey, P. (1990). Central actions of interleukin-1β on fever and thermogenesis. *Prog. Leukocyte Biol.*, **108**, 307–9
57. Rothwell, N. J. (1990). Central actions of CRF on energy expenditure and body weight regulation. *Neurosci. Biobehav. Rev.*, **14**, 263–6
58. De Simoni, M. G., Sironi, M., De Luigi, A., Manfridi, A., Montovani, A. and Ghezzi, P.

(1990). Intracerebroventricular injection of interleukin 1 induces high circulating levels of interleukin 6. *J. Exp. Med.*, **171**, 1773–8
59. LeMay, L. G., Vander, A. J. and Klugger, M. J. (1990). Role of interleukin 6 in fever in rats. *Am. J. Physiol.*, **258**, R798–R803
60. Naitoh, Y., Fukata, J., Tominaga, T., Nakai, Y., Tamai, S., Mori, K. and Immura, H. (1988). Interleukin-6 stimulates the section of adrenocorticotrophic hormone in conscious, freely-moving rats. *Biochem. Biophys. Res. Commun.*, **155**, 1459–63
61. Bernton, E. W., Beach, J. E., Holaday, J. W., Smallridge, R. C. and Fein, H. G. (1987). Release of multiple hormones by a direct action of interleukin 1 on pituitary cells. *Science*, **238**, 519–21
62. Roh, M. S., Drazenovich, K. A., Barbose, J. J., Dinarello, C. A. and Cobb, C. F. (1987). Direct stimulation of the adrenal cortex by interleukin 1. *Surgery*, **102**, 140–6
63. Salas, M. A., Evans, S. W., Levell, M. J. and Whicher, J. T. (1990). *In vitro* effects of rIL 1 and rIL 6 on corticosterone release by isolated rat adrenal gland cells. In Oppenheim, J. J. *et al.* (eds), *Molecular and Cellular Biology of Cytokines*, pp. 427–32 (New York: Wiley–Liss)
64. Barton, R. N. and Stoner, H. B. (1987). Why does a high cortisol concentration persist after a fracture of the femoral neck in the elderly? *Circ. Shock*, **21**, 292
65. Suzuki, C., Okano, A., Takatsuki, F., Miyasaka, Y., Hirano, T., Kishimoto, T., Ejima, D. and Akiyama, Y. (1989). Continuous perfusion with interleukin 6 (IL-6) enhances production of hematopoietic stem cells (CFU-S). *Biochem. Biophys. Res. Commun.*, **159**, 933–8
66. Caracciolo, D., Clark, S. C. and Rovera, G. (1989). Human interleukin 6 suports granulocytic differentiation of hemopoietic progenitor cells and acts synergistically with GM-CSF. *Blood*, **73**, 666–70
67. Chiu, C. P. and Lee, F. (1989). IL 6 is a differentiation factor for M1 and WEHI 3B myeloid leukemic cells. *J. Immunol.*, **142**, 1922–8
68. Shabo, Y., Lotem, J. and Sachs, L. (1989). Regulation of genes for interleukin 6 and granulocyte–macrophage colony stimulating factor by different inducers of differentiation in myeloid leukemic cells. *Leukemia*, **3**, 859–65
69. Rennick, D., Jackson, J., Yang, G., Wideman, J., Lee, F. and Hudak, S. (1989). Interleukin-6 interacts with interleukin-4 and other hematopoietic growth factors to selectively enhance the growth of megakaryocytic, erythroid, meyloid, and multipotential progenitor cells. *Blood*, **73**, 1828–35
70. Ishibashi, T., Kimura, H., Shikama, Y., Uchida, T., Kariyone, S., Hirano, T., Kishimoto, T., Takatsuki, F. and Akiyama, Y. (1989). Interleukin-6 is a potent thrombopoietic factor *in vivo* in mice. *Blood*, **74**, 1241–4
71. Suematus, S., Matsuda, T., Aozasa, K., Akira, S., Nakao, N., Ohno, S., Miyazaki, J., Jamamura, K., Hirano, T. and Kishimotto, T. (1989). IgG1 plasmacytoma in interleukin 6 transgenic mice. *Proc. Natl. Acad. Sci. USA*, **86**, 7547–51
72. Bertolini, J. N. and Benson, E. M. (1990). The role of human interleukin-6 in B-cell isotype regulation and differentiation. *Cell. Immunol.*, **125**, 197–209
73. Van-Snick, J. (1989). From hybridoma and plasmacytoma growth factors to interleukin 6. *Contrib. Microbiol. Immunol.*, **11**, 73–95
74. Kawamo, M., Hirano, T., Masuda, T., Taga, T., Horii, Y., Iwato, K., Asaoku, H., Tang, B., Tanabe, O., Kuramoto, A. and Kishimoto, T. (1988). Autocrine generation and essential requirement of BSF-2/IL-6 for human multiple myelomas. *Nature*, **332**, 83–6
75. Richter, W., Eiermann, T. H. and Scherbaum, W. A. (1990). Effect of cytokines on proliferation of Epstein Barr virus-transformed B lymphocytes. *Hybridoma*, **9**, 1–8
76. Yoshizaki, K., Matsuda, T., Nishimoto, N., Kuritani, T., Taeho, L., Aozasa, K., Nakahata, T., Kawai, H., Tagoh, H., Komori, T. *et al.* (1989). Pathogenic significance of interleukin-6 (IL-6/BSF-2) in Castleman's disease. *Blood*, **74**, 1360–7
77. Mule, J. J., McIntosh, J. K., Jablons, D. M. and Rosenberg, S. A. (1990). Antitumor activity of recombinant interleukin 6 in mice. *J. Exp. Med.*, **171**, 629–36
78. Luger, T. A., Krutmann, J., Kirnbauer, R., Urbanski, A., Schwarz, T., Klappacher, G., Kock, A., Micksche, M., Malejczyk, J., Schauer, E. *et al.* (1989). IFN-beta2/IL-6 augments the activity of human natural killer cells. *J. Immunol.*, **143**, 1206–9
79. Gallagher, G., Stimson, W. H., Findlay, J. and Al-Azzawi, F. (1990). Interleukin-6 enhances the induction of human lymphokine-activated killer cells. *Cancer Immunol. Immunother.*, **31**, 49–52

80. Ming, J. E., Cernetti, C., Steinman, R. M. and Granelli-Piperno, A. (1989). Interleukin 6 is the principal cytolytic T lymphocyte differentiation factor for thymocytes in human leukocyte conditioned medium. *J. Mol. Cell. Immunol.*, **4**, 203–11
81. Stringfellow, M. M., Wilson, R. E. and Hermann, S. H. (1989). Production of interleukin-6 in vitro parallels development of cytotoxic T lymphocytes from murine thymocytes. *Surgery*, **106**, 332–8
82. Utsumi, K., Takai, Y., Tada, T., Ohzeki, S., Fujiwara, H. and Hamaoka, T. (1990). Enhanced production of IL-6 in tumor-bearing mice and determination of cells responsible for its augmented production. *J. Immunol.*, **145**, 397–403
83. Parekh, R., Isenberg, D., Rook, G., Roitt, I., Dweck, R. and Rademacher, T. (1989). A comparative analysis of disease-associated changes in the galactosylation of serum IgG. *J. Autoimmun.*, **2**, 101–14
84. Pos, O., van-Dijk, W., Landiques, N., Linthorst, C., Sala, M., van-Tiel, D. and Boers, W. (1988). Glycosylation of four acute-phase glycoproteins secreted by rat liver cells *in vivo* and *in vitro*. Effects of inflammation and dexamethasone. *Eur. J. Cell. Biol.*, **46**, 121–8
85. Greaves, D., Whicher, J. T., Bhoola, K. D. *et al.* (1989). Anionic salivary proteins associated with connective tissue disorders: sialated tissue kallikreins. *Ann. Rheum. Dis.*, **48**, 753–9
86. Tomana, M., Schrohenloher, R. E., Koopman, W. J., Alarcon, G. S. and Paul, W. A. (1988). Abnormal glycosylation of serum IgG from patients with chronic inflammatory bowel diseases. *Arthritis Rheum.*, **31**, 333–8
87. Rademacher, T. W., Parekh, R. B., Dwek, R., Isenberg, D. A., Rook, G. A. W., Axford, J. S. and Roitt, I. (1988). The role of AgG glycoforms in the pathogenesis of rheumatoid arthritis. *Springer Semin. Immunopathol.*, **10**, 231–49
88. Axford, J. S., Makenzie, L., Lydyard, P. M., Hay, F. C., Isenberg, D. A. and Roitt, I. M. (1987). Decreased B cell galactosyl transferase in rheumatoid arthritis. *Lancet*, **2**, 1486–8
89. Thompson, S., Kelly, C. A., Griffiths, I. D. and Turner, G. A. (1989). Abnormally-fucosylated serum haptoglobins in patients with inflammatory joint disease. *Clin. Chim. Acta*, **184**, 251–8
90. Thompson, S., Guthrie, D. and Turner, G. A. (1988). Fucosylated forms of alpha-1-antichymotrypsin that predict unresponsiveness to chemotherapy in ovarian cancer. *Br. J. Cancer*, **58**, 589–93
91. Mackeiweiz, A., Pawlowski, T., Wiktorowicz, K. A. and Mackiewicz, S. (1986). Microheterogeneity forms of alpha-1-acid glycoprotein, alpha-1-antichymotrypsin and alpha-1-antitrypsin rheumatoid arthritis. In Bog-Hanse, T. C. and van Diessche, E. (eds), *Lectins*, vol. V, pp. 623–30 (Berlin: Walter de Gruyter)
92. Mackiewicz, A., Khan, M. A., Reynolds, T. L., van der Liden, S. and Kuschner, I. (1989). Serum IgA, acute phase proteins, and glycosylation of α1-acid glycoprotein in ankylosing spondylitis. *Ann. Rheum. Dis.*, **42**, 99–103
93. Moule, S. K., Peak, M., Thompson, S. and Turner, G. A. (1987). Studies of the sialation and microheterogeneity of human serum α1-acid glycoprotein in health and disease. *Clin. Chim. Acta*, **166**, 177–85
94. Carter, S. W., Tompkins, R. G. and Burke, J. F. (1988). Increase of sialyltransferase activity in the small intestine following thermal injury in rats. *Biochem. Biophys. Res. Commun.*, **141**, 1665–9
95. Hirayama, Y., Inaba, K., Inaba, M., *et al.* (1988). Neuraminidase treated macrophages stimulate allogenic CD8+ cells in the presence of exogenous interleukin 2. *J. Exp. Med.*, 1443–56
96. *Nabi, Z. F., Zucker-Franklin, D. and Basten, A.* (1989). *Phorbol ester-induced loss of membrane sialic acid: implications for tumor cytolysis by natural killer cells. J. Leuk. Biol.*, **45**, 183–8
97. King, P. D., Batchelor, A. H., Lawlor, P. and Katz, D. R. (1990). The role of CD44, CD45, CD45RO, CD46 and CD55 as potential anti-adhesion molecules involved in the binding of human tonsillar T cells to phorbol 12 myrisate 13 acetate differentiated U937 cells. *Eur. J. Immunol.*, **20**, 363–8
98. Beries, P. N., Feger, J., Benberneu, N., Reuzeau, J. D., Agneray, J. and Durand, G. (1990). Prevalence of tri- and tetra-antennary glycans of human alpha 1-acid glycoprotein in release of macrophage inhibitor of interleukin 1 activity. *Inflammation*, **14**, 315–23
99. Morris, M. A. and Preddy, L. (1986). Glycosylation accelerates albumin degradation in normal and diabetic dogs. *Biochem. Med. Metab. Biol.*, **35**, 267–70

100. Dube, R., Rook, G. A., Steele, J., Brealey, R., Dwek, R., Rademacher, T. and Lennard-Jones, J. (1990). Agalactosyl C-reactive protein. *Gut*, **31**, 431–4
101 Guo, Y., Dickerson, C., Chrest, F. J., Adler, W. L., Hunster, A. M. and Winchurch, R. A. (1990). Increased levels of circulating interleukin 6 in burns patients. *Clin. Immunol. Immunopathol.*, **54**, 361–71
102. Murata, A., Ogawa, M., Yasuda, T., Nishijima, J., Oka, Y., Ohmachi, Y., Hiraoka, N., Niinobu, T., Uda, K. and Mori, T. (1990). Serum interleukin 6, C-reactive protein and pancreatic secretory trypsin inhibitor (PSTI) as acute phase reactants after major thoraco-abdominal surgery. *Immunol. Invest.*, **19**, 271–8
103. Cruickshank, A. M., Fraser, W. D., Burns, H. T., Van-Damme, J. and Shjenkin, A. (1990). Response of serum interleukin 6 in patients undergoing elective surgery of varying severity. *Clin. Sci.*, **79**, 161–5
104. Van-Oers, M. H., Van-der-Heyden, A. A. and Aarden, L. A. (1988). Interleukin 6 (IL-6) in the serum and urine of renal transplant recipients. *Clin. Exp. Immunol.*, **71**, 314–19
105. Lobo, A. J., Jones, S. C., Evans, S. W., Banks, R., Rathbone, B. J. and Axon, A. T. R. (1990). Plasma interleukin 6 in inflammatory bowel disease. *Gut*, **31**, A1194
106. Fong, Y., Moldawer, L. L., Marano, M., Wei, H., Tatter, S. B., Clarick, R. H., Santhanam, U., Sherris, D., May, L. T. and Sehgal, P. B. (1989). Endotoxemia elicits increased circulating beta 2-IFN/IL 6 in man. *J. Immunol.*, **142**, 2321–4
107. Hack, C. E., De-Groot, E. R., Feit-Bersma, R. J., Nuijens, J. H., Strack-Van-Schijndel, R. J., Eerenberg-Belmer, A. J. and Thijs, L. G. (1989). Interleukin 6 in sepsis. *Blood*, **74**, 1704–10
108. Houssiau, F. A., Devogeler, J. P., Van-Damme, J., de-Deuxchaisnes, C. N. and Van-Snick, J. (1988). Interleukin 6 in synovial fluid and serum of patients with rheumatoid arthritis and other inflammatory arthritides. *Arthritis Rheum.*, **31**, 784–8
109. Herrman, E., Fleischer, B., Mayet, W. J., Poralla, T. and Mayerzum-Buschenfelde, K. H. (1989). Correlation of synovial fluid interleukin 6 (IL 6) activities with IgG concentrations in patients with inflammatory joint disease and osteoarthritis. *Clin. Exp. Rheumatol.*, **7**, 411–14

13
The acute phase response

J. T. WHICHER and C. I. WESTACOTT

INTRODUCTION

Inflammation comprises a series of cellular changes which ultimately facilitate phagocytosis and either the killing of microorganisms or the digestion of cell debris. This is followed by proliferation of connective tissue cells and repair of the intercellular matrix. Both of these events require the complex control of various cell types at a local level. There is increasing evidence that, while many molecules may mediate effects such as vascular permeability and chemotaxis, cytokines exert control in a very sophisticated way with remarkable duplication of key elements and complex negative and positive interaction with each other and other hormones.

The local processes of inflammation are facilitated by systemic metabolic changes that mobilize energy in the form of glucose and fatty acids and amino acid building blocks. Fever up-regulates several enzymatic reactions in inflammatory and tissue cells which, perhaps being potentially hazardous, operate at a suboptimal level at normal body temperature. Leukocytosis provides an increased supply of phagocytic cells. Counter-regulatory effects such as the release of cortisol come into play, and curtail the potentially destructive effects of inflammation. Liver production of acute phase proteins provides an increased tissue supply of certain inflammatory mediators and inhibitors. All these events are, in part, controlled by the same pleotropic cytokines which exert key local controls.

The constellation of systemic responses which accompany trauma and inflammation, regardless of cause, are known as the acute phase response[1]. The response is remarkably stereotyped regardless of the localized or systemic nature of the underlying inflammation. Many threads of evidence support the notion, put forward by several workers over the past 40 years, that this is an adaptive response conditioning the 'milieu interieur' so that inflammation and healing may progress optimally.

A complex array of hormones and cytokines induce and control the components of the response and it is rapidly becoming clear that these two systems and the nervous system are closely integrated (Figure 13.1).

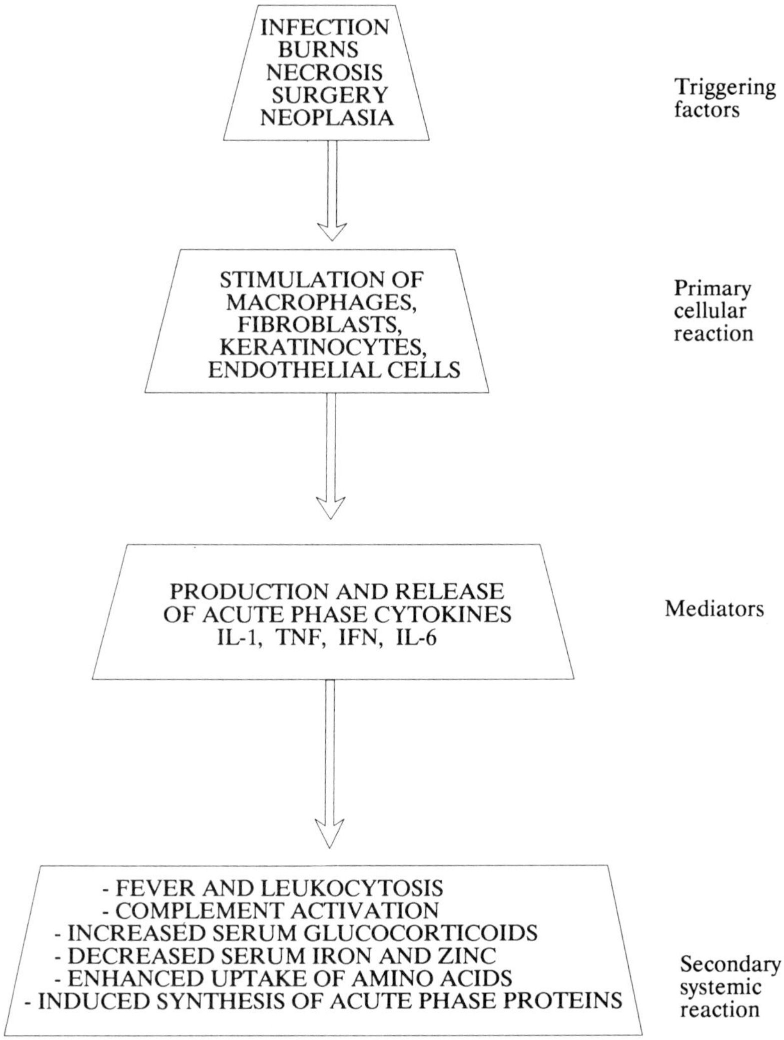

Figure 13.1 Cascade of events and systemic responses of the acute phase response.

NEUROENDOCRINE COMPONENTS OF THE ACUTE PHASE RESPONSE

Fever

Experimentally it has been shown that increased temperature, within the physiological range of fever, greatly enhances a number of cellular functions integral to inflammation and host survival. Indeed it has been suggested that some aspects of the immune response and inflammation do not function optimally at normal body temperature in homeotherms. By optimizing these responses at temperatures reached only in 'disease' these powerful systems can be brought into play when their protective effect is required, thus minimizing the deleterious aspects of autoimmunity and host damage by inflammation[2].

Some examples of *in vitro* effects enhanced by temperatures at or above 40°C serve to underline the potential power of this response. Incubation at 40°C has been shown to enhance the bactericidal activity of human PMNL against certain Gram-negative bacteria and the antiviral effects of IFN[3]. Temperatures corresponding to mild to moderate fevers in humans enhance and accelerate the proliferative response of T cells to mitogen, IL 1, and IL 2[4,5]. B cell antibody production in response to T cell cytokines is also greatly enhanced[6]. Thus phagocytosis, bacterial and viral killing and immune responses are potentiated. In addition, metabolic changes in other cells such as prostaglandin production, muscle proteolysis and oxygen radical production have shown enhancement in *in vitro* systems.

In vivo many experiments have shown the beneficial effect of fever in poikilotherms and homeotherms against viral and bacterial infection. In lizards increased survival against bacterial infection[7] was shown to be due to more rapid recruitment of leukocytes to the site of infection and containment of spread[8]. If fever was abrogated by administration of sodium salicylate the mortality increased. Fever is characteristic of infected fish, and under these conditions survival was significantly enhanced[9]. In homeotherms enhanced survival to infection at increased body temperature has been shown for mice infected with herpes simplex and other viruses[10], puppies infected with herpes virus[11], piglets with gastroenteritis virus[12], rabbits with pneumococal pneumonia[13], and humans with bacterial peritonitis[14].

In poikilotherms the genesis of fever is behavioural, with the animal seeking hotter environments. In homeotherms the thermoregulatory centre in the hypothalamus controls temperature by a combination of peripheral vasoconstriction and increased muscle metabolism which, at its extreme, is manifested as shivering[15].

A vast body of experimental work has shown that fever is mediated by peptides released from inflammatory cells, collectively known as endogenous pyrogen. The 'IL 1 boom' of the early 1980s rapidly defined this cytokine as a potent endogenous pyrogen and indeed it was soon seen as *the* pyrogen. However, since then other pyrogenic cytokines have been discovered, namely TNF and IL 6. Dinarello[16], in attempting to identify the pyrogen in leukocyte supernatants, has concluded that activity is due to a mixture of all of them.

A 1°C fever in rabbits is induced by about 20 ng/kg of IL 1, 200 ng/kg of TNF and 1 μg/kg of IL 6. As all the molecules have a similar molecular weight IL 1 is more potent on a molar basis, and in fever IL 1 rises to 1 ng/ml in plasma, TNF to 3 ng/ml and IL 6 to 300 pg/ml.

Studies on the injection of EP into the brain show that the sole site of action is the anterior hypothalamus. Certain prostaglandins, notably PGE_1, induce an immediate fever when injected into the same areas but are not blocked by PG synthetase inhibitors, such as aspirin, while EP is. This has led to the conclusion that PGE_1 is acting as the final common pathway in pyrogenesis. Some evidence suggests that several monoamines, including catecholamines and serotinin, may also be pyrogenic[17].

Sleep and analgesia

IL 1 acts on the brain to induce slow-wave sleep and analgesia. Injection into the cerebral ventricle of rats and rabbits enhances slow-wave sleep in the EEG which is not blocked by salicylates which prevent the concomitant fever[18,19]. In human plasma IL 1 is greater during slow-wave sleep than in waking[20]. In addition IL 1 is secreted by astrocytes in response to bacterial products, probably explaining the sleep-inducing effects of endotoxin and muramyl dipeptide[21].

Purified human IFN causes naloxone-reversible analgesia when injected into the cerebral ventricles of mice[22] and when injected intraperitonally in morphine-dependent rats[23]. Thus IFN seems to have opiate agonist effects. rH-IL 1α and rH-IL 1β have analgesic actions which are not naloxone-reversible but are partly prevented by intravenous injection of antibody against corticotrophin releasing factor, suggesting that opioid peptides may be induced. It is also interesting that virally infected or endotoxin-treated peripheral blood leukocytes can synthesize β-endorphin[24].

The pituitary adrenal axis and cortisol release

Exposure to bacterial toxins has long been known to stimulate release of ACTH from the anterior pituitary. Indeed the administration of endotoxin was used as a clinical test of anterior pituitary function. Experiments with hypophysectomized animals show that the major part of the corticosterone release caused by endotoxin is mediated by ACTH but that a significant extrapituitary mechanism also exists.

Besedovsky first showed in 1986[25] that rH-IL 1β increased ACTH and cortisol levels in C3H/HeJ mice. Further studies of corticotrophic cells from pituitaries incubated with IL 1 confirm that it is a potent secretagogue for ACTH[26]. *In vivo* increases in ACTH and corticosterone were blocked by antibodies to CRF, implying a hypothalamic site of action, though indomethacin had no effect, implying a different mechanism from pyrogenicity[27].

It has also been reported that IL 1 is able to induce corticosterone release directly from adrenal gland cells[29,30]. More recently it has been shown that rIL 6 is even more potent in this respect[30] and that it synergizes with low concentrations of ACTH[31]. In addition it has been shown that virally infected human peripheral blood leukocytes can be induced by CRF[32].

Glucocorticoids have strong 'anti-shock' and 'anti-endotoxin' effects and critically ill patients who fail to manifest an appropriate response have a poor prognosis[33]. The immediate cortisol increase of trauma is undoubtedly mediated by neural pathways, CRF and ACTH; however, IL 1 may play an important role in CRF release sepsis. In addition, there is a marked lack of correlation between levels of ACTH and continuing high levels of corticosteroid several days after the onset of trauma. Interestingly the stimulatory effect of IL 1β and IL 6 on adrenal cell steroid release was not present within the first 12 h of culture but only at 24 h[30]. Since serum levels of IL 1 and especially IL 6 have been shown to rise and remain elevated for several days following severe trauma these cytokines are strong candidates as factors controlling the long-term adrenal response.

EFFECTS ON INTERMEDIARY METABOLISM

Nitrogen balance

It has been known since the turn of the century that sepsis is accompanied by excess urinary nitrogen excretion. In the 1930s Cuthbertson and others[34] showed that the increased nitrogen excretion was accompanied by potassium, sulphur, phosphorus and zinc, implying a cellular origin. It was correctly assumed that the major source was muscle, as loss of muscle mass is a common clinical observation in severe trauma and sepsis far exceeding that seen in starvation.

It was thus of great interest when it was shown that stimulated leukocyte supernatants (EP) were able to induce muscle proteolysis by a prostaglandin-dependent mechanism[35]. Further studies showed that this activity was present in purified IL 1[36] and a putative 4 kD fragment of it[37]. However, despite these promising findings more recent studies with rH-IL 1 and other cytokines have completely failed to reproduce the effect. It is either only present in natural IL 1 or a contaminating factor was responsible. Whatever the mechanism, it is evident that amino acids released from muscle are used by the lymphoid tissue for cellular proliferation and antibody synthesis, and by the liver for acute phase protein synthesis.

Energy metabolism

Studies of the hyperlipidaemia accompanying parasitic infection have led to the observation that TNF, and to a lesser extent IL 1, inhibit lipoprotein lipase and enzymes responsible for the conversion of glucose to fatty acid[37,38]. Decreased glucose utilization for fat synthesis results in greater availability of glucose for metabolism by peripheral tissues and the unopposed action of fat cell lipase releases fatty acids from fat stores for similar use. The resulting weight loss and cachexia gives the name cachectin to TNF alpha.

There is evidence for cytokine mediated effects on the hormones of intermediary metabolism in the acute phase response but it is conflicting. The early work showed the leukocyte supernatants caused insulin and glucagon release in the pancreas[39], though more recently IL 1 appears to be cytotoxic for pancreatic islet cells[40]. Other work suggests that IL 1 may increase production of both insulin and glucagon[41].

LEUKOCYTOSIS

There is a well-known association between increased numbers of immature peripheral blood PMNLs and the acute response to infection, trauma and inflammation, such that this may be thought of as part of the acute phase response. PMNL enter the circulation from the marginal pool in response to many signals such as complement factors, catecholamines, prostaglandins and cytokines, while release from the bone marrow of immature cells and accelerated turnover are mediated by cytokines.

IL 1 induces PMNL released from the marrow[42], and in addition can induce production of specific granulocyte and macrophage replication factors (colony stimulating factors, CSFs) from various cell types[43]. IL 6 can induce production of GM-CSF and expression of receptors for GM-CSF, IL 3 and G-CSF.

METALS

Inflammation is often associated with decreased levels of iron and zinc and increased levels of copper. The mechanisms of these effects are entirely different, as is suggested by their kinetics[44].

Plasma iron levels fall within the first hour following operative trauma, paralleling the rapid fall in transferrin to which all iron in plasma is bound. This initial response, which is observed for many proteins and protein-bound substances, is probably due to alteration in vascular permeability mediated by a multiplicity of factors[44]. Iron levels, however, continue to fall and transferrin saturation decreases, reaching a nadir of about an 80% reduction 12 h following the onset of acute trauma. Iron is rapidly sequestered in damaged tissue, probably as a result of complexing to lactoferrin, an iron binding protein released from PMNL[45]. The iron lactoferrin complex is thus sequestered in macrophages as haemosiderin, a complex with ferritin. This iron is in a dynamic state and will subsequently re-enter the transferrin-bound pool for participation in haemopoesis.

Degranulation of neutrophils, releasing lactoferrin, can be induced by purified preparations of EP and the activity may well reside within IL 1[46]. Iron is essential for bacterial growth and the rapid sequestration of iron at inflammatory sites may serve as an antimicrobial mechanism and even the low plasma iron may confer a protective effect[47].

Following acute trauma in humans, plasma zinc levels fall by about 40% during the first 8 h. The initial fall parallels that of albumin (the major zinc binding protein of plasma) which stops falling at about 2 h, whilst zinc continues, reducing the amount carried on the protein. As with iron the first phase is due to loss of albumin from the vascular to the extravascular compartment.

The second phase of zinc reduction which persists for the duration of inflammation can be induced *in vivo* by EP administration[48]. *In vitro* rH-IL 6 but not rH-IL 1 was found to increase hepatocyte levels of metalothionine[49]. Under normal conditions metalothionine expression is transcriptionally regulated by dietary zinc. Induction of metalothionine synthesis by glucocorticoids, catecholamines, glucagon and IL 6 results in rapid transfer of zinc from plasma to the liver. The role of the response is unclear, although

Table 13.1 The acute phase proteins of inflammation

Protein	*Function*
Mediators	
C-reactive protein	Ligand binding complement activation
Complement components C1s, C2, C3, C4, C5, C9, Factor B	Opsonization, chemotaxis, mast cell degranulation
Kininogenase (kallikrein) Kininogen	Vascular permeability and dilatation
Factor VIII Fibrinogen Prothrombin	Clotting formation of fibrin matrix for repair
Plasminogen	Proteolytic activation of complement and clotting
Inhibitors	
Antithrombin III C1 INH Factor I, Factor H	Control of mediator pathways
α_1-Antitrypsin	Collagenase, elastase
α_1-Antichymotrypsin	Cathepsin G
Haptoglobin	Cathepsins B, H, L
Scavengers	
Haptoglobin	Haemoglobin
Serum amyloid A protein	Cholesterol
Ceruloplasmin	$[O_2^-]$?
Immune regulation	
C-reactive protein	Interactions with T and B cells. Expressed on
Orosomucoid	lymphocyte surface, T cell inhibitor
Repair and resolution	
Orosumucoid	Promotes fibroblast growth, interacts with collagen
α_1-Antitrypsin α_1-Antichymotrypsin C1 INH	Bound to surface of new elastic fibres

cytoprotection of liver cells from the toxic effects of carbon tetrachloride is enhanced by intracellular zinc accumulation. Zinc is also necessary for microbial growth.

The increase in copper as seen in inflammation is a consequence of cytokine-induced expression and secretion from the liver into the plasma of the copper containing protein caruloplasmin (see below).

ACUTE PHASE PROTEINS

Acute phase proteins are a family of approximately 30 plasma proteins produced in increased amounts by the liver in inflammation. When classified according to function it is clear that they may all have roles to play in inflammation or the healing process which follows (Table 13.1). The rate of increase in their plasma concentration, and the incremental change which occurs following inflammation, varies considerably between the acute phase proteins and reflects their induction by different cytokines and their molecular size, volume of distribution and rate of catabolism, both in the circulation and at the site of inflammation. Inflammation complicated by other processes such as intravascular coagulation may thus induce a different pattern of serum acute phase proteins, though in simple acute inflammation it is very characteristic for a particular species of animal.

Kushner[50] has defined acute phase proteins as those whose concentration rises by 25% or more following inflammation, and has divided them into three groups[51], on the basis of the magnitude of the increase (Table 13.2). The blood concentrations of several other proteins and enzymes, such as ferritin and serum alkaline phosphatase, frequently increase during inflammation,

Table 13.2 Major human acute phase proteins

Protein	*Normal plasma concentration* (g/l)	*Plasma concentration in inflammation* (g/l)	*Response time* (h)
Group III, up to 1000 × increase			
C-reactive protein	0.00007–0.008	0.4	6–10
Serum amyloid A	0.001–0.030	2.5	6–10
Group II, 2–4 × increase			
α_1-Antichymotrypsin	0.3–0.8	3.0	10
α_1-Antitrypsin	1.0–2.0	7.0	
α_1-Acid glycoprotein	0.5–1.4	3.0	24
Haptoglobin	1.0–3.0	6.0	
Fibrinogen	2.0–4.5	10	
Group I, about 50% increase			
Caeruloplasmin	0.15–0.6	2.0	
C3	0.55–1.2	3.0	48–72
C4	0.2–0.5	1.0	

Adapted from ref. 51.

possibly by mechanisms which differ from those of the acute phase response, whilst others such as transport proteins decrease in concentration. This latter group, often termed negative acute phase reactants, include albumin, prealbumin, transferrin, α_2-HS glycoprotein and α- and β-lipoproteins. While the positive acute phase proteins almost certainly play important roles in inflammation, there is little evidence to suggest that the negative reactants play an active part in inflammation and may simply reflect redistribution into the extravascular space[52] or cytokine-mediated decreases in gene transcription[53] which may help to conserve hepatic metabolites for the production of essential acute phase proteins.

Functions of acute phase proteins

Mediators

The acute phase proteins have a role in inflammation as mediators and inhibitors and also as scavengers of cell-derived products released from damaged tissue or macrophages. In addition some members of the family may influence the immune response which often accompanies inflammation and the release of autologous antigens. The acute phase protein response is thus a physiological mechanism providing increased serum and tissue levels of proteins modulating inflammation, and it is probable that it affects both the nature of the inflammatory lesion and the healing process which follows it.

Inflammation may be thought of as a series of biochemical and cellular events resulting in the phagocytosis of foreign material or damaged host cells. It occurs directly as a result of trauma or invasion by microorganisms, or it may result from the immune response (Figure 13.2).

The acute phase proteins responsible for the mediation of inflammation are shown in Table 13.1. A number of mechanisms are probably responsible for initiating the process. Trauma to tissue results in lysosomal enzyme release from damaged cells, in particular capillary endothelium, together with the production of cell membrane fragments and the exposure of capillary basement membrane collagen to plasma. Figure 13.2 shows the way in which these events activate the four proteolytic mediator systems of inflammation; the coagulation pathway, the complement system, the kallikrein kinin system and plasmin. This interacting network of proteases produces the complement effector molecules and kinins which result in the cellular events of inflammation[54].

Infecting microorganisms are able to initiate inflammation directly as a result of activation of the alternative pathway of complement or due to the binding of C-reactive protein to cell surface phosphorylcholine or galactosamine (see below).

Immune reactions result in complement activation by antibody complexed with antigen. IgG Fc results in macrophage adherence and phagocytosis. It is possible that cationic proteins, such as major basic protein, released by eosinophils, and heparin at sites of IgE-mediated mast cell degranulation may result in the binding of C-reactive protein.

Phagocytosing macrophages and polymorphonuclear leukocytes release acid lysosomal proteases and neutral proteases which are very important in

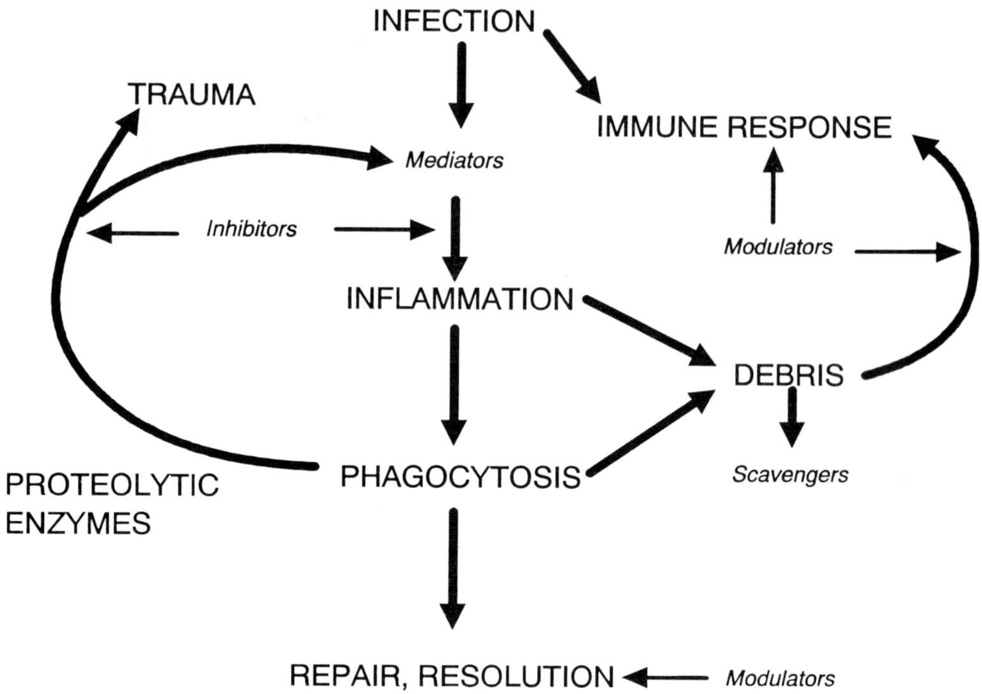

Figure 13.2 The processes of inflammation and the role of the acute phase proteins (in italics).

perpetuating inflammation by proteolytic activation of the mediators. They may also cause damage in the areas surrounding the inflammatory process. Other leukocytic products such as leukocytic cationic protein may bind C-reactive protein and thus activate complement. These 'feedback loops' are controlled by a number of inhibitory acute phase proteins (see below).

It is clear from this outline that *C-reactive protein* (CRP) may be emerging as an important inflammatory mediator able to initiate complement activation in a number of circumstances. Although Tillet and Francis showed the binding of CRP to pneumococcal C-polysaccharide in 1930[55] it was not until the early 1970s that this was shown to be due to binding to phosphorylcholine[56]. This calcium-dependent binding specificity is probably of great importance as this protein may bind to a number of micro organisms such as streptococci, *Proteus* and *Aspergillus*[57], and also to damaged autologous cell membranes[58]. There is probably also calcium-dependent binding to galactosamine[59]. Besides this CRP shows non-calcium-dependent binding to cationic molecules such as protamine, heparin, leukocytic cationic protein and histones[60]. The importance of these binding specificities is in the ability of bound CRP to activate complement via Clq and thus to initiate inflammation and phagocytosis[57]. That these phenomena are likely to be important *in vivo* is supported by the findings of CRP deposited on damaged cells soon after injury[61] and CRP-mediated complement-dependent opsonic clearance in the mouse[62]. Complexed CRP has also been shown to bind to T, B and null cells bearing IgG FcR[63] and also to platelets[64], thus giving rise to speculation about further activities for this protein in inflammation.

The inhibitors

Plasma contains two important groups of protease inhibitors involved in inflammation. First the mediator pathways themselves are controlled by a number of inhibitors several of which have been shown to be acute phase proteins (Table 13.1). It is important that although antithrombin III does not show an increase in plasma concentration its synthesis is increased in inflammation, but this is counteracted by increased consumption[65]. It is thus possible that other obvious candidates for acute phase behaviour, such as α-antiplasmin and α_2-macroglobulin have their response masked in this way. The pathway inhibitors show a spectrum of specificity for their substrates, some of them acting at several places in the four mediator systems. For example, C1 INH is a potent inhibitor of both C1s and kallikrein.

The second group of protease inhibitors are primarily concerned with inhibiting the products of phagocytosing cells. Alpha$_1$-antitrypsin has a specificity for the neutral proteases released from leucocytic granules, collagenase and elastase. Alpha$_1$-antichymotrypsin acts on the granule-derived cathepsin G. Haptoglobin has been shown to inhibit the lysosomal thiol proteases, cathepsins B, H and L[66]. Alpha$_2$-macroglobulin is a broad-spectrum inhibitor which is probably able to accept proteases from α_1-antitrypsin for clearance by receptor-mediated pinocytic uptake into macrophages. The ability of the neutral and acidic proteases to act on substrates within the mediator pathways make this group of protease inhibitors particularly important, not only in limiting proteolytic damage to surrounding tissues in inflammation but also in controlling the positive feedback effect.

The scavengers

Several proteins are probably concerned with the clearance of the products of inflammation. Caeruloplasmin may act as both a scavenger of damaging superoxide radicals released during phagocytosis and also to prevent autoxidation of lipids in damaged cell membranes[67]. Haptoglobin has an important role in conserving haemoglobin iron released as a result of microvascular damage and coagulation occurring during inflammation. Serum amyloid A protein (SAA) is an apolipoprotein present largely in HDL_3, the subset of HDL particles with a particularly rapid clearance from the circulation[68]. It is probable that SAA is acting as a recognition site for removal of HDL bound cholesterol from the circulation. Its acute phase behaviour may thus be related to the clearance of cholesterol from macrophages at the site of inflammation where cell membrane cholesterol accumulates as a result of phagocytosis of cell debris.

C-reactive protein, as already mentioned, binds to an FcR bearing subset of B, T and null cells, and although the role of this function is unknown it is tempting to speculate that it may exert a controlling influence on the immune reaction. Similarly orosomucoid (α_1-acid glycoprotein) has many characteristics implicating it as an immunodulatory protein. It shows sequence homology with the immunoglobulins; it is expressed on the lymphocyte cell membrane and the purified protein may inhibit T cells[69]. It is certainly clear that, quite apart from immune defence against invading organisms, the immune response may play a part in the clearance of autologous material from the sites of tissue damage by the formation of autoantibodies and its removal as immune complexes. Immune complexes are present in elevated concentrations in the blood in many acute and chronic inflammatory conditions, and may well form part of the physiological clearance mechanisms without necessarily having further pathogenic significance.

Repair and resolution

The biochemistry of repair and resolution following inflammation is little understood, but such evidence as there is strongly suggests that some of the acute phase proteins may have a role to play. Orosomucoid has been shown to promote fibroblast growth and to bind to collagen; α_1-antitrypsin, α_1-antichymotrypsin and C1 INH have been shown to be deposited in a sequential fashion on the surface of newly formed elastic fibres, perhaps controlling the remodelling of connective tissue resulting from locally produced proteases[70]. This is clearly an important area for further research.

Other acute phase reactants

Fibronectin and ferritin, both primarily tissue proteins, show acute phase behaviour under some circumstances. They differ, however, in having major sites of synthesis outside the liver, and are probably not induced in their hepatic synthesis by IL 1. It is probable that they do not form functional members of the true acute phase protein family. More puzzling, however, are the negative acute phase reactants, albumin, prealbumin, transferrin and retinol binding protein, the plasma levels of which fall in parallel with the acute phase response. The evidence suggests that their hepatic synthesis does in fact fall as a direct effect of IL 1. Is this of functional significance in the acute phase response, or does it merely reflect a switching of protein synthesis towards the acute phase reactants themselves?

Interspecies differences

The acute phase proteins have been studied most comprehensively in humans, rat and mouse, all of which have α-acid glycoprotein, haptoglobin and fibrinogen in common as acute phase reactants. Serum amyloid A protein (SAA), serum amyloid P protein (SAP), C-reactive protein (CRP) and α_2-macroglobulin, however, show marked interspecies differences in acute phase response (Table 13.3).

Table 13.3 Subsets of acute phase proteins induced by different cytokines

Type I – induced by IL 1β, TNF and IL 6	α_1-acid glycoprotein Complement C3 Complement factor B	Haptoglobin SAA SAP?
Type II – induced only only by IL 6	α_1-Protease inhibitor α_1-Antichromotrypsin α_1-Macroglobulin Caeruloplasmin	C-reactive protein Cysteine protease inhibitor Fibrinogen Haemopexin
Dependent on both IL 1β and IL 6	*Synergy* α_1-Acid glycoprotein Complement C3 Haptoglobin	*Inhibition* Cysteine protease inhibitor Fibrinogen Fibrinogen

Adapted from ref. 9.

CRP and SAP have been shown to possess substantial homology of amino acid sequence, subunit composition and calcium-dependent binding to specific ligands[71,72]. In humans the genes encoding them are both found on the long arm of chromosome 1[73], suggesting ancestral gene duplication.

When pentaxins (the term used to describe the common five-subunit composition) are isolated from the plasma of a wide variety of other species proteins resembling either human CRP or SAP or both may be present[74]. In other species, although the pentaxins demonstrate an acute phase response to inflammation, the order of magnitude is not as great as CRP in humans, and either CRP or SAP respond. Therefore, the acute phase response of human, monkey, rabbit, rat and plaice involve CRP, whereas in the mouse SAP is the acute phase reactant. Molecules which resemble CRP or SAP have been identified from all vertebrates which have been studied, including the marine toad, flounder, dogfish, cow, donkey, goat, sheep, chicken, pig, dog and also from the horseshoe crab[75]. In the Syrian hamster the pentaxin, known as female protein, is present in a high concentration in females. During the acute phase response the concentration in females decreases, and in males increases[76].

In the mouse SAA is the most sensitive acute phase protein, though antisera are difficult to raise. SAP is therefore the measurement of choice as this protein is easily purified and now commercially available. The mouse shows a strong strain-dependency in endogenous plasma SAP concentration and acute phase responsiveness. The choice of strain for experiments utilizing the acute phase response is therefore extremely important[77,78]. C57BL have been shown to exhibit the lowest baseline SAP levels with the largest incremental response to inflammation, DBA/2 the highest baseline and the least response, whereas Balb/c were intermediate in character as were C3H/He, the endotoxin-unresponsive mouse. The response is primarily influenced by the non-H-2 genotype and to a lesser extent by the H-2 haplotype of the strain, and possibly reflects the ability of macrophages to release SAP-inducing cytokines[79].

Haptoglobin has also been used successfully to monitor inflamamtion in the mouse, although in humans it is not regarded as the ideal protein to measure, due to the possibility of genetic defects and the low levels due to consumption which may occur during haemolysis.

In rabbit CRP and SAA are the major acute phase proteins although α_2-macroglobulin and transferrin also demonstrate moderate increases.

Kinetics of the acute phase response

In humans, CRP and SAA show the greatest response to injury, although the rate of increase in plasma concentration and the incremental change achieved following the inflammatory stimulus varies considerbly between the acute phase proteins. These variations possibly reflect the differential sensitivity to induction of synthesis, although in a particular species the pattern of response to acute inflammation is constant[80,81]. In chronic inflammation different patterns of response may be seen following different stimuli, in different inflammatory diseases, and following the same stimulus in different species or individuals of the same species. This complex situation may reflect alterations in the rate of synthesis of individual proteins in response to changes in regulating mediator patterns. Glibetic and Baumann[82] showed that during the progression from acute (less than 24 h after injury) to chronic inflammation in the mouse, there was a switch from a predominant expression of the gene for α_1-acid glycoprotein 1 to the gene for α_1-acid glycoprotein 2. In addition, the concentration of albumin mRNA returned to normal levels after an initial reduction of 50%, whereas the mRNA for SAA, α_1-acid glycoprotein, haptoglobin and fibrinogen was maximal at 24 h and decreased afterwards despite continuing inflammation. These findings afford some evidence that a change in regulation of protein synthesis for different proteins occurs during chronic inflammation.

Sites of acute phase protein production

The presence of CxRP (now known as CRP) in necrotic myofibres at the injection site some 8–10 h after typhoid vaccination in rabbits led Kushner and co-workers[61,83] to postulate that the protein was released into the circulation by dead and dying tissue. Gottleib[84] suggested that a precursor which existed in tissue was converted into active CRP at the site of inflammation. However, work by Thorbecke *et al.*[85] and Asofsky *et al.*[86] demonstrated the presence of CRP only in liver tissue from animals stimulated to produce acute phase proteins. Later experiments by Hurlimann, Thorbecke and Hochwald[87] were able to demonstrate incorporation of radiolabelled amino acids into albumin, haptoglobin and transferrin as well as CRP, produced by cultured rabbit, monkey and human liver preparations. Further work using minced hepatic tissue and isolated animal liver preparations confirmed that CRP and many other acute phase proteins are produced by the liver[88].

The cellular source of CRP was investigated by Kushner and Feldman[89]. CRP was found to be contained within hepatocytes adjacent to portal areas 24–38 h after administration of inflammatory stimulus, with successive time-related recruitment of cells to protein production[90,91], thereby supporting the concept of circulating mediators of the acute phase response.

Some evidence for extrahepatic synthesis of acute phase proteins also exists. Production of α_1-antitrypsin protein has been shown by rat and human monocyte/macrophages[92,93] and gene expression demonstrated in human monocytes[94]. NK effector cells have been shown to synthesize and express CRP on the cell surface[95], whereas secretion of CRP from T cells has been reported to increase in the presence of supernatants from phorbol myristate acetate-stimulated monocytes[96]. Several groups have reported the production of complement components by monocytes[97–100] and C2 production was found to be enhanced by supernatants from antigen-stimulated lymphocytes[101], possibly due to interferon activity[102].

Extrahepatic synthesis of SAA has also been demonstrated[103]. Specific mRNAs have been detected in various mouse and hamster organs including spleen, lung, kidney and intestine, although the reason for production of this molecule at such diverse sites is not known.

Whilst there is no comparison of the scale of production of these extrahepatic proteins with hepatic synthesis, it raises the interesting possibility of their production at sites of inflammation, perhaps in response to activated cell products. Cells at inflammatory foci may well form part of a front-line defence mechanism whereby acute phase proteins are released locally to limit the spread of inflammation and initiate tissue repair prior to the onset of the systemic acute phase response.

Cytokines and the acute phase response *in vivo*

Evidence of correlations between plasma IL 1 levels and acute phase reactants in humans are not apparent despite the recent availability of sensitive immunoassay detection methods. Using bioassay methods raised serum levels of IL 6 have been detected in patients with burns[104], and following surgical procedures [105]. Nijsten *et al.*[104] showed that IL 6 detected in plasma within hours after burn injuries was 2–100 times the normal level, while increases in CRP and α_1 AT followed more gradually. In postoperative patients IL 6 was detectable in serum within 3 h, had reached a maximum at 24 h and levelled off by 48 h, whereas CRP could not be detected during the first 6 h but gradually increased over the next 48 h. Other acute phase proteins measured, haptoglobin, α_1-antitrypsin and orosomucoid, increased gradually over a longer time course.

IL 6 has also been reported in the serum and synovial fluid of patients with various rheumatic diseases[106]. Synovial fluid levels of IL 6 were found to be 1000-fold higher and to correlate positively with those in serum, suggesting localized production in the joint. Synovial fluid levels of IL 6 could also be correlated with articular index, a clinical measure of local inflammation, whereas serum IL 6 levels were positively correlated with CRP and negatively correlated with albumin in rheumatoid arthritis. Raised levels of IL 6 in serum, urine and CSF have also been reported in various other inflammatory conditions involving acute phase responses[107–110].

Cytokine control of acute phase protein production

Since the liver was discovered to be the major site of acute phase protein synthesis a vast amount of experimental work has been directed towards elicudation of the chemical messengers involved in synthesis and regulation. Although several cytokines have been implicated, the complexity of the acute phase response is only just becoming apparent, and it is likely that synergistic interaction takes place not only between cytokines, but also between cytokines, hormones and other molecules.

IL 1

In the 1980s IL 1 was generally believed to be the major inducer of acute phase protein production. *In vivo* experiments using the newly available recombinant IL 1[111] appeared to substantiate the role of IL 1 implied by experiments using purified material[112] and direct action on the liver was suggested[113]. Although evidence pointed to similarities in inducibility of complement components and α_1AGP by rIL 1 in animal and human cells[53,114–119] IL 1-induced SAA production could not be demonstrated in human hepatocytes[120,121] and other discrepancies soon became clear due either to differences in cell systems or to gene responsiveness to different species. Lack of correlation between *in vivo* and *in vitro* activity has also become apparent. *In vivo* administration of purified or rH-IL 1 causes the induction of fibrinogen in all species tested[112,122] although fibrinogen expression is not induced by IL 1 at the mRNA or protein level in hepatocytes or hepatoma cells from either rat, mouse, rabbit or human[117,123–125]. It is now apparent that IL 1 can induce a limited number of acute phase protein genes, and it has also been shown to act in a negative manner by suppressing the induction of a number of acute phase proteins (including fibrinogen in rat and human as well as α_2M and cysteine proteinase inhibitor in the rat) caused by other mediators such as IL 6[117,123,126]. Apart from suggestions of differential production of α_1AGP[119] both the α and β forms of IL 1, encoded by separate genes, are equipotent in their actions on hepatocytes, and their receptors on human and murine lymphocytes have been shown to be identical[127].

TNFα

In some circumstances TNFα and IL 1β, molecules with the same spectrum of activities at other cellular target sites, have similar acute phase protein inducing capabilities. In various rat hepatoma cell lines both molecules have been shown to increase synthesis of α_1AGP, haptoglobin and C3[125], inhibit production of fibrinogen, thiostatin and α_2M[128].

In some cell systems and *in vivo*, rTNF is not as potent as rIL 1 on the induction of acute phase proteins[113,117,123], although it is generally thought that the same genes are affected.

Attempts to elucidate the regulatory mechanisms used by IL 1 and/or TNFα revealed that these cytokines could elicit only a partial acute phase response in cultured liver cells compared to hepatocytes treated with crude supernatants from COLO 16 tumour cells[117,123,129], and pointed to the existence of other mediators of the acute phase response.

IL 6

The monocyte-derived hepatocyte stimulating factor first described by Ritchie and Fuller[130,131] and later by other groups[123,132–134] proved to be identical to interferon-β_2, hybridoma growth factor, 26 kD protein and B-cell stimulating factor[129], and synonymous with monocyte granulocyte inducer type 2 and ILHP-1, and subsequently named IL 6. This molecule has since been recognized as the major inducer of acute phase protein synthesis, and the hepatocyte thought to be the main physiological target of the molecule.

Gauldie and others[135] established that IL 6, in combination with IL 1β and glucocorticoid, accounts for all the hepatic specific stimulation released by monocytes, and Baumann and co-workers have described an additive effect of IL 6, IL 1 and glucocorticoids on AGP and haptoglobin synthesis in rat hepatoma H-35 cells. In contrast, IL 1 was found to have a negative additive effect on IL 6 induction of fibrinogen in rat and human cells, and on thiostatin and α_2M in the rat[135]. These effects – the collated results using several cell lines – are summarized in Table 13.3, which shows the acute phase proteins as distinct subsets based on differential induction by combinations of cytokines.

IL 6 is known to be produced by a wide variety of cells including fibroblasts, synovial cells, endothelial cells and hepatocytes themselves[136], and reports of significant expression of IL 6 in normal human hepatocytes[137] and IL 1-stimulated hepatoma cells[104] suggests an autocrine mechanism may be involved in liver stimulation. However, IL 6 mRNA expression was not detected in the liver of normal rats or those undergoing an acute phase response[138], which suggests the use of caution when interpreting data using isolated hepatocytes cultured under non-physiological conditions such as in the absence of corticosteroids.

IFNγ

Conflicting evidence exists regarding the effect of IFNγ on the acute phase response and both lack of effect[135] and inhibitory activity for some proteins and enhancement of others[139] have been reported in the HepG2 cell line. Although the genes of complement components appear to be sensitive to IFNγ when transfected into fibroblasts, the greatest contribution of IFNγ to the acute phase response is likely to be via modulation of macrophage production of IL 1 and TNFα[140].

Cytokine and hormone interactions

Although the direct effects of IL 1, TNFα and IFNγ on the liver appear to be rather limited these cytokines affect other cells involved in the acute phase response, most notably endothelial cells and fibroblasts. IL 1 and TNFα have been shown to induce the production of IL 6 in fibroblasts[141], each is involved in the production of the other[142,143] and IL 1 can also induce its own gene expression[144]. In addition IL 1 acting directly on the pituitary to release adrenocorticotrophic hormone (ACTH), or indirectly through the hypothalamus to induce corticotrophin-releasing hormone, can cause the increase in glucocorticoid necessary for the hepatic responses[145,25,146].

The network of cytokines may well be viewed as an amplification system which conrols acute phase protein production. Although the pattern of proteins synthesized is genetically programmed it may be 'finely tuned' by the cytokines – IL 6 being the main signal – with other cytokines and hormones acting as accessory modulators (Figure 13.2). Proteins synthesized would therefore be determined by the sequence of exposure of the hepatocyte to the various regulating molecules. In this way the most effective homeostatic response to infection, inflammation or tissue damage may be achieved.

Prostaglandins

Although the interactions described above are generally believed to regulate the majority of acute phase proteins synthesized there is some evidence to suggest the involvement of prostaglandins (PG) in animal models of the acute phase response[147–149].

Whilst these observations are of interest, the mechanisms involved are not known and are likely to be complex. Arachidonic acid metabolites are produced by most cells involved in tissue repair, and serve to act as mediators of alterations in vascular permeability, oedema formation and fever production[150]. However, direct action on hepatocytes seems unlikely in view of the observation that CRP synthesis in isolated rabbit hepatocytes was not affected by addition of prostaglandin, and that the acute phase reaction to turpentine in rabbits was not affected by indomethacin[151]. Direct induction of cytokine synthesis in macrophages is also unlikely, as prostaglandins increase intracellular cAMP which has been shown by Dinarello[152] to decrease translation of IL 1, and gene expression of TNFα can be suppressed by PGE_2[153]. However, prostaglandins are thought to be chemotactic for granulocytes[140], of which neutrophils have been shown to be capable of IL 1 production[154].

Inhibitors of cytokine activity

Apparent defects in the acute phase response may in fact be due to the presence of cytokine inhibitors. Specific inhibitors of IL 1 activity have been reported in a variety of normal and pathological preparations in the presence or absence of various stimuli, and the subject is comprehensively reviewed by Seckinger *et al.*[155]. Inhibitory molecules of various size have been described, and all have been shown to be inhibitory in the lymphocyte activating factor assay; two were also able to block IL 1-induced collagenase production by human synovial cells and fibroblasts[156,157]. The 18–25 kD inhibitor purified from the urine of patients with monocytic leukaemia[157] was also able to block fibroblast proliferation, was effective against both IL 1α and IL 1β, and acted at the cell surface or at the receptor.

More recent are reports of the existence of IL 1 receptor antagonists – 22 kD molecule purified from human monocyte conditioned medium[158,159] and a similar 25 kD molecule purified from the cells of the human U937 monocyte cell line. This latter antagonist has been found to bind selectively to the high-affinity IL 1 receptor on T lymphocytes and fibroblasts, but not to the receptor of slightly lower affinity on bone marrow granulocytes, pre-B cells and macrophages[160]. *In vitro* the receptor antagonist has been shown to inhibit IL 1-induced adhesion of neutrophils and eosinophils to endothelial cells in a concentration-dependent fashion and to inhibit both IL 1α and IL 1β activities in the LAF assay. *In vivo* the receptor antagonist has been found to suppress corticosterone release when injected subcutaneously into mouse hind paw together with IL 1α and IL 1β. Soluble extracellular portions of the IL 1 receptor have also been demonstrated to neutralize *in vivo* IL 1 activity in mice[161]. A 40–60 kD inhibitor specific for TNF has also been isolated from the urine of febrile patients[155]. It has been shown to be neither a precursor nor denatured TNF, and is non-species specific as it also acts on a murine cell line. The cellular source of the IL 1 and TNF inhibitors is postulated to be the monocyte, and it is likely that negative feedback regulators of other cytokines are waiting to be revealed.

Defective acute phase responses in disease

Anomalies in the acute phase protein response have been reported in vartious diseases. Studies in systemic lupus erythematosus, dermatomyositis, systemic sclerosis, mixed connective disease, ulcerative colitis, primary biliary cirrhosis and chronic active hepatitis have shown low acute phase protein responses for the amount of inflammatory activity present[162]. This may be due either to disease-related unresponsiveness or to 'down-regulation' of the acute phase response in chronic inflammation[163,90]. Patients with systemic sclerosis did not mount an appreciable acute phase response to therapeutic infusion of PGE, compared with patients with atherosclerosis[149].

Unresponsiveness in scleroderma was later shown to be associated with disease duration[164]. Increased spontaneous IL 1 activity[165] and production of an IL 1 inhibitor have been shown in patients with this disease[166], although decreased monocyte IL 1 production has been observed in a number of chronic disease states such as cancer, leprosy and SLE[167]. Chellingsworth *et al.*[168] reported a 'normal' rapid increase in CRP levels in response to staphylococcal infection in a scleroderma patient despite low levels detected in active disease, whilst patients with osteoarthritis, SLE and scleroderma were found to respond to urate crystal injection in a manner comparable to that in controls[169].

Decreased monocyte production of TNF also has been reported in SLE[170], and decreased IL 6 production in patients with chronic lymphocytic leukaemia, whilst Yorston *et al.*[171] showed that patients with recurrent iritis are progressively less likely to show acute phase responses with increasing numbers of previous attacks. In some conditions the acute phase response mechanism may become refractory to certain stimuli, or it may be that a greater degree of stimulation is required in chronic disease. Defective host response to tissue damage or injury could therefore enhance or perpetuate inflammation.

References

1. Dinarello, C. A. (1984). Interleukin-1 and the pathogenesis of the acute phase response. *N. Eng. J. Med.*, **311**, 1413–18
2. Roberts, N. J. Jr and Steigbigel, R. T. (1977). Hyperthermia and human leukocyte functions: effects on response of lymphocytes to mitogen and antigen and bactericidal capacity of monocytes and neutrophils. *Infect. Immun.*, **18**, 673–9
3. Heron, I. and Berg, K. (1978). The actions of interferon are potentiated at elevated temperature. *Nature (Lond.)*, **274**, 508–10
4. Borodkin, P. A. (1972). Vliianie temperatury na mitoticheskuiu aktivnost' limfotsitov perifer icheskoikrovi cheleveka v kul'ture. *Bul. Exp. Biol. Med.*, **73**, 87–8
5. Duff, G. W. and Durum, S. K. (1982). Fever and immunoregulation hyperthermia, interleukin 1 and 2 and T cell proliferation. *Yale J. Biol. Med.*, **55**, 437–42
6. Hanson, D. F., Murphy, P. A., Silicano, R. and Shin, H. S. (1983). The effect of temperature on the activation of thymocytes by interleukins I and II. *J. Immunol.*, **130**, 216–21
7. Kluger, M. J., Ringler, D. H. and Anver, M. R. (1975). Fever and survival. *Science*, **188**, 166–8
8. Bernheim, H. A., Bodel, P. T., Askenase, P. W. and Atkins, E. (1978). Effects of fever on host defense mechanisms after infection in the lizard *Dipsosaurus dorsalis*. *Br. J. Exp. Pathol.*, **59**, 76–84
9. Covert, J. B. and Reynolds, W. W. (1977). Survival value of fever in fish. *Nature (Lond.)*, **267**, 43–5
10. Schmidt, J. R. and Rasmussen, A. F. (1960). The influence of environmental temperature on the course of experimental herpes simplex infection. *J. Infect. Dis.*, **107**, 356–60
11. Carmichael, L. E., Barnes, F. D. and Percy, D. H. (1966). Temperature as a factor in resistance of young puppies to canine herpesvirus. *J. Infect. Dis.*, **120**, 669–78
12. Furuuchi, S. and Shimizu, Y. (1976). Effect of ambient temperatures on multiplication of attenuated transmissable gastroenteritis virus in the bodies of newborn piglets. *Infect. Immun.*, **13**, 990–2
13. Rich, A. R. and McKee, C. M. (1936). The mechanism of a hitherto unexplained form of native immunity to the type III pneumococcus. *Bull. Johns Hopkins Hosp.*, **59**, 171–204
14. Weinstein, M. P., Iannini, P. B., Stratton, C. W. and Eikhoff, T. C. (1978). Spontaneous bacterial peritonitis. A review of 28 cases with emphasis on improved survival and factors influencing prognosis. *Am. J. Med.*, **64**, 592–8
15. Atkins, E. and Bodel, P. J. (1972). Fever. *N. Engl. J. Med.*, **286**, 27–34
16. Dinarello, C. A. (1989). Was the original endogenous pyrogen Interleukin 1? In Bomford R. and Henderson, B. (eds) *Interleukin 1 Inflammation and Disease*, pp. 17–28 (New York: Elsevier)
17. Atkins, E. (1989). Fever: historical aspects. In Bomford, R. and Henderson, B. (eds), *Interleukin 1 Inflammation and Disease*, pp. 13–15 (New York: Elsevier)
18. Tobler, I., Borbely, A. A., Schwyzer, M. and Fontana, A. (1984). Interleukin-1 derived from astrocytes enhances slow wave activity in sleep EEG of the rat. *Eur. J. Pharmacol.*, **104**, 191–2
19. Krueger, J. M., Dinarello, C. A. and Chedid, L. (1983). Promotion of slow wave sleep (SWS) by a purified interleukin I (IL-1) preparation. *Fed. Proc.*, **42**, 356
20. Moldofsky, H., Lue, F. A., Eisen, J., Keystone, E. and Gorczynski, R. M. (1986). The relationship of interleukin 1 and immune functions to sleep in humans. *Psychosomat. Med.*, **48**, 309–18
21. Fontana, A., Weber, E. and Dayer, J. M. (1984). Synthesis of interleukin 1/endogenous pyrogen in the brain of endotoxin-treated mice: a step in fever induction. *J. Immunol.*, **133**, 1696–8
22. Blalock, J. E. and Smith, E. M. (1981). Human leukocyte interferon (HuIFN-α): potent endorphin-like opioid activity. *Biochem. Biophys. Res. Commun.*, **101**, 472–8

23. Nakamura, H., Nakanishi, K., Kita, A. and Kadokawa, T. (1988). Interleukin 1 induces analgesia in mice by a central action. *Eur. J. Pharmacol.*, **149**, 49–54
24. Blalock, J. E. and Smith, E. M. (1985). A complete regulatory loop between the immune and neuroendocine systems. *Fed. Proc.*, **44**, 108–11
25. Besadovsky, H., Delrey, A., Sorkin, E. and Dinarello, C. A. (1986). Immuno regulatory feedback between interleukin 1 and glucocorticoid horomones. *Science*, **233**, 652–4
26. Bernton, E. W., Beech, J. E., Holaday, G. W., Smallridge, R. C. and Fein, H. G. (1987). Release of multiple hormones by a direct action of interleukin 1 on pituitary cells. *Science*, **238**, 519–21
27. Sapolsky, R., Rivier, C., Yamamoto, G., Plotsky, P. and Vale, W. (1987). Interleukin 1 stimulates the secretion of hypothalamic corticotrophin-releasing factor. *Science*, **238**, 522–4
28. Whitcomb, R. W., Linehan, W. H., Wahl, L. M. and Knazek, R. A. (1988). Monocytes stimulate cortisol production by cultured human adrenocortical cells. *J. Clin. Endocrinol. Metab.*, **66**, 33–8
29. Salas, M. A., Evans, S. W., Levell, M. J. and Whicher, J. T. (1990). *In vitro* effect of rIL-1 and rIL-6 on corticosterone release by isolated rat adrenal cells. In Oppenheim, J. J., Powanda, M. C., Kluger, M. J. and Dinarello, C. A. (eds), *Molecular and Cellular Biology of Cytokines*, pp. 427–32 (New York: Wiley–Liss)
30. Salas, M. A., Evans, S. W., Levell, M. J. and Whicher, J. T. (1990). Interleukin 6 and ACTH acts synergistically to stimulate the release of corticosterone from adrenal gland cells. *Clin. Exp. Immunol.*, **79**, 470–3
31. Smith, E. M., Morrill, A. C., Meyer, W. J. and Blalock, J. E. (1986). Corticotrophin releasing factor induction of leucocyte-derived immunoreactive ACTH and endorphins. *Nature*, **321**, 881–2
32. Mills, L. C. (1971). Corticosteroids in endotoxic shock. *Proc. Soc. Exp. Biol. Med.*, **138**, 507–11
33. Finlay, W. E. I. and McKee, J. I. (1982). Serum cortisol levels in severely stressed patients. *Lancet*, **1**, 1414–15
34. Cuthbertson, D. P. (1931). The distribution of nitrogen and sulphur in the urine during conditions of increased catabolism. *Biochem. J.*, **25**, 236–44
35. Baracos, V., Rodemann, H. P., Dinarello, C. A. and Goldberg, A. L. (1983). Stimulation of muscle protein breakdown and prostaglandin E2 release by leucocytic pyrogen (interleukin 1). A mechanism for the increased degradation of muscle proteins during fever. *N. Engl. J. Med.*, **308**, 553–8
36. Clowes, G. H. A. Jr, George, B. C. and Bigatello, L. M. (1985). Regulation of protein metabolism by proteolysis inducing factor (PIF) the stable circulating fragment of interleukin 1. *Br. J. Rheumatol.*, **24**, (Suppl.), 113–17
37. Beutler, B. and Cerami, A. (1986). Cachectin and tumour necrosis factor as two sides of the same biological coin. *Nature*, **320**, 584–8
38. Beutler, B. and Cerami, A. (1985). Recombinant interleukin 1 suppresses lipoprotein lipase activity in 3T3-L1 cells (1985). *Immunology*, **135**, 3969–71
39. George, D. T., Abeles, F. B., Mapes, C. A., Sobocinsky, P. Z., Zenser, T. V. and Powanda, M. C. (1977). Effect of leucocytic endogenous mediators on endocrine pancreas secretory responses. *Am. J. Physiol.*, **233**, E240
40. Dinarello, C. A. (1986). Interleukin 1, amino acids, sequences, multiple biological activities and comparison with tumor necrosis factor. *Year Immunol.*, **86**, 68–89
41. Besadovsky, N. and Del Rey, A. (1987). Neuroendocrine and metabolic responses induced by interleukin-1. *J. Neurosci. Res.*, **18**, 172–8
42. Ulich, T. R., Castillo, J., Keys, M., Granger, G. A. and Ni, R. X. (1987). Kinetics and mechanisms of recombinant interleukin 1 and tumour necrosis factor-α induced changes in circulating numbers of neutrophils and lymphocytes. *J. Immunol.*, **139**, 3406–15
43. Shabo, Y., Lotem, J. and Sachs, L. (1989). Regulation of the genes for interleukin 6 and granulocyte macrophage colony stimulating factor by different inducers of differentiation in myeloid leukaemic cells. *Leukaemia*, **3**, 859–65
44. Myers, M. A., Fleck, A., Sampson, B., Colley, C. M., Bent, J. and Hall, G. (1984). Early plasma protein and mineral changes after surgery: a two stage process. *J. Clin. Pathol.*, **37**, 862–6
45. Van Snick, J. L., Masson, P. L. and Heremans, J. F. (1974). Involvement of lactoferrin in the hyposideremia of acute inflammation. *J. Exp. Med.*, **140**, 1068–84
46. Klempner, M. S., Dinarello, C. A. and Gallin, J. I. (1978). Human leucocytic pyrogen

induces release of specific granule contents from human neutrophils. *J. Clin. Invest.*, **61**, 1330–6
47. Bullen, J. J. (1981). Significance of iron in infection. *Rev. Infect. Dis.*, **3**, 1127–38
48. Kampschmidt, R. F. and Pulliam, L. A. (1978). Effect of human monocyte pyrogen on plasma iron plasma zinc and blood neutrophils in rabbits and rats. *Proc. Soc. Exp. Biol. Med.*, **158**, 32–5
49. Schroeder, J. J. and Cousins, R. J. (1990). Interleukin 6 regulates metalothionine gene expression and zinc metabolism in hepatocyte monolayer cultures. *Proc. Natl. Acad. Sci. USA*, **87**, 3137–41
50. Kushner, I. (1982). The phenomenon of the acute phase response. *Ann. N.Y. Acad. Sci.*, **389**, 39–48
51. Kushner, I. and Mackiewicz, A. (1987). Acute phase proteins as disease markers. *Dis. Markers*, **5**, 1–11
52. Ballantyne, F. C., Tilstone, W. J. and Fleck, A. (1973). Effect of injury on albumin synthesis in the rabbit. *Br. J. Exp. Pathol.*, **54**, 409–15
53. Ramadori, G., Sipe, J. D., Dinarello, C. A., Mizel, S. B. and Colten, H. R. (1985). Pretranslational modulation of acute phase hepatic protein synthesis by murine recombinant interleukin-1 (IL1-1) and purified human IL-1. *J. Exp. Med.*, **162**, 930–42
54. Ratnoff, Q. D. (1971). A tangled web. The interdependence of mechanisms of blood clotting, fibrinolysis, immunity and inflammation. *Thromb. Diath. Haemorrh.*, (Suppl. 45), 109–18
55. Tillet, W. S. and Francis, T. (1930). Serological reactions in pneumonia with a non-protein somatic fraction of the pneumococcus. *J. Exp. Med.*, **52**, 561–71
56. Volanakis, J. E. and Kaplan, M. H. (1971). Specificity of C-reactive proteins for choline phosphate residues of pneumoccal C-polysaccharide. *Proc. Soc. Exp. Biol. Med.*, **136**, 612–14
57. Volanakis, J. E. (1982). Complement activation by C-reactive protein complexes. *Ann. NY Acad. Sci.*, **389**, 235–50
58. Mold, C., Rodgers, C. P., Richards, R. L., Alving, C. R. and Gewurz, H. (1981). Interaction of C-reactive protein with liposomes. III Membrane requirements for binding. *J. Immunol.*, **126**, 856–60
59. Volanakis, J. E. and Narkates, A. J. (1981). Interaction of C-reactive protein with artificial phosphatidylcholine bilayers and complement. *J. Immunol.*, **126**, 1820–5
60. Siegel, J., Osmand, A. P., Wilson, M. F. and Gewurz, H. (1975). Interaction of C-reactive proteins with the complement system. *J. Exp. Med.*, **142**, 709–21
61. Kushner, I. and Kaplan, M. H. (1961). Studies of acute phase protein. *J. Exp. Med.*, **114**, 961–74
62. Nakayama, S., Mold, C., Gewurz, H. and Du Clos, T. (1981). Opsonic properties of C-reactive protein in vivo. *Fed. Proc.*, **40**, 1046
63. James, K., Hansen, B. and Gewurz, H. (1980). Further studies on the binding of C-reactive protein (CRP) to human lymphocytes. Development of a radioassay and requirement for a multivalent binding specificity. *Fed. Proc.*, **39**, 941
64. Fiedel, B. A., Simpson, R. M. and Gewurz, H. (1982). Interaction between C-reactive protein (CRP) and platelets. In Allen, R. C., Bienvenu, J., Laurent, P. and Suskind, R. M. (eds), *Marker Proteins in Inflammation*, pp. 112–30 (Berlin: Walter de Gruyter)
65. Koj, A. and Regoeczi, E. (1979). Effect of experimental inflammation on the synthesis and distribution of antithrombin III and α_1-antitrypsin in rabbits. *Br. J. Exp. Pathol.*, **59**, 473–81
66. Pagano, M., Engler, R., Gelin, M. and Jayle, M. F. (1980). Kinetic study of the interaction between rat haptoglobin and rat liver cathepsin B. *Can. J. Biochem.*, **58**, 410–17
67. Goldstein, I. M., Kaplan, H. B., Edelson, H. S. and Weissmann, G. (1982). Ceruloplasmin: An acute phase reactant that scavenges oxygen-derived free radicals. *Ann. N.Y. Acad. Sci.*, **389**, 368–79
68. Benditt, E. P., Hoffman, J. S. and Eriksen, N. (1982). SAA, an apoprotein of HPL: its structure and function. *Ann. N.Y. Acad. Sci.*, **389**, 183–9
69. Arnaud, P. and Gianazza, E. (1982). Alpha-1 acid glycoprotein – structure, genetics and biological significance. In Allen, R. C., Bienvenu, J., Laurent, P. and Suskind, R. M. (eds), *Marker Proteins in Inflammation*, pp. 157–69 (Berlin: Walter de Gruyter)
70. Davies, J. D., Barnard, K., Whicher, J. T. and Young, W. (1982). Breast elastosis: association with lysozyme and certain protease inhibitors. *Proc. Pathol. Soc.*, **145**, 38
71. Osmand, A. P., Friedenson, B., Gewurz, H., Painter, R. H., Hofmann, T. and Shelton, E. (1977). The characterisation of C-reactive protein and the CIT subcomponent of CI as pentraxine: homogenous proteins displaying cyclic pentameric symmetry. *Proc. Natl. Acad. Sci. USA*, **74**, 739–43

72. Pepys, M. B. and Baltz, M. L. (1983). Acute phase proteins with special reference to C-reactive protein and related proteins (pentaxins) and serum amyloid A protein. *Adv. Immunol.*, **34**, 141–212
73. Floyd-Smith, G., Whitehead, A. S., Colten, H. R. and Francke, U. (1986). The human C-reactive protein gene (CRP) and serum amyloid P component gene (APCS) are located on the proximal long arm of chromosome 1. *Immunogenetics*, **24**, 171–6
74. Pepys, M. B., Dash, A. C., Fletcher, F. C., Richardson, N., Munn, E. A. and Feinstein, A. (1978). Analogues in other mammals and in fish of human plasma protein C-reactive protein and amyloid P component. *Nature*, **273**, 168–70
75. Robey, F. A. and Liu, T. Y. (1981). Limulin: a C-reactive protein from *Limulus polyphemus*. *J. Biol. Chem.*, **256**, 969–75
76. Coe, J. F. (1983). Analogues of CRP: a diverse family or proteins with similar structure. *Contemp. Topics Mol. Immunol.*, **9**, 211–38
77. Le, P. T., Muller, M. T. and Mortenson, R. F. (1982). Acute phase reactants of mice. I: production of serum amyloid P-component (SAP) and its induction by a monokine. *J. Immunol.*, **129**, 665–72
78. Pepys, M. B. (1979). Isolation of serum, amyloid P-component (protein SAP) in the mouse. *Immunology*, **37**, 637–41
79. Mortensen, R. F., Beisel, K., Zelezik, N. J. and Le, P. T. (1983). Acute phase reactants of mice. II: strain dependence of serum amyloid P-component (SAP) levels and response to inflammation. *J. Immunol.*, **130**, 885–9
80. Aronsen, K. F., Ekelund, G., Kindmark, C. O. and Laurell, C. B. (1972). Sequential changes of plasma proteins after surgical trauma. *Scand. J. Clin. Lab. Invest.*, **29** (Suppl. 124), 127–36
81. Colley, C. M., Fleck, A., Goode, A. W., Muller, B. R. and Myers, M. A. (1983). Early time course of the acute phase protein response in man. *J. Clin. Pathol.*, **36**, 203–7
82. Glibetic, M. D. and Baumann, H. (1986). Influence of chronic inflammation on the level of mRNA for acute phase reactants in the mouse liver. *J. Immunol.*, **137**, 1616–22
83. Kushner, I., Rakita, L. and Kaplan, M. H. (1963). Studies of acute phase proteins. II. Localisation of CX-reactive protein in heart in induced myocardial infarction in rabbits. *J. Clin. Invest.*, **42**, 286–92
84. Gottleib, A. A. (1962). Kinetics of formation of C-reactive protein. *Proc. Soc. Exp. Biol. Med.*, **110**, 568–71
85. Thorbecke, C. J., Asofsky, R., Hochwald, C. M. and Jacobson, E. B. (1963). Autoradiography of immunoelectrophoresis in the study of 14C amino acid incorporation into serum proteins by tissues in vitro and in vivo. *Prot. Biol. Fluids Proc. Colloq.*, **11**, 125–7
86. Asofsky, R., Thorbecke, G. J., Hochwald, G. M. and Williams, C. A. (1963). Formation in vitro of plasma protein by tissues from normal and infected animals. *Fed. Proc.*, **22**, 264 (abstract)
87. Hurlimann, J., Thorbecke, G. J. and Hochwald, G. M. (1966). The liver as the site of C-reactive protein formation. *J. Exp. Med.*, **123**, 365–78
88. Koj, A. (1974). Acute-phase reactants, their synthesis, turnover and biological significance. In Allison, A. C. (ed.), *Structure and Function of Plasma Proteins*, Vol. 1, pp. 73–125 (London: Plenum Press).
89. Kusner, I. and Feldmann, G. (1978). Control of the acute phase response. Demonstration of C-reactive protein synthesis and secretion by hepatocytes during acute inflammation in the rabbit. *J. Exp. Med.*, **148**, 466–77
90. Macintyre, S. S., Schultz, D. and Kushner, I. (1982). Biosynthesis of C-reactive protein. *Ann. N.Y. Acad. Sci.*, **389**, 76–87
91. Baumann, H., Firestone, G. L., Gross, K. W., Yamamoto, H. R. and Held, W. A. (1983). Dexamethosone regulation of alpha-1-acid glycoprotein and other acute phase reactants in rat liver and hepatoma cells. *J. Biol. Chem.*, **258**, 563–70
92. Lamontagne, L. R., Stadnyk, A. W. and Gauldie, J. (1985). Synthesis of alpha-1-protease inhibitor by resident and activated mouse alveolar macrophages. *Am. Rev. Respir. Dis.*, **131**, 321–5
93. Van Furth, R., Kramps, J. A. and Diesselhof-DenDulk, M. M. C. (1983). Synthesis of alpha-1 antitrypsin by human monocytes. *Clin. Exp. Immunol.*, **51**, 551–7.
94. Perlmutter, D. H., Cole, F. S., Kilbridge, P., Rossing, T. H. and Colten, H. R. (1985). Expression of alpha-1-protease inhibitor gene in human monocytes and macrophages. *Proc. Natl. Acad. Sci. USA*, **82**, 795–9

95. Kuta, A. E. and Baum, L. L. (1986). CRP is produced by a small number of normal peripheral blood lymphocytes. *J. Exp. Med.*, **164**, 321–6
96. Ikuta, T., Okuboh, Ishibashi, H., Okumura, Y. and Hayashida, K. (1986). Human lymphocytes synthesise C-reactive protein. *Inflammation*, **10**, 223–32
97. Colten, H. R. (1974). Synthesis and metabolism of complement proteins. *Transplant. Proc.*, **6**, 33–8
98. Colten, H. R. (1982). Biosynthesis of MHC-linked complement proteins C2, C4 and factor B by mononuclear phagocytes. *Mol. Immunol.*, **19**, 1279–85
99. Cole, E. S., Auerbach, H. S., Goldberger, G. and Colten, H. R. (1985). Tissue specific pretranslational regulation of complement production in human mononuclear phagocytes. *J. Immunol.*, **134**, 2610–16
100. Einstein, L. P., Hansen, P. J., Ballow, M., Davies, A. E., Davis, J. S., Alper, C. A., Rosen, F. S. and Colten, H. R. (1977). Biosynthesis of the third component of complement (C3) in vitro by both normal and homogenous C3 deficient monocytes. *J. Clin. Invest.*, **60**, 963–9
101. Littman, B. H. and Ruddy, S. (1977). Production of the second component of complement by human monocytes: stimulation by antigen activated lymphocytes or lymphokines. *J. Exp. Med.*, **145**, 1344–52
102. Perlmutter, D. H., Strunk, R. C., Goldberger, G. and Cole, F. S. (1986). Regulation of complement proteins C2 and factor B by interleukin-1 and interferon-gamma acting on transfected L-cells. *Mol. Immunol.*, **23**, 1263–6
103. Ramadori, G., Sipe, J. D. and Colten, H. R. (1985). Expression and regulation of the murine serum amyloid A (SAA) gene in extrahepatic sites. *J. Immunol.*, **135**, 3645–7
104. Nijsten, M. W. N., DeGroot, E. R., Ten Duis, H. J., Klaren, J. H., Hack, C. E. and Aarden, L. A. (1987). Serum levels of interleukin-6 and acute phase responses. *Lancet*, **2**, 921
105. Nishimoto, N., Yoshizaki, K. and Tagoh, H. (1989). Elevation of serum interleukin-6 prior to acute phase proteins on the inflammation by surgical operation. *Clin. Immunol. Immunopathol.*, **50**, 399–401
106. Swaak, A. J., Van Rooyen, A., Nieuwenhuis, E. and Aarden, L. A. (1988). Interleukin-6 in synovial fluid and serum of patients with rheumatic disease. *Scand. J. Rheumatol.*, **17**, 469–74
107. Houssiau, F. A., Bukasa, K., Sindic, C. J. M., Van Damme, J. and Van Snick, J. (1988). Elevated levels of 26k human hybridoma growth factor (interleukin 6) in cerebrospinal fluid of patients with acute infection of the central nervous system. *Clin. Exp. Immunol.*, **71**, 320–3
108. Houssiau, F. A., Devogelaer, J. P., Van Damme, J., Nagant de Deuxchaisnes, C. and Van Snick, J. (1988). Interleukin 6 in synovial fluid and serum of patients with rheumatoid arthritis and other inflammatory arthritides. *Arthritis Rheum.*, **31**, 784–8
109. Helfgott, D. C., Tatter, S. B., Santhanam, U., Claric, R. H., Bhardwaj, N., May, L. T. and Sehgal, P. B. (1989). Multiple forms of IFNβ2/IL-6 in serum, and body fluids during acute bacterial infection. *J. Immunol.*, **142**, 948–53
110. Van Oers, M. J. H., Van Der Heyden, A. A. P. A. M. and Aarden, L. A. (1988). Interleukin-6 in serum and urine of renal transplant recipients. *Clin. Exp. Immunol.*, **71**, 314–19
111. Sipe, J. D. and Ramadori, G. (1986). In Marrink, J. and Van Rijswijk, M. H. (eds), *Amyloidosis*, pp. 319–28 (Dordrecht: Martinus Mijhoff)
112. Kampschmidt, R. F. and Mesecher, M. (1985). Interleukin 1 from P388D$_1$: effects upon neutrophils, plasma iron and fibrinogen in rats, mice and rabbits. *Proc. Soc. Exp. Biol. Med.*, **179**, 197–200
113. Sipe, J. D., Johns, M. A., Ghjezzi, P. and Knapschaefer, G. (1988). Modulation of serum amyloid A gene expression by cytokines and bacterial cell wall components. *Adv. Exp. Med. Biol.*, **243**, 193–201
114. Perlmutter, D. H., Dinarello, C. A., Punsal, P. I. and Colten, H. R. (1986). Cachectin/tumour necrosis factor regulates hepatic acute phase gene expression. *J. Clin. Invest.*, **78**, 1349–54
115. Marinkovic, S., Jahreis, G. P., Wong, G. G. and Baumann, H. (1988). IL-6 modulates the synthesis of a specific set of acute phase plasma proteins in vivo. *J. Immunol.*, **142**, 808–12
116. Gauldie, J., Sauder, D. N., McAdam, K. P. W. J., and Dinarello, C. A. (1987). Purified interleukin (IL-1) from human monocytes stimulates acute phase protein synthesis by rodent hepatocytes *in vitro*. *Immunology*, **60**, 203–7
117. Koj, A., Kurdowska, A., Magielska-Zero, D., Rokita, H., Sipe, J. D., Dayer, J. H., Demczuk, S. and Gaudlie, J. (1987). Limited effects of recombinant human and murine interleukin-1 and tumour necrosis factor on production of acute phase proteins by cultured rat

hepatocytes. *Biochem. Int.*, **14**, 553–60

118. Baumann, H., Richards, C. and Gauldie, J. (1987). Interaction among hepatocyte stimulating factors, interleukin-1 and glucocorticoids for regulation of cute phase plasma proteins in human hepatoma (HepG2) cells. *J. Immunol.*, **139**, 4122–8
119. Geiger, T., Andus, T., Klapporth, J., Northoff, H. and Heinrich, P. C. (1988). Induction of alpha-1-acid glycoprotein by recombinant human interleukin-1 in rat hepatoma cells. *J. Biol. Chem.*, **263**, 7141–6
120. Perlmutter, D. H., Goldberger, G., Dinarello, C. A., Mizel, S. B. and Colten, H. R. (1986). Regulation of class III major histocompatibility complex gene products by interleukin-1. *Science*, **232**, 850–2
121. Ganapathi, M. K., Schultz, D., Mackiewicz, A., Samols, D., Hu, S.-I., Brabenec, A., Macintyre, S. S. and Kushner, I. (1988). Heterogenous nature of the acute phase response. Differential regulation of human serum amyloid A, C-reactive protein, and other acute phase proteins by cytokines in Hep3B cells. *J. Immunol.*, **141**, 564–9
122. Dinarello, C. A. (1988). Biology of interleukin-1. *FASEB J.*, **2**, 108–15
123. Darlington, G. J., Wilson, D. R. and Lachman, L. B. (1986). Monocyte-conditioned medium, interleukin-1 and tumour necrosis factor stimulate the acute phase response in human hepatoma cells in vitro. *J. Cell Biol.*, **103**, 787–93
124. Evans, E., Courtois, G. M., Killian, P. L., Fuller, G. M. and Crabtree, G. R. (1987). Induction of fibrinogen and a subset of acute phase response genes involves a novel monokine which is mimicked by phorbol esters. *J. Biol. Chem.*, **262**, 10850–4
125. Baumann, H., Onorato, V., Gauldie, J. and Jahreis, G. P. (1987). Distinct sets of acute phase plasma proteins are stimulated by separate human hepatocyte-stimulating factors and monokines in rat hepatoma cells. *J. Biol. Chem.*, **262**, 9756–68
126. Andus, T., Geiger, T., Hirano, T., Kishimoto, T., Tran-Thi, T. A., Decker, K. and Heinrich, P. C. (1988). Regulation of synthesis and secretion of major rat acute phase proteins by recombinant human interleukin-6 (BSF-2/IL-6) in hepatocyte primary cultures. *Eur. J. Biochem.*, **173**, 287–93
127. Dower, S. K., Kronheim, S. R., Hopp, T. P., Cantrell, M., Deeley, M., Gillis, S., Henney, C. S. and Urdal, D. L. (1986). The cell surface receptors for interleukin-1 alpha and interleukin-1 beta are identical. *Nature*, **324**, 266–8
128. Whicher, J. T., Thompson, D., Billingham, M. E. J. and Kitchen, E. A. (1989). Acute phase proteins. In Chang, J. Y. and Lewis, A. J. (eds), *Pharmacological Methods in the Control of Inflammation*, pp. 101–28 (New York: Liss)
129. Gauldie, J., Richards, C., Harnish, D., Landsdorp, P. and Baumann, H. (1987). Interferon β2/B-cell stimulatory factor type 2 shares identity with monocyte-derived hepatocyte stimulating factor and regulates the major acute phase protein response in liver cells. *Proc. Natl. Acad. Sci. USA*, **84**, 7251–5
130. Ritchie, D. G. and Fuller, G. M. (1981). An *in vitro* bioassay for leukocytic endogenous mediator(s) using cultured rat hepatocytes. *Inflammation*, **5**, 287–9
131. Ritchie, D. G. and Fuller, G. M. (1983). Hepatocyte stimulating factor: a monocyte-derived acute phase regulatory protein. *Ann. N.Y. Acad. Sci.*, **408**, 490–502
132. Baummann, H., Jahreis, G. P., Sauder, D. N. and Koj, A. (1984). Human keratinocytes and monocytes release factors which regulate the synthesis of acute phase plasma proteins in hepatic cells from man, rat and mouse. *J. Biol. Chem.*, **259**, 7331–42
133. Koj, A., Gauldie, J., Regoeczi, E., Sauder, D. N. and Sweeney, G. D. (1984). The acute phase response of cultured rat hepatocytes. System characterisation and the effect of human cytokines. *Biochem. J.*, **224**, 505–14
134. Bauer, J., Trans-Thi, T. A., Northoff, H., Hirsch, F., Schalyer, H. J., Gerok, W. and Heinrich, P. C. (1986). The acute-phase induction of alpha 2-macroglobulin in rat hepatocyte primary cultures: action of a hepatocyte-stimulating factor, triiodothyronine and dexamethasone. *Eur. J. Cell Biol.*, **40**, 86–93
135. Gauldie, J., Richards, C., Harnish, D. and Baumann, H. (1988). Interferon-beta-2 is identical to monocytic HSF and regulates the full acute phase protein response in liver cells. In Powanda, M. C. *et al.* (eds), *Monokines and Other Non-lymphatic Cytokines*, pp. 15–20 (New York: Liss)
136. Lotz, M., Zuraw, B. L., Carson, D. A. and Jirik, F. R. (1989). Hepatocytes produce interleukin 6. *Ann. NY Acad. Sci.*, **557**, 509–11

137. Tovey, M. G., Content, J., Gresser, I., Gugenheim, J., Blanchard, B., Guymarho, J., Poupart, P., Gigou, M., Shaw, A. and Fiers, W. (1988). Genes for IFN-beta-2(IL-6) tumour necrosis factor and IL-1 are expressed at high levels in the organs of normal individuals. *J. Immunol.*, **141**, 3106–10
138. Baumann, H. and Gauldie, J. (1990). Regulation of hepatic acute phase plasma protein genes by hepatocyte stimulating factors and other mediators of inflammation. *Mol. Biol. Med.*, **7**, 147–59
139. Magielska-Zero, D., Bereta, J., Czuba-Pelech, P. V., Gauldie, J. and Koj, A. (1988). Inhibitory effect of recombinant human interferon-gamma on synthesis of some acute phase proteins in human hepatoma HepG2 cells. *Biochem. Int.*, **17**, 17–23
140. Dowton, S. B. and Colten, H. R. (1988). Acute phase reactants in inflammation and infection. *Semin. Hematol.*, **25**, 84–90
141. Kohase, M., May, L. T., Tamm, I., Vilcik, J. and Seghal, P. B. (1987). A cytokine network in human diploid fibroblasts: interactions of beta-interferons, tumour necrosis factor, platelet-derived growth factor and interleukin-1. *Mol. Cell. Biol.*, **7**, 273–80
142. Dinarello, C. A., Cannon, J. G. and Wolff, S. M. (1986). Tumour necrosis factor (cachectin) is an endogenous pyrogen and induces production of interleukin-1. *J. Exp. Med.*, **163**, 1433–49
143. Bachwich, P. R., Chensue, S. W., Larrick, J. W. and Kunkel, S. (1986). Tumour necrosis factor stimulates interleukin-1 and prostaglandin E2 production in resting macrophages. *Biochem. Biophys. Res. Commun.*, **136**, 94–101
144. Warner, S. J., Auger, K. R. and Libby, P. (1987). Human interleukin-1 induces interleukin-1 gene expression in human vascular smooth muscle cells. *J. Exp. Med.*, **165**. 1316–51
145. Lumpkin, M. D. (1987). The regulation of ACTH secretion by interleukin-1. *Science*, **238**, 452–4
146. Bernardini, R., Kamilaris, T. C., Calogero, A. E., Johnson, E. D., Gomez, M. T., Gold, P. W. and Chrousos, G. P. (1990). Interactions between tumor necrosis factor-alpha, hypothalamic corticotropin-releasing hormone, and adrenocorticotropin secretion in the rat. *Endocrinology*, **126**, 2876–81
147. Shim, B.-S. (1976). Increases in serum haptoglobin stimulated by prostaglandins. *Nature*, **259**, 326–27
148. Whicher, J. T., Bell, A. M., Unwin, J., Martin, M. and Dieppe, P. (1982). The prostaglandin-induced acute phase response is defective in endotoxin tolerant mice and in humans with scleroderma. *Ann. N.Y. Acad. Sci.*, **289**, 474–5
149. Whicher, J. T., Bell, A. M., Martin, M. F. R., Marshall, L. A. and Dieppe, P. A. (1984). Prostaglandins cause an increase in serum acute-phase proteins in man, which is diminished in systemic sclerosis. *Clin. Sci.*, **66**, 165–71
150. Davies, P., Bailey, P. J., Goldenberg, M. M. and Ford-Hutchinson, A. W. (1984). The role of arachidonic acid oxygenation products in pain and inflammation. *Ann. Rev. Immunol.*, **2**, 335–57
151. Schultz, D., Macintyre, S., Chelladuri, M. and Kushner, I. (1982). Biosynthesis of C-reactive protein. *Ann. N.Y. Acad. Sci.*, **389**, 465–6
152. Dinarello, C. A. (1984). Interleukin-1 and the pathogenesis of the acute phase response. *N. Engl. J. Med.*, **311**, 1413–18
153. Kunkel, S. L., Spengler, M., May, M. A., Spengler, R., Larrick, J. and Remick, D. (1988). Prostaglandin E2 regulates macrophage derived tumor necrosis factor gene expression. *J. Biol. Chem.*, **263**, 5380–4
154. Tiku, K., Tiku, M. L. and Skosey, J. L. (1986). Interleukin-1 production by human polymorphonuclear neutrophils. *J. Immunol.*, **136**, 3675–77
155. Seckinger, P., Isaac, S. and Dayer, J.-M. (1988). A human inhibitor of tumour necrosis factor alpha. *J. Exp. Med.*, **167**, 1511–16
156. Arend, W. P., Joslin, F. G. and Massone, R. J. (1985). Effects of immune complexes on production of human monocytes of interleukin-1 or an interleukin-1 inhibitor. *J. Immunol.*, **134**, 3868–75
157. Balavoine, J.-F., De Rochemonteix, B., Williamson, K., Seckinger, P., Cruchaud, A. and Dayer, J.-M. (1986). Prostaglandin E2 and collagenase production of fibroblasts and synovial cells is regulated by urine-derived human interleukin-1 inhibitor(s). *J. Clin. Invest.*, **78**, 1120–4
158. Hannum, C. H., Wilcox, C. J. and Arend, W. P. (1990). Interleukin-1 receptor antagonist activity of a human interleukin-1 inhibitor. *Nature*, **343**, 336–40

159. Eisenberg, S. P., Evans, R. J., Arend, W. P., Verderber, E., Brewer, M. T., Hannum, C. H. and Thompson, R. C. (1990). Primary structure and functional expression from cDNA of a human interleukin-1 receptor antagonist. *Nature*, **343**, 341–6
160. Carter, D. B., Deibel, M. R., Dunn, C. J., Tomich, C. S. C., Laborde, A. L., Slighton, J. L., Berger, A. E., Bienkowski, M. J., Sun, F. F., McEwan, R. N., Harris, P. K. W., Yem, A. W., Waszak, C. A., Chosay, J. G., Sieu, L. C., Hardee, M. M., Zurcher-Neely, H. A., Reardon, I. M., Heinrikson, R. L., Truesdell, S. E., Shelly, J. A., Eessalu, T. E., Taylor, B. M. and Tracey, D. E. (1990). Purification, cloning, expression and biological characterisation of an interleukin-1 receptor antagonist protein. *Nature*, **344**, 633–8
161. Fanslow, W. C., Sims, J. E., Sasseneld, H., Morissey, P. J., Gillis, S., Dower, S. K. and Widmer, M. B. (1990). Regulation of alloreactivity *in vivo* by a soluble form of interleukin-1 receptor. *Science*, **248**, 739–42
162. Pepys, M. B. (1981). Serum C-reactive protein, serum amyloid P-component and serum amyloid A protein in autoimmune disease. *Clin. Immunol. Allergy*, **1981**, 77–101
163. Weimer, H. E. and Humelbaugh, C. (1966). The effects of periodic challenge on the response of alpha2-AP globulin and other acute-phase reactants of rat serum to tissue injury. *Can. J. Physiol. Pharmacol.*, **45**, 241–7
164. Smith, E. A., Kahalen, M. B. and LeRoy, E. C. (1986). The acute phase response in scleroderma: differing responses to intravenous PGE1. *Clin. Exp. Rheumatol.*, **4**, 341–5
165. Sandborg, C. I., Berman, M. A., Andrews, B. S. and Friou, G. J. (1983). Interleukin-1 production of mononuclear cells from patients with scleroderma. *Arthritis Rheum.*, **26** (Suppl.), 116 (abstract)
166. Sandborg, C. I., Berman, M. A., Andrews, B. S. and Friou, G. J. (1985). Interleukin-1 production by mononuclear cells from patients with scleroderma. *Clin. Exp. Immunol.*, **60**, 294–302
167. Whicher, J. T., Westacott, C. I. and Dieppe, P. A. (1986). Defective acute phase responses in systemic sclerosis: disease mechanisms and consequences. *Prot. Biol. Fluids Proc. Colloq.*, **34**, 605–9
168. Chellingsworth, M., Scott, M. G. I., Crockson, P. A. and Bacon, P. A. (1984). 'Normal' acute phase response in systemic sclerosis. *Br. Med. J.*, **289**, 946–7
169. Hutton, C. W., Collins, A. J., Chambers, R. E., Whicher, J. and Dieppe, P. A. (1985). Systemic response to local urate crystal induced inflammation in man: a possible model to study acute phase response. *Ann. Rheum. Dis.*, **44**, 533–6
170. Yu, C.-L., Chang, K.-L., Chiu, C.-C., Chiang, B. N., Hans, S.-H. and Wang, S.-R. (1989). Defective phagocytosis, decreased tumour necrosis factor-alpha production and lymphocyte hyporesponsiveness predispose patients with system lupus erythematosus to infections. *Scand. J. Rheumatol.*, **18**, 97–105
171. Yorston, D., Whicher, J. T., Chambers, R., Klouda, P. and Easty, D. (1988). The acute phase response in acute anterior uveitis. *Trans. Opththalmol. Soc. UK*, **104**, 166–70

14
The role of leukocyte chemotaxis in inflammation

A. ROT

INTRODUCTION

The movement of leukocytes from blood into the tissues in response to inflammatory stimuli was observed and described as early as 1891 by Metchnikoff[1] and 1888 by Leber[2]; however, only within the past few decades has some light been shed on the cellular and molecular mechanisms involved in the process of leukocyte emigration. During inflammation, blood leukocytes: (1) marginate and adhere to the endothelial cells of the postcapillary venules, (2) migrate across the endothelial cell layer and basal membrane, and (3) move in the tissues towards the source of inflammation where they fulfil their function in host defence. Whereas altered parameters of circulation and the expression of recently identified adhesion molecules by the leukocytes and endothelial cells are responsible for margination and adhesion, the chemotaxis of leukocytes (their capacity of directed movement along a concentration gradient of molecules referred to as chemotaxins or chemoattractants) is considered essential for leukocyte emigration and movement in extravascular tissues.

Leukocyte chemotaxis is a complex process which includes receptor-mediated gradient perception, signal transduction via a second messenger pathway, conformational changes of cytoplasmic contractile elements leading to polarized behaviour, including development of morphological asymmetry, coordinated attachment to the surface at the leading edge and detachment at the back end resulting in continuous unidirectional movement. In spite of the rapidly growing body of knowledge on the biochemistry and cell biology of leukocyte chemotaxis, the molecular mechanism of none of the described steps is fully understood.

During the past two decades numerous new leukocyte chemotaxins have been discovered. These include factors produced by microorganisms, generated in the blood from serum proteins or by platelets, derived from extracellular matrix, produced by endothelial cells, smooth muscle cells, leukocytes, fibroblasts and the nervous system. The differences in the origin of chemotaxins, their potency and target cell population result in the variability and pleomorphic appearance of cellular exudate in different locations and in different stages of the inflammatory response.

This chapter gives a brief overview of the methods used for studying leukocyte chemotaxis, molecular mechanisms involved in signal transduction and cell movement, factors influencing chemotaxis, differences and common features of chemoattractants, and the possible role of chemotaxis in the inflammatory processes.

MEASUREMENT OF LEUKOCYTE CHEMOTAXIS

The *in vivo* injection of a chemoattractant induces the accumulation of leukocytes at the site of the injection. Emigration of leukocytes in response to the chemoattractants can also be observed *in vivo* using either the Rebuck skin window technique[3] or the blister chamber technique[4]. Thus, chemoattractants and chemotaxis can be studied *in vivo*, which would seem ideal since the response of mixed and physiologically proportionate leukocyte populations can be observed in their 'natural habitat' under the influence of the same factors as in health and disease. However, the factors influencing the leukocyte emigration *in vivo* are also related to phenomena other than leukocyte chemotaxis. Altered parameters of circulation, endothelial cell adhesion and vascular permeability can affect leukocyte emigration and the results of *in vivo* chemotaxis assays. A number of non-chemotactic molecules, e.g. endotoxin, interleukin 1 (IL 1), tumour necrosis factor alpha (TNFα), interferon-gamma (INFγ), etc., will cause leukocyte emigration *in vivo*. It is likely that *in vivo* all such compounds induce the production of chemotactic cytokine(s) which in turn cause the emigration of leukocytes. In addition, the stimulation of responding or bystanding cells with one chemotaxin can lead to the production and release of another chemotaxin with a different spectrum of activities. Thus, the criterion for chemotactic activity of the molecule must be its ability to induce the directed migration of leukocytes *in vitro*. In general, leukocyte migration and chemotaxis, like other phenomena, are better understood when studied separate from other biological processes, namely *in vitro*.

The early investigators studied *in vitro* leukocyte chemotaxis with great devotion but lacked pure, well-defined attractants, pure responding cell populations and reproducible *in vitro* methods for measuring chemotaxis. Therefore, it is difficult to state in modern terms the results of their efforts, which are documented in a detailed review by H. Harris[5]. In the 1960s two papers signalled the beginning of the new age of *in vitro* leukocyte chemotaxis studies. A. Böyum described a simple leukocyte separation technique[6] and S. Boyden a method to ascertain *in vitro* leukocyte chemotaxis using a device of new design[7]. Though several other methods for studying leukocyte chemotaxis *in vitro* have since been described (reviewed by P. C. Wilkinson[8]), including migration under agarose[9], migration into three-dimensional gels[10], Zigmond chamber[11], time-lapse techniques[12,13], etc., the Boyden-type chamber technique remains the easiest, most reproducible and most widely used method for measuring cell migration *in vitro*. The chamber consists of cell-containing (upper) and attractant-containing (lower) compartments separated by a membrane. Upon assembly of the chamber, the gradient of chemoattractant becomes established across the membrane. Either thick membrane (a mesh of cellulose ester fibre[7]) or thin membrane (a polycarbonate nucleopore sheet with uniform, randomly distributed pores[14]) can be used. In the case of a thick filter the distance which the cells migrated is defined either for the representative population of all the cells in the filter[15,16] or only for cells which moved the longest distance (leading front method[17]). In the case of a thin membrane the cells migrate through the pores and their number is defined by counting them on the lower surface of the filter or measuring in the lower compartment of the chamber the cell-associated radiological[18], physicochemical[19] or biochemical[20] parameters. Numerous modifications of the Boyden chamber exist; the 48-well chamber[21] is one of the most successful among them. Due to the small well volume the chamber's attractant and cell requirement is minimal and the fast assembly allows the simultaneous use of several chambers[22]. Both nucleopore and millipore[23] filters can be used for studying chemotaxis of all leukocyte types[24,25] (Figure 14.1) and other cells[26,27]. However, even the Boyden-type chamber is not ideal, either for simulation of the *in vivo* situation or for strict control of *in vitro* physicochemical and biological parameters[28].

LEUKOCYTE CHEMOATTRACTANTS

The use of the Boyden-type chamber, the development of modern biochemistry and new separation techniques, and the recent advances in recombinant technology greatly facilitated the discovery of a number of well-defined leukocyte chemoattractants. Table 14.1 lists only those most frequently studied. Few chemoattractants are specific for one leukocyte type; the majority of them attract more than one type, and some are capable of inducing chemotaxis of all the leukocyte types (panchemotaxins). Due to the differences in chemotaxin potency (concentration of chemotaxin causing optimal response) and efficacy (the magnitude of the response at the optimal concentration) for different leukocytes, even panchemotaxins at a given concentration predominantly attract only one or two types of leukocytes. The specificity of chemotaxins for a certain leukocyte type might be one of the causes of a differential appearance of leukocytes in inflammatory exudates. The proportions of different leukocytes in blood can also have an impact on the composition of the cellular infiltrate. For example, the infiltrate induced by a hypothetical chemotaxin with identical potency and efficacy for neutrophils and lymphocytes in humans would, theoretically, contain twice as many neutrophils as

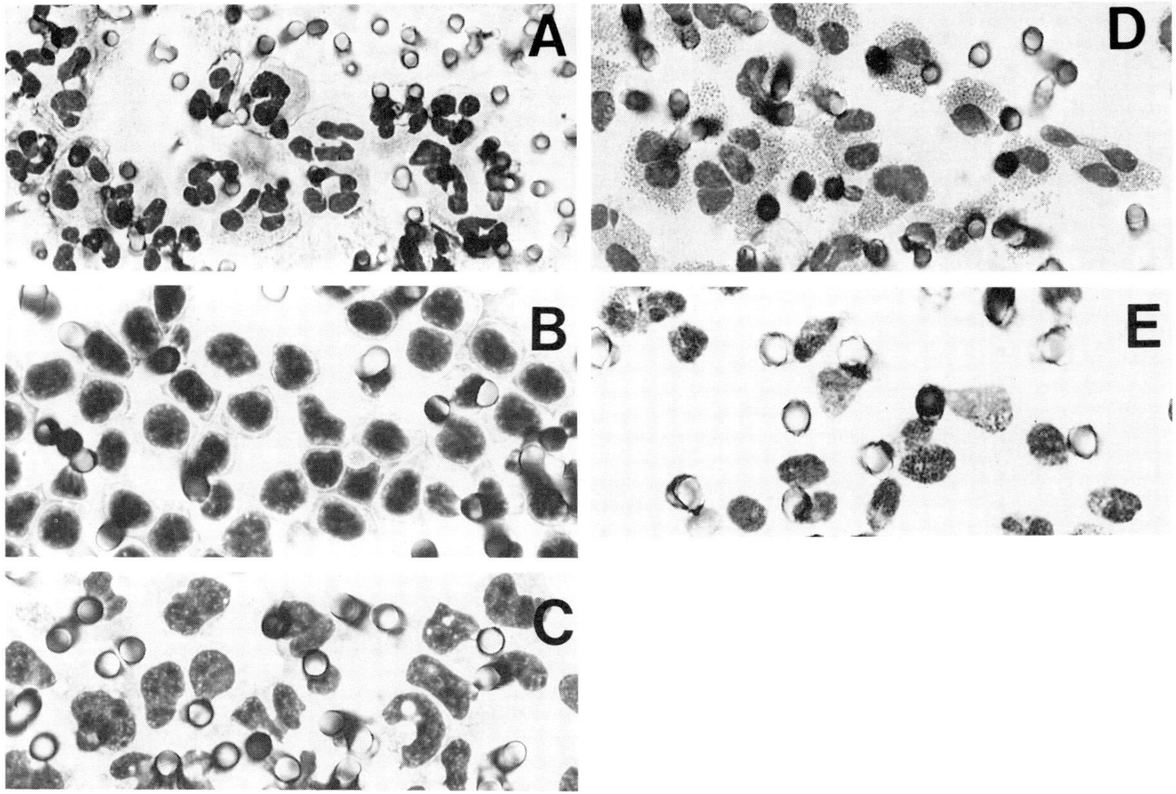

Figure 14.1 Human leukocytes adherent to the lower surfaces of Nucleopore filters in Boyden-type chemotaxis assays. **A**: neutrophils; **B**: lymphocytes; **C**: monocytes; **D**: eosinophils; **E**: basophils. The use of different responding cells requires modifications of the assay. A polyvinylpyrrolidone (PVP)-coated filter was used in the monocyte chemotaxis assay, whereas PVP-free membranes were used for measurement of neutrophil, eosinophil and basophil chemotaxis. To prevent cell fall-off from the lower surface of the filter in the T-lymphocyte chemotaxis assay, the PVP-free filter was precoated with collagen type IV. Filters with 3 μm pores were used in neutrophil and eosinophil assays, and filters with 5 μm pores were used in lymphocyte, monocyte and basophil chemotaxis assays.

Table 14.1 Leukocyte chemoattractants

Exogenous
Formyl peptides[29]
Endogenous: plasma-derived
C5a[30]
Thrombin[31]
Fibrinopeptide[32]
Endogenous: leukocyte-derived
Leukotriene B4 (LTB4)[33]
Platelet activating factor (PAF)[34]
Urate crystal-induced chemotactic factor (CCF)[35]
Eosinophil chemotactic factor of anaphylaxis (ECF-A)[36]
Neutrophil activating/attracting peptide (NAP-1/IL-8)[37–41]
Monocyte chemotactic peptide (MCP-1)[42]
Transforming growth factor β (TGFβ)[43]
Intercellular matrix proteins and their fragments
Collagen[44]
Elastin fragments[45]
Fibronectin fragments[46]
Laminin[47]
Neuropeptides and their synthetic analogues
β-Endorphin and met-enkephalin[48]
Bombesin[49]
Benzodiazepines[50]
Substance P[51]

lymphocytes, whereas in the rat the lymphocytes would outnumber neutrophils 50 to 1.

The major event modifying the outcome of leukocyte chemotactic response *in vivo* is the requirement (and the differential ability) of leukocytes to adhere to the endothelial cells prior to emigration. Thus, the induction of selective adherence between endothelial cells and different leukocyte types at the different stages of inflammation, a phenomenon unrelated to chemotaxis but promoted by a variety of cytokines[52] and, possibly, chemotaxins, can also contribute to the pleomorphic appearance of the inflammatory cell infiltrate. Whereas several neutrophil- and monocyte-specific chemotaxins have been described[31,32,37–41,42,48–51], little is known about lymphocyte-, eosinophil-, and basophil-specific chemotaxins, although these almost certainly exist. This is partly due to the fact that basophils and eosinophils constitute only a small proportion of peripheral blood leukocytes and are difficult to purify in large numbers. The problems associated with studying lymphocyte chemotaxis include the use of a heterogeneous responding cell population, very low efficacy of lymphocyte chemotaxins, and slow speed of cell movement[53]. Formyl peptides, C5a, and several not fully defined cytokines derived from different cells participating in chronic inflammation are amongst the factors thought to induce lymphocyte locomotion[53]. Eosinophils respond chemotactically to LTB_4, formyl peptides, and C5a, but factors with preferential activity for eosinophils are also known. PAF is the most potent among them. Others include ECF-A[36] and the recently identified chemotactic lipoxygenase product, eosinophil-derived eosinophil chemotactic lipid (ECL)[54]. Basophils appear rarely in human inflammatory infiltrates, e.g. occasionally in the late stages of acute hypersensitivity and in delayed-type hypersensitivity. Chemotaxins stimulating basophil migration include C5a and NAP-1, but no specific basophil chemotaxins are known.

CHEMOKINESIS AND HAPTOTAXIS

Chemotaxis can be distinguished from other defined and significant forms of leukocyte movement. Unstimulated leukocytes exhibit spontaneous random migration. The higher-speed random movement of the cells caused by chemical substances is called chemokinesis.

Chemokinesis can be studied by placing the tested substance with the responding cells in the top compartment or simultaneously in the top and bottom compartments of the Boyden-type chamber. Almost all known chemoattractants also have a chemokinetic effect. In some cases the contribution of chemokinesis to the overall cell locomotion could be overestimated due to the experimental artifact related to the capability of leukocytes to rapidly degrade and inactivate chemotaxins[55,56].

The gradient of a surface-bound substance can also cause directed movement of the cells. This phenomenon is called haptotaxis[57]. The role of haptotaxis is well documented in the case of tumour cell migration along the substrate-attached gradients of extracellular matrix components[58]. Since the leukocytes, unlike bacteria, have to adhere to the surface in order to migrate, and chemoattractants, often being hydrophobic molecules, also tend to bind to the biological surfaces, it would be sensible if leukocytes could recognize the gradients of the substrate-bound ligand and migrate along them. The significance of haptotaxis in inflammation is not yet fully established, since most of the conventional methods for studying leukocyte migration do not permit the differentiation between directed migration in response to soluble and insolubilized gradients. Nevertheless, when using some attractants, e.g. C5a or casein, the phenomenon of leukocyte haptotaxis can be seen[59,60] but when using others, e.g. formyl peptide, haptotaxis is not observed[61].

LEUKOCYTE ACTIVATION BY CHEMOATTRACTANTS

Besides stimulating directed and random cell movement, chemoattractants also enhance phagocyte aggregation and adherence to foreign surfaces, initiate the release of lysosomal enzymes and the production and release of superoxide and hydrogen peroxide resulting, in turn, in chemiluminescence[62–65]. For several chemoattractants the concentration required to elicit optimal metabolic burst and enzyme release was reported to be several-fold higher than the concentration required for optimal chemotactic response[63]; therefore it was postulated that the production of oxygen radicals and degranulation *in vivo* does not begin until the leukocytes reach the area with the highest chemoattractant concentration. The *in vitro* chemotactic and secretory potencies of some attractants, e.g. NAP-1, are very similar, but no signs of either degranulation or endothelial cell damage can be observed in the process of massive emigration of neutrophils in response to an *in vivo* injection of NAP-1 (Rot and Paku, unpublished). This suggests the existence of *in vivo* mechanisms or factors that suppress the leukocyte secretory functions while they are still in blood or migrating across the vessel wall. One such factor could be adenosine, which at physiological blood concentrations inhibits oxygen radical production in leukocytes but enhances chemotaxis[66]. Some chemotaxins, e.g. formyl peptides and C5a, are potent inducers of lysosomal enzyme and oxygen radical secretion; others, like LTB_4 or PAF, in spite of being potent chemoattractants, are very weak inducers of secretory functions[67–70]. The chemotactic potency of different formyl peptides correlates well with their secretory potency[63,68]. In contrast to this, the chemotactic efficacy of the formyl peptides from the same series shows no correlation with their secretory efficacy[68]. Chemoattractant-induced enhanced leukocyte aggregation and adherence to substrate are probably achieved by up-regulation of leukocyte adhesion molecule expression which also promotes the adherence of leukocytes to endothelial cells.

CHEMOATTRACTANT RECEPTORS

Chemoattractants exert their effect on leukocytes via specific cell surface receptors which have been described for most of the defined chemoattractants[69–72] and constitute the subject of several reviews[73,74]. Following ligand binding, receptors are aggregated and internalized[75]. Receptor internalization and possibly changes in receptor affinity result in the decrease of further chemotaxin binding[76,77] (receptor down-regulation). The internalized formyl peptide receptors are rapidly replaced, possibly from the intracellular 'reserve' pool which was initially thought to be present on the membrane of secondary granules[78]. The recent discovery of a new cellular compartment, which can fuse with the cell membrane and cause the up-regulation of the formyl peptide receptor and Mac-1 (a molecule also previously thought to be present exclusively in secondary granules), suggests an alternative site of intracellular storage for formyl peptide receptors[79]. In contrast to formyl peptide receptors, C5a and LTB_4 receptors probably have no intracellular storage pool and are re-expressed on the surface membrane more slowly by recycling, possibly via the Golgi complex[80,81]. The neutrophil formyl peptide receptor was shown to have three different affinity states[82]. The interconvertible change from higher to lower affinity can be achieved by GTP and analogues[83] which act via a guanine nucleotide-binding protein (G-protein). The receptor is shifted to its third, highest affinity (non-dissociable state) shortly after binding the chemotactic ligand[82]. This G-protein independent affinity shift is the first step of receptor internalization, and may involve interaction with the cytoskeleton since it is inhibited by cytochalasin B[82]. The interconversion of the receptor's affinity can play a role in leukocyte adaptation to the chemotactic stimulus (cells lose responsiveness to restimulation with the same concentration of a chemoattractant, whereas a higher concentration elicits the full response)[13,84,85]. Adaptation also allows the leukocytes to respond to chemotactic gradients in a wide range of attractant concentrations. Several factors, including the ubiquitous LPS, up-regulate the receptor number and decrease the affinity of chemoattractant receptors[86]. The mobilization of receptors, the conversion of their affinities before or during the receptor binding assay, different temperatures of cell isolation and assay, the use of different labelled ligands, and also the fact that some studies were done on intact cells and others on membrane preparations, can account for the wide variation in the published number of receptors per cell and their affinity[73,74] and also the results consistent with either one subset[72,87] or two affinity subsets of chemoattractant receptors[88–90].

The notion that low concentrations of formyl peptides stimulate leukocyte chemotaxis and high concentrations stimulate the metabolic burst prompted the development of two hypotheses attempting to explain the transduction of multiple cell function by formyl peptide receptors. According to one hypothesis the high-affinity chemotaxin receptors transduce locomotory signals, whereas low-affinity receptors transduce secretory signals (experimental evidence suggesting that dual receptor affinity reflects dual receptor function is reviewed in ref. 73). The alternative hypothesis[74] postulates that all receptors are capable of transducing all signals, and the elicited cellular response (locomotion or secretion) depends on the level of receptor occupancy determined by chemotaxin concentration. The ligand binding to 1% of a cell's total chemotaxin receptors stimulates chemotaxis; ligand binding to all receptors is required for induction of the metabolic burst. If either of these hypotheses is correct, one has to assume that additional factors regulate the differential signalling for various cellular functions in the case of chemotaxins with similar locomotory and secretory potencies (e.g. NAP-1).

SIGNAL TRANSDUCTION AND CYTOSKELETAL ACTIVATION

The transduction of the chemotactic signal to the contractile cytoskeletal elements probably happens via the G-protein coupled phosphatidylinositol pathway. According to the prevailing concept[74,91–94], the occupancy of a chemoattractant receptor will cause the binding of GTP to, and the release of GDP from, cholera and pertussis toxin-sensitive G-protein, resulting in its subsequent activation. The G-protein GTP complex activates inositol phospholipid specific phospholipase C (PLC) which hydrolyses phosphatidylinositol-4,5-biphosphate (PIP_2) into inositol-1,4,5-triphosphate (IP_3) and 1,2-diacylglycerol (DAG). IP_3 mobilizes intracellular calcium (Ca^{2+}) which promotes the influxes of extracellular Ca^{2+}, whereas DAG can stimulate protein kinase C (PKC) which, in turn, activates NADPH oxidase and the respiratory burst. PIP_2-derived DAG was recently shown to be insufficient to fully activate PKC[96]. IP_3 metabolites may play a role[97] in the further mobilization of Ca^{2+}. Free cytosolic Ca^{2+} stimulates the additional production of DAG from an alternative to the PIP_2 source, possibly phosphatidylcholine (PC). Methylation of phosphatidylethanolamine and generation of PC, a transduction pathway of several signals in a variety of cells[98], has also been implicated in the transduction of chemotactic signals[99,100]. Phospholipase D, activated by PKC, Ca^{2+}, and also by an independent pathway, can amplify the chemoattractant-induced metabolic burst of the leukocytes by generation of phosphatidic acid which stimulates NADPH oxidase[101]. The involvement of phospholipase A2 in the transduction of locomotory signals, in addition to the generation of LTB_4 and PAF precursors, has also been suggested[102].

Two negative feedback loops can terminate the biological response: (a) the stimulation of PKC leads to the down-regulation of chemoattractant surface receptors[103] and the inhibition of G-protein coupling to PLC[104,105]; and (b) the intracellular Ca^{2+} induces an elevation of cAMP levels, leading to inactivation of PLC probably via its phosphorylation by the cAMP-dependent protein kinase[92]. No pieces are missing from the jigsaw puzzle picture of the transduction pathway leading from chemotaxin–receptor interaction to activation of metabolic burst, while the Ca^{2+} influx and PKC were identified as signals necessary for degranulation[91]. Conversely, it is not easy to pinpoint the mediators initiating leukocyte locomotion. Leukocyte movement is thought to be driven by the contractions of cytoskeletal elements which are induced, in turn, by rapid polymerization–depolymerization of actin[106,107]. The analogy with other contractile systems would suggest that Ca^{2+} can stimulate cytoskeletal protein polymerization directly or by acting via Ca^{2+} or calmodulin-dependent protein kinases. However, it has been shown that neither Ca^{2+} influx and the consequential cytoplasmic pH drop nor the oxidative burst play a signalling role in the initiation of actin polymerization elicited by chemoattractants[108]. Another possible mediator capable of initiating actin polymerization is PIP_2, a substrate rather than a product of the phosphoinositol pathway[109]. It was shown that PIP_2 can induce *in vitro* actin polymerization by releasing actin from its complex with the actin binding protein profilin[110] and inhibiting the severing function of gelsolin[111]. In this respect it could be significant that besides the stimulation of PIP_2 hydrolysis by PLC, chemotaxins also induce very rapid activation of phosphatidylinositol-4-phosphate kinase (PIP kinase), the enzyme responsible for PIP_2 synthesis[112]. PKC could also influence actin polymerization by phosphorylating cytoskeletal proteins such as vimentin and myosin[91]. The role of PKC in mediating leukocyte chemotaxis is emphasized by the fact that PKC inhibitors can selectively inhibit neutrophil chemotaxis[113]. Also, DAG could be involved in locomotory signal transduction; DAG metabolites can alter the lipid composition of membranes leading to redistribution of the attached contractile elements[91]. DAG itself was found to be chemotactic for human neutrophils[114]. This means either that cell surface receptors and their adaptational changes are not required for gradient perception and chemotaxis or that DAG is not chemotactic but stimulates the randomly migrated neutrophils to release a chemotactic factor.

MECHANISM OF LEUKOCYTE LOCOMOTION

The mechanism by which the contraction of cytoskeletal elements causes leukocyte migration is envisaged in several different models. According to the attractive hypothesis introduced by Bray and White[115], cortical tension created by actin-containing cytoskeletal elements relaxes at the front of the cell, creating a pseudopod, whereas the rest of the membrane-associated cytoskeletal apparatus contracts towards the back of the cell in a form of 'constriction rings'. Transmembrane components of the rings are attached to the substratum and remain stationary in respect to it, whereas the rest of the membrane and the cytoplasm float forward 'through' the constriction rings; the uropod periodically detaches from the substrate and retracts into the cell. As a result, directed migration of the cell is achieved. For prolonged movement the building blocks of the constriction rings (cytoskeletal elements, adhesion molecules) must recirculate forward. This happens either by cytoplasm flow or the recently demonstrated rapid forward transport of the molecules on the surface of a locomoting cell[116]. According to an alternative theory of cell locomotion[117], the surface membrane of a moving cell moves backward, gets pinocytosed at the tail end, and recycled via cytoplasm to the front where the vesicles get inserted into the surface membrane. The driving force of the cell locomotion is the backwards movement of membrane-incorporated adhesion molecules which are attached to the substrate. Evidence against this 'retrograde lipid flow' theory of leukocyte locomotion recently came from two experimental studies. One used gold particle labelling and showed that some of the surface membrane-bound particles, and the glycoprotein molecules by which they attach, diffuse randomly, whereas only those attached to the cytoskeleton move rearwards[118]. The other study, using photobleaching and digital image processing, showed that the membrane lipid moves at the speed of cell locomotion forward and not backward[119].

A biophysical approach to the question of leukocyte locomotion resulted in the development of an 'osmotic pressure' theory[120]. According to this theory, cytoskeletal actin cannot be a source of protrusive force which moves the cell forward. Instead, osmotic pressure created by the appearance of osmotically active particles produces the protrusion, whereas actin polymerization only fills the protrusion up, preventing its collapse.

GRADIENT PERCEPTION BY LEUKOCYTES

Upon stimulation by a chemoattractant gradient, leukocytes undergo a characteristic shape change: they become elongated and develop a wide pseudopod oriented in the direction of the gradient[11]. This is accompanied by polarization of their ultrastructure, including actin filaments, centriole, microtubules and nucleus[121]. When the direction of the chemotactic gradient is changed, the leukocyte either retracts the pseudopod and develops a new one at its tail end[12,122] or 'walks around' in a circle but continues to develop a pseudopod at its leading edge[121,123]. It is noteworthy that the morphological polarity of leukocytes does not develop as a result of stimulation by a chemotactic gradient, but is probably a function of cell motility. Leukocytes moving in the absence of a chemotactic gradient also show polarized morphology and continue to extend pseudopods from their front end[13]. The polarized morphology could enhance the detection accuracy of a chemotactic gradient by the cell if, according to the prevailing 'spatial' hypothesis of gradient perception, leukocytes 'read' the chemotactic gradients by sensing the differences in chemoattractant receptor occupancy along their axes[11,124]. In contrast to this, bacteria compare their present 'after-the-move' chemoattractant receptor occupancy with the previous 'before-the-move' one ('temporal' gradient sensing)[125]. As a result of this comparison the bacterial cell either tumbles and swims a short lap (direction: down the gradient) or suppresses tumbling and swims a long lap (direction: up the gradient). The essential part of this mechanism of gradient detection is bacteria's intermittent 'trial-and-error' movement in all directions, which finally adds up in the migration along the gradient. The 'temporal' mechanism of gradient perception has also been postulated for leukocyte chemotaxis. Since the gradient detection by leukocytes does not require their movement[124], the morphological substrate for the 'temporal' gradient detection would be the pseudopod which acts as a probe by rapidly advancing in different directions[123]. Depending on the encountered concentration of chemotactic ligand, the receptors on the pseudopod would experience a different degree of saturation. The cell would follow the movement of the pseudopod along the gradient but would retract the pseudopod and would not move down the gradient. The 'temporal' mechanism of gradient-sensing by leukocytes would also be possible if the cells could detect impulse ('temporal') but not stable ('spatial') gradients of chemoattractants[126]. Experimental evidence is insufficient to decide between the 'spatial' and 'temporal' theories of gradient detection by leukocytes.

FACTORS INFLUENCING LEUKOCYTE CHEMOTAXIS

Leukocyte heterogeneity

Not all leukocytes of one type are capable of migrating to the same chemotaxin. This is partly because leukocyte populations are not homogeneous in their chemotaxin receptor expression. Less than 10% of lymphocytes have receptors for C5a[127] and NAP-1. Only about 60% of human monocytes have formyl-peptide receptors[128] and 68% of them have receptors for C5a[127]. The monocyte subpopulation with the receptors for one chemoattractant also has a receptor for others, leaving the population without chemotactic receptors incapable of chemotactic response[129,130]. However, it was recently demonstrated that some of the monocytes from a population previously shown to be devoid of chemotactic receptors may have C5a and formyl-peptide receptors but in very low numbers[131].

The presence of a cell surface receptor for a particular chemotaxin does not necessarily mean that the leukocyte will show a chemotactic response to it. Though almost all neutrophils have receptors for C5a, only a fraction of them migrate in response to this chemotaxin[127,132]. The high efficacy formyl methionyl peptides cause the migration of almost all the neutrophils and all the monocytes with the formyl peptide receptor[68], whereas formyl tripeptide chemoattractants, though binding to the same receptors, stimulate the migration of only a fraction of the receptor-bearing cells[128,132]. Thus, the poor response of some leukocytes is not an experimental artifact related to an apparent inability of all leukocytes in the suspension to initiate their migration simultaneously[28]. Some receptor-bearing leukocytes do not migrate but respond only with respiratory burst and degranulation following stimulation with chemoattractant. For example, the binding of formylated peptide to its receptor on equine neutrophils and LTB_4 to its receptor on rat neutrophils causes cell activation but not chemotaxis[133,134]. These examples also reflect the profound species-specific differences in leukocyte responsiveness to different chemoattractants. Whereas formylated peptides are chemotactic for mouse, rat, rabbit and monkey neutrophils, they are not chemotactic for horse, cow, cat, dog, pig and goat neutrophils, chicken heterophils, mouse monocytes and macrophages[135].

Deactivation

Pre-exposure of leukocytes to a chemoattractant can cause an inhibition of chemotaxis towards the same attractant. This deactivation is attractant-specific since other chemoattractants are able to elicit full chemotactic response, and is probably induced by down-regulation of the surface receptors. Pre-exposure of leukocytes to high concentrations of an attractant abolishes the chemotactic responsiveness of the cells to all chemotaxins. This 'unspecific' deactivation is probably caused by exhaustion of a second messenger component common to all attractants, or by a negative feedback in signal transduction pathways, e.g. inhibition of PLC by PKC[105]. When leukocyte chemotaxis is studied *in vitro*, chemoattractants usually produce a bell-shaped dose–response curve (Figure 14.2). Rapid specific and, maybe, unspecific deactivation causes the low-level migration in response to high concentrations of chemoattractant. The practical consequence of this phenomenon is that in order to establish the chemotactic potency and efficacy of an attractant it is important to test its full concentration range.

Besides the specific deactivation of the responding leukocytes by chemoattractants, specific *in vivo* deactivation of the inflammatory site has also been described. Injection of a chemoattractant into the skin site of

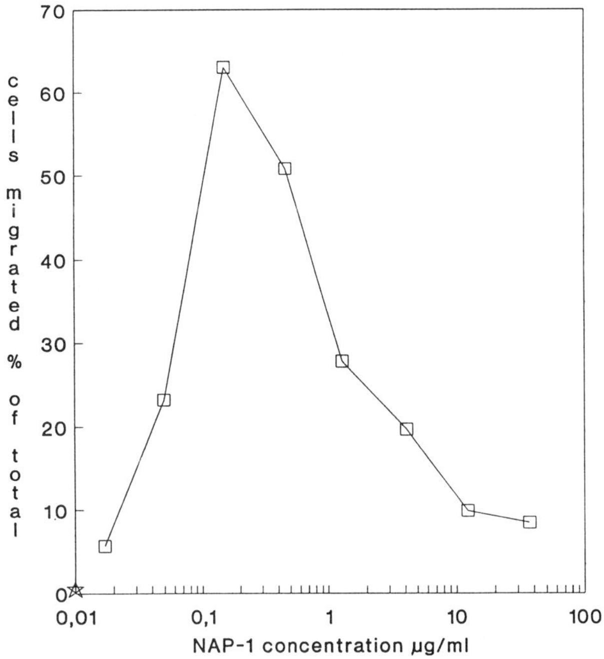

Figure 14.2 *In vitro* human neutrophil chemotaxis to NAP-1. Note the bell shape of the dose–response curve. The star marks the level of neutrophil migration to the buffer control.

experimental rabbits was shown to deactivate the site for restimulation with the same attractant but not an alternative attractant[136,137]. The failure of leukocytes to emigrate following the repeated injection of the same attractant into the identical site was not a result of either altered blood and lymph circulation or systemic desensitization of neutrophils, but was possibly related to down-regulation of hypothetical receptors involved in the control of neutrophil extravasation and located on endothelial cells of postcapillary venules[138].

Inhibition

In addition to the fast degradation or inactivation of chemotaxin by responding cells and environmental factors[55,56,139,140], the leukocyte chemotactic response can also be terminated by inhibitors of chemotactic movement. Physiological chemotactic inhibitors such as retroviral p15E and related proteins, which are also present in human tumour effusions[141] and are produced by endothelial cells in response to IL 1 stimulation, possibly play a role in the termination of leukocyte emigration[142]. A number of cytokines can inhibit leukocyte migration and/or chemotaxis. These include the first known cytokine, the recently cloned migration inhibitory factor[143], INFγ[144], interleukin 4[145], TNF[146] and granulocyte monocyte colony stimulating factor[147]. Pharmacological inhibitors of *in vitro* chemotaxis include antibiotics, sulphonamides, sulphones, bacterial toxins, various anti-inflammatory agents, lipoxygenase inhibitors, etc.[148].

EXOGENOUS CHEMOATTRACTANTS

The notion that exogenous factors, including bacteria, can be a source of chemoattractant comes from the founding fathers of leukocyte chemotaxis[1,2]. The application of modern protein chemistry and quantitative *in vitro* measurement of chemotaxis to this problem began with the work of Keller and Sorkin[149] and also Ward, Lepow and Newman, who showed that a number of bacteria elaborated small peptides with chemoattractant activity for neutrophils[150]. E. Schiffmann and co-workers purified chemotactic activity from *Escherichia coli* (*E. coli*) culture supernatants and found that it is associated with several N-terminally blocked peptides[151]. Unable to directly identify the structure of these peptides, Schiffmann postulated that these molecules must have characteristically prokaryotic markers which can be recognized by the eukaryotic host during infection. Since bacteria initiate their protein synthesis with formylmethionin (an amino acid in eukaryotes found only in mitochondria), the hypothesis was developed that chemotactic N-terminally blocked peptides in *E. coli* supernatants were formylmethionyl oligopeptides derived from N-terminal regions of bacterial proteins[29]. To test this hypothesis a series of N-formylmethionyl peptides was synthesized and found to be chemotactic for neutrophils and macrophages[29]. In a larger series of synthetic formylmethionyl tripeptides, fMLF was the most potent[63].

The family of synthetic formyl peptides provided an ideal opportunity to study chemotaxin structure – biological activity correlations (reviewed by E. L. Becker[152]), whereas fMLF became the most commonly used experimental chemoattractant. Several recent attempts were made to separate and identify bacterial chemoattractants and thus directly prove Schiffmann's hypothesis. Since bacterial chemotaxins are present in culture filtrates in very small amounts, and the chemotactic potency of the filtrate is a sum of activities of multiple related but different peptides, all attempts to purify to homogeneity and sequence these chemotaxins have failed[153–155]. Despite the failure to purify and sequence bacterial chemotactic peptides, one can conclude on the basis of an overwhelming body of indirect evidence that formyl oligopeptides are indeed the major bacterial chemoattractants. Their ability to attract cells as diverse as leukocytes, spermatozoa[26] and tumour cells[27] reflects the important role these peptides played in the process of phylogenesis.

Bacteria-derived chemoattractants other than formyl peptides also exist. It was recently shown that bacterial pheromones, small non-formyl peptides, have chemotactic activity for leukocytes[156]. These molecules are not very potent chemoattractants since they act via the formyl peptide receptor to which they show very low-affinity binding[156]. Lipid and glycopeptide molecules with chemotactic activity for neutrophils were also isolated from *E. coli* filtrates, but their structure was not defined[157].

Apart from producing leukocyte chemoattractants, bacteria initiate several mechanisms of endogenous chemoattractant production. Bacteria and LPS activate complement and cause the generation of chemotactic complement factor C5a[157]; either the phagocytosis of bacteria or several bacterial products initiate LTB_4 release from leukocytes[158,159]. Bacterial LPS also induces the production of chemotactic cytokines like NAP-1 or MCP-1 by several cell types[160,161]. Fungi also produce leukocyte chemotaxins[162], but the attraction of leukocytes to the site of fungal infection can be achieved by alternative mechanisms involving either complement activation and generation of C5a[157] or the release of LTB_4 by monocytes following the stimulation of their β-glucan receptors[163].

COMPLEMENT-DERIVED CHEMOTACTIC ACTIVITY

When S. Boyden introduced a new *in vitro* method for measuring leukocyte chemotaxis as an attractant he used antigen–antiserum mixtures[7]. In retrospect it is likely that he was studying complement-derived chemotactic activity since antigen–antibody complexes are known to activate complement via the 'classical' pathway. The chemotactic activity of complement fragments was described by Ward *et al.*[30]. Initially it was thought that both small anaphylatoxic complement fragments C5a and C3a have chemotactic activity for leukocytes; but it was shown later that only C5a has significant chemotactic activity[164]. In 'classical' and 'alternative' pathways of complement activation, C5a is generated via the proteolytic cleavage of native C5 by two different complexes of C3b. Different cellular enzymes can also cleave C5 and generate C5a[165]. The leukocyte chemotactic activity attributed to two plasma-derived factors, kallikrein and plasminogen activator[166,167], is possibly due to their ability to generate C5a[168]. The limited proteolysis of C5 can also result in the generation of a large molecular weight chemoattractant without the release of C5a[169,170]. C5a is a more potent anaphylatoxin than chemotaxin. At concentrations as low as 10^{-15} mol/l it induces the release of histamine and other vasoactive mediators[171] which, in turn, act via their receptors on the endothelial cells of postcapillary venules to induce the plasma leakage essential for further generation of C5a in the extravascular tissue. The anaphylatoxin activity of C5a is rapidly and completely abolished by carboxypeptidase N cleavage of C-terminal arginine, thus creating C5a des-Arg[139]. C5a des-Arg is 15 times less potent than C5a chemoattractant for neutrophils, but has the same chemotactic potency for monocytes as C5a[172]. Chemotactic activity of C5a and C5a des-Arg is enhanced by a serum factor initially called 'cochemotaxin'[173] and recently identified as a vitamin D-binding protein (group-specific component globulin, GcG)[174,175]. Because the conversion of C5a to C5a des-Arg is almost instantaneous in the presence of serum, it is likely that all *in vivo* complement-derived chemotactic activity is due to C5a des-Arg + GcG. In addition, the serum contains a protein, named chemotactic factor inactivator, which is capable of decreasing C5a-related chemotactic activity[176]. Initially it was thought to enzymatically cleave chemotaxins[177], but recently was reported to bind to GcG and inhibit its cochemotaxin function[140].

The complement cascade can be activated by a number of substances, such as immunoglobulin–antigen complexes, LPS, and polysaccharides, or by foreign surfaces, such as intact bacteria and fungi. Also, C5a can be cleaved directly from C5 by proteases. It is hard to imagine an inflammatory reaction to which C5a would not contribute. In contrast to C5a, C5a des-Arg is a more potent chemoattractant for monocytes than for neutrophils; therefore, the conversion of C5a to C5a des-Arg may contribute to the shift from neutrophil to monocyte emigration in the process of acute inflammation.

LTB_4 and PAF

Leukotrienes are products of lipoxygenase-catalyzed oxygenation of arachidonic acid induced in leukocytes by a variety of stimuli, including chemoattractants. One of the major products of this pathway, LTB_4, which is generated by hydrolysis of the unstable intermediate LTA_4, is chemokinetic and chemotactic for neutrophils[33,178,179]. Besides activated leukocytes, resident macrophages, mast cells and endothelial cells can also release LTB_4 following their activation by several stimuli. LTB_4 can attract neutrophils, eosinophils and monocytes while its chemotactic activity for lymphocytes and basophils is not documented. In contrast to other potent chemotaxins, LTB_4's high *in vitro* chemotactic potency and efficacy is combined with its very low *in vitro* secretory potency and efficacy. This notion was utilized in recent studies which, by comparing the effects of LTB_4 and formyl peptide, were an attempt to dissect signal transduction pathways responsible for chemotaxis and secretion.

PAF was initially identified in supernatants of IgE-challenged basophils[180]. Later its chemical structure was determined to be acetyl-alkylglyceryl phosphorylcholine[181], and it was shown to be produced by endothelial cells and several types of leukocytes[182,183]. Besides stimulating platelet aggregation and secretion, and exerting half a dozen other pro-inflammatory activities[184], it was shown to be chemotactic for monocytes[185], neutrophils[34] and eosinophils[186]. Whereas PAF is a much less potent chemoattractant for human neutrophils than LTB_4 or formyl peptides, its potency and efficacy for human eosinophils is higher than that of any known eosinophil chemoattractant[186,187] and its chemotactic potency for the most dense eosinophils is higher than for any other leukocyte type[188]. Since LTB_4 and PAF are released from leukocytes upon stimulation with other chemoattractants, both could play a major role in amplification of *in vivo* leukocyte emigration and chemotactic response.

NAP-1, MCP-1 AND RELATED CHEMOTACTIC CYTOKINES

The ability of leukocytes to produce chemotactic cytokines was noted at the beginning of the cytokine era when the activity of several factors had been described but their chemical structures were not identified[53,189]. It is likely that some of these factors are either identical or related to the chemotactic cytokines NAP-1 (also referred to as interleukin 8) and MCP-1, which have been recently characterized by several research groups. Because six recent reviews[160,161,190–193] discuss in detail the structure and activities of NAP-1, MCP-1 and related peptides, only the most important chemical and biological features of these molecules are mentioned here. NAP-1 is a member of a cytokine family which includes human molecules such as platelet factor-4 (PF-4), β-thromboglobulin, IP-10, connective tissue activating peptide-III (CTAP-III) and its derivative NAP-2, melanoma growth stimulating activity (also identified as GRO and NAP-3)[194], and several animal cytokines, e.g. mouse macrophage inflammatory protein 2. The common 'family feature' is that the member molecules can be aligned according to the four cysteine residues which are in the same position relative to each other within every molecule. Since the first two cysteines have an amino acid between them, the NAP-1 cytokine family is also called the 'C–X–C family'; whereas the MCP-1 family, members of which have the first two cysteines adjacent to each other, is called the 'C–C family'. The 'C–C family' includes MCP-1, I-309, ACT-2, RANTES and several animal cytokines such as mouse macrophage inflammatory protein 1 α and β and JE. The chemotactic members of the 'C–X–C' family, which are NAP-1, NAP-2 and NAP-3 (CTAP-III and PF-4 have very low chemotactic potency)[195,196], utilize the same neutrophil surface receptor[196].

NAP-1, the most potent chemotaxin of the 'C–X–C family', has several different N-terminal variants. It is expressed as a 99 amino acid precursor and secreted upon cleavage of the signal peptide as the 79 amino acid variant (NAP-1α); the 77 and 72 amino acid variants (NAP-1β and NAP-1γ) are generated by extracellular cleavage of NAP-1α[161]. NAP-1γ is relatively resistant to further proteolysis and is a more potent chemotaxin than NAP-1β and NAP-1α[197]. Fibroblasts and endothelial cells produce mostly NAP-1α and NAP-1β[197,198] and mononuclear cells produce predominantly NAP-1γ, which probably reflects the different proteolytic activity present. NAP-1 is produced in monocytes (MONAP) and endothelial cells (ENAP) upon LPS, IL 1 or TNF stimulation; in lymphocytes (LYNAP) after PHA stimulation; in alveolar macrophages (AMNAP)[199] after LPS stimulation; in fibroblasts (FINAP) and chondrocytes (CONAP)[200] after IL 1 or TNF stimulation; and in keratinocytes (KENAP) after IL 1 stimulation[161]. NAP-2 is generated by truncation of CTAP-III and/or platelet basic protein[195]. NAP-3 is produced by monocytes[194]. Human MCP-1 is generated by lymphocytes, endothelial cells and fibroblasts[160]. While MCP-1 was demonstrated to attract only monocytes, NAP-1 initially was considered to be specific for neutrophils until it was also shown to attract lymphocytes[201] and basophils[25], but not monocytes or eosinophils[25]. However, chemotactic efficacy of NAP-1 for lymphocytes and basophils is low compared to that for neutrophils, whereas its potency for these cells is similar. Therefore, one can conclude that in acute inflammation the primary action of NAP-1 in humans can be only on neutrophils[25], whereas in several chronic inflammatory diseases, where NAP-1 possibly also plays a pathoethiological role (e.g. psoriasis, rheumatoid arthritis, idiopathic pulmonary fibrosis and different types of pneumoconiosis, all characterized by the periodic appearance of neutrophil-rich exudate), it also can attract lymphocytes. Human NAP-1 was shown to have a proinflammatory effect in different experimental animal species. While neutrophils of 10 different species migrate *in vitro* in response to human NAP-1, its chemotactic potency varies in the range of three orders of magnitude; monkey neutrophils are the most, and rat neutrophils are the least, sensitive.

The generation of NAP-1 and MCP-1 by cells infected with different viruses[202,203] suggests that in viral infection either neutrophil and lymphocyte or monocyte infiltrate can be induced before the immune system is stimulated by viral antigens. Thus, both chemotactic cytokines may play an important role in aiding the afferent phase of the immune response to viruses. The secretion of NAP-3 (MGSA) and MCP-1 by different types of tumour cells suggests that these cytokines can be responsible for infiltration of tumours by neutrophils and monocytes, respectively.

OTHER LEUKOCYTE CHEMOATTRACTANTS

Intercellular matrix proteins

Several matrix proteins and their fragments were found to have chemotactic activity for neutrophils and monocytes[44–47]. In order to form soluble chemotactic gradients these proteins or their fragments have to be disattached, e.g. cleaved by proteolytic enzymes present at the site of inflammation. Alternatively, the leukocytes could recognize and move along a surface-attached chemotactic gradient which enzymatically modified matrix protein molecules are more likely to form. Tumour cells were shown to respond to the substrate-bound gradients of matrix proteins[58]. Haptotaxis to matrix proteins would deserve a thorough exploration also in the case of leukocytes.

Mitochondrial formyl peptides

Similarly to bacteria, mitochondrial protein synthesis is initiated with formylmethionine; therefore, one can imagine that N-formylmethionyl peptides or proteins with chemotactic activity for leukocytes are also generated in mitochrondria. This hypothesis was tested and proven correct by H. Carp[204]; thus, mitochondria can be an additional source of chemotactic activity for leukocytes at the site of tissue damage.

Crystal-induced chemotactic factor

The ingestion of urate and other crystals by neutrophils and monocytes stimulates the release of chemotactic for neutrophils factor, which can play an important role in the induction of cellular infiltrate around tissue deposits of various crystals. Crystal-induced chemotactic factor (CCF) has been isolated and partially characterized[35], and its biological activities and receptor binding have been studied; however, recent findings suggest that leukocytes also generate NAP-1 following the ingestion of crystals. In addition, anti-NAP-1 antibodies almost completely neutralize the urate crystal-induced chemotactic activity released by monocytes (R. Terkeltaub, personal communication), suggesting that CCF and NAP-1 could be related.

Neuropeptides

A series of neuropeptides and their synthetic derivatives were shown to possess chemotactic activity for monocytes[48–51]. Whereas the role of these factors in different types of inflammation is only hypothetical, their activity hints that, in addition to regulation of inflammatory vascular responses, the nervous system can be directly involved in the generation of cellular exudate.

Finally, several inflammatory cytokines have been featured in reports implying their chemotactic activity for leukocytes, and deserve to be mentioned. In spite of the fact that it was the recognition that IL 1 and TNF lack chemotactic activity for neutrophils[205] and monocytes (Leonard and Rot, unpublished) which led to the discovery of NAP-1 and MCP-1, several recent studies have reported the *in vitro* leukocyte chemotactic activity of natural and recombinant preparations of IL 1 and/or TNF. At the same time, reports from different laboratories acknowledged the lack of chemotactic activity of one or both of these cytokines (discussed in refs 146 and 206). It is puzzling why these two well-defined cytokines show such different behaviour in the hands of different investigators. The answer probably lies either in the differences of IL 1 and TNF preparations, or in the additional cellular responses these cytokines can elicit. It is well established that both IL 1 and TNF have potent *in vivo* leukocyte emigration-inducing activity[207], which together with their ability to induce *in vitro* NAP-1 and MCP-1 production establishes both IL 1 and TNF as potent chemotaxinogens. It is likely that during the *in vitro* chemotaxis assay IL 1 and TNF can induce the release of LTB_4 or chemotactic cytokines from leukocytes activated in the process of separation. The released chemotaxin can stimulate leukocyte chemotaxis and chemokinesis. In addition, even the highly purified natural cytokines can contain small amounts of contaminants with chemotactic activity, whereas recombinant cytokines expressed in bacteria may have formylated amino terminals which directly, or upon cleavage, can initiate leukocyte chemotaxis via the formyl peptide receptor. Thus, while IL 1 and TNF are most likely not chemotactic, the factors mentioned above can be responsible for the observations of leukocyte migration stimulated by these cytokines and also others, e.g. GM-CSF and PDGF, found to be either chemotactic or not chemotactic for leukocytes[147,208].

CHEMOTAXINS IN ACUTE AND CHRONIC INFLAMMATION

The initiating event of acute inflammation is most often the tissue damage caused by physical, chemical or biological agents. Endothelial cell damage initiates coagulation, clot formation and platelet aggregation which – together with infectious agents and their products, foreign objects, etc. – lead to complement activation via the 'alternative' pathway and generation of chemotactic C5a. C5a appears in extravascular tissues since tissue damage also results in an increase of vascular permeability due to disruption of vascular integrity or the release of vasoactive mediators from perivascular mast cells. Either the engulfment of microorganisms or stimulation by their products, such as LPS, leads to the immediate production and release of LTB_4 by resident macrophages. In addition, LTB_4 is also produced by endothelial and mast cells. Exogenous chemotaxins, like formyl peptides, can also be present at the early phases of acute inflammation induced by microorganisms.

Clot formation and platelet aggregation provides an additional source of chemotactic activity for monocytes (attributable to thrombin[31]), and for neutrophils (attributable to fibrinogen derivatives[32] and NAP-2[195]). Thus, panchemotaxins with the highest potency and efficacy for neutrophils and monocytes and specific neutrophil and monocyte chemotaxins are generated in the initial phase of acute inflammation. Conclusively, a mixed cellular infiltrate consisting of various proportions of neutrophils and monocytes is characteristic for most forms of acute inflammation. Neutrophils usually appear in the tissues first, and are followed by monocytes. This is possibly due to the slower speed of monocyte migration[14] and their reduced ability to traverse intercellular junctions[209]. The production and release of LTB_4, and possibly PAF, by emigrated leukocytes in response to chemotaxins provides the possibility of amplification of phagocyte eggression.

Another positive feedback loop involves the increase in vascular permeability caused by PAF or C5a (via degranulation of mast cells) resulting in plasma leakage and C5a generation in extravascular tissues. Neutrophil degranulation provides an additional source of chemotactic activity for leukocytes, since their granules contain chemotaxins[210] and enzymes capable of forming chemotactic complexes with plasma proteins[211] or cleaving chemotactic fragments of complement and extracellular matrix proteins. Chemotaxin-induced phagocyte oxygen radical production can cause further chemotaxin generation by activation of an unidentified plasma chemotactic factor[112] or via tissue damage and possible stimulation of nerve endings which can lead to the release of neuromediators with chemotactic[48–51] or chemotaxis-potentiating activity. LPS induces the production of NAP-1 by endothelial cells, macrophages, and MCP-1 by macrophages; additional massive production of MONAP begins upon emigration of monocytes. LPS-induced ENAP and MONAP can initiate the second wave of neutrophil emigration, whereas MCP-1 causes monocyte emigration. Inflammatory cytokines such as IL 1 and TNF can stimulate the additional production of NAP-1 and MCP-1 by fibroblasts and endothelial cells, but since two consecutive steps of protein synthesis are involved, IL 1 and TNF-induced ENAP, FINAP, and MCP-1 generation reaches its peak days after the initiation of inflammation. In addition, ENAP and FINAP consist of the low-potency NAP-1α and NAP-1β variants which, in order to achieve optimal chemotactic potency, require the presence of proteolytic activity at the site of inflammation. Similarly, leukocyte enzymes can aid NAP-2 generation by cleaving it from chemotactically inactive precursors.

Immune mechanisms also can initiate or contribute to the development of leukocyte emigration in acute inflammation. In the immediate-type hypersensitivity, which is characteristic for allergic reactions, IgE can induce mast cell and basophil degranulation leading to the release of vasoactive mediators and chemotaxins with the highest potency for eosinophils (PAF, ECF-A) or neutrophils (LTB_4). Emigrated eosinophils promote further eosinophil egress by releasing ECL. IgG and IgM antibodies binding to either infectious agents or normal host cell antigens can activate complement via its 'classical' pathway. This leads to target cell lysis and also C5a generation which results, in turn, in infiltrates dominated by monocytes and neutrophils. The circulating antibody–antigen complexes following their deposition in the walls of blood vessels or kidney glomeruli can also initiate complement activation and C5a generation with consequent tissue destruction and phagocyte accumulation exemplified by systemic vasculitis and glomerulonephritis. IgG–antigen complexes also can bind to basophils or mast cells and stimulate PAF release, possibly resulting in eosinophil emigration characteristic for allergic angiitis. The amazing redundancy of chemotactic factors, and the variety of ways in which they can be generated, ensures continuous leukocyte chemotaxis to inflammatory sites.

The above-described 'grand avalanche' of chemotactic factor generation and consequent leukocyte emigration can come to a halt and inflammation can end upon elimination of the initial cause or source of chemotactic activity, rapid destruction of released chemotaxins, deactivation of leukocytes and inflammatory sites and release of inhibitory mediators. Alternatively, acute inflammation can progress into chronic inflammation. This happens when the source of tissue damage either persists or recurs and prevents healing, the leukocytes are not able to eliminate either the infectious agent or foreign body, and cellular immune reactions are induced by the antigens present in the inflammatory lesion (delayed-type hypersensitivity). As much as neutrophil presence is a hallmark of acute inflammation, lymphocytes are the characteristic feature of chronic inflammatory infiltrate which can consist of widely differing proportions of all leukocyte types, as well as fibroblasts and proliferating endothelial cells. However, the predominant cell in chronic inflammatory infiltrates usually is a monocyte-derived macrophage, which can undergo profound morphological transformations (into epithelioid cells and giant cells) and also gain the ability to proliferate on site. Nevertheless, leukocyte recruitment from blood, especially by chemotactic cytokines, continues to play an important role in the development of cellular infiltrate. Produced by sensitized lymphocytes, MCP-1 is thought to be responsible for the influx of monocytes; whereas NAP-1 (MONAP, LYNAP, FINAP, ENAP) probably plays a role in the periodic recruitment of neutrophils, characteristic for several types of chronic inflammation. Lymphocytes are also likely to be attracted into the sites of chronic inflammation by chemotactic cytokines, including NAP-1.

MECHANISM OF LEUKOCYTE CHEMOTAXIS *IN VIVO*

In the extravascular tissues, leukocyte chemotaxis probably happens the same way as it does *in vitro*, and is the only major mechanism of unidirectional leukocyte movement, although alternative mechanisms such as cell- and mediator-specific matrix-driven cell translocation have also been suggested[213]. Conversely, in addition to chemotaxis, several processes contribute to leukocyte emigration from the blood vessels (reviewed by I. Colditz[137]). Since adherence is a prerequisite of leukocyte chemotaxis, in order to respond to the transendothelial chemotactic gradients, leukocytes have to marginate from the mainstream of circulation and adhere to endothelial cells.

In the process of inflammation, and following the injection of chemotaxin, leukocytes selectively adhere to the endothelial cell lining of the postcapillary venules, small veins and, in some instances, small arteries (Figure 14.3). Chemoattractants can promote *in vitro* adherence of leukocytes to endothelial cells[214,215] by up-regulating the surface expression and activating the leukocyte integrin heterodimers CD11/CD18[79,216]. CD11/CD18 molecules are also involved in mediating leukocyte aggregation, another factor contributing to leukocyte retention in the microvasculature. Lack of neutrophil accumulation in the inflammatory sites of patients with leukocyte adherence deficiency, a human hereditary disease characterized by the absence of CD18 molecules from the leukocyte surface, indicates the significance of CD18 heterodimers in leukocyte emigration[217]. However, experimental evidence suggests that CD18 complex does not initiate endothelial adhesion *in vivo* under the influence of a lateral shear force similar to that created by the blood flow[218]. The binding of leukocyte CD11/CD18 to the endothelial counterligand ICAM-1 can only secure the leukocyte adherence already established by selectins, adhesion molecules present on leukocytes (L-selectin or LAM-1) and endothelial cells (E-selectin or ELAM-1 and P-selectin or GMP-140)[214,219]. Selectins bind to carbohydrate counterligands, such as sialyl-Lewis X, and mediate leukocyte 'rolling' which *in vivo*, under the conditions of venous lateral shear stress, is the first step of the adhesion interaction between leukocytes and endothelial cells[214,219]. Chemoattractants cause shedding of L-selectin from the leukocyte surface and, therefore, can inhibit the initial adhesive interaction between leukocytes and the endothelium[214]. Thus, chemoattractants can either promote or inhibit the leukocyte adherence to the endothelium depending on them acting either on the leukocyte already adherent by selectin-dependent mechanism or the one still in circulation. Several cytokines, including IL 1 and TNF, as well as LPS, up-regulate the expression of E-selectin and ICAM-1 on the surface of endothelial cells[220,221]. This provides the possibility of targeting leukocytes to the segments of blood vessel lining affected by inflammation; but since the expression of E-selectin and ICAM-1 is protein synthesis-dependent and takes 2–4 h[221], whereas neutrophils begin to adhere to the endothelium of postcapillary venules and small veins as early as minutes following the injection of a chemoattractant, one has to postulate the existence of an alternative mechanism of targeted endothelial cell-dependent leukocyte adherence.

It was shown that thrombin, histamine, and non-chemotactic leukotrienes

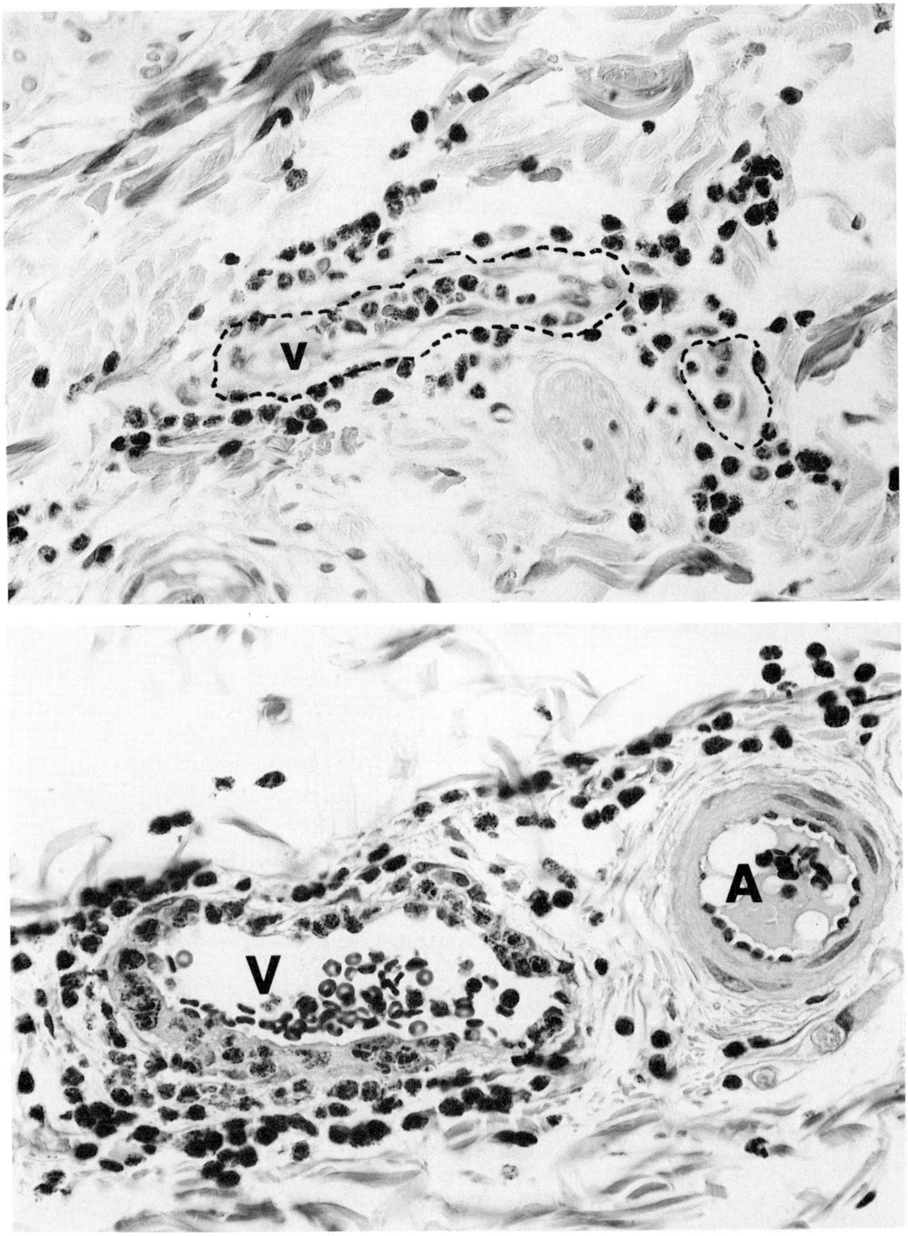

Figure 14.3 Rabbit neutrophil margination and emigration from postcapillary venule (**A**) and small vein (**B**) in response to intradermal injection of NAP-1. **A**. The outline of the venule (V) is marked by a dashed line. The lumen contains several marginating neutrophils; a few of the neutrophils are in the process of traversing the vessel wall, while more of them have already emigrated. **B**. Neutrophils are either in the process of emigrating across the wall of the small vein (V) or already infiltrating the connective tissue around the vessel. The small artery (A) contains marginating lymphocytes.

C4 and D4 can induce rapid endothelial cell-dependent neutrophil adherence either by stimulating the expression of endogenous PAF on the endothelial cell surface[222] and by translocation of P-selectin from Weibel-Palade bodies of the endothelial cells onto their surface[223]. However, there is no indication that chemoattractants can initiate leukocyte adherence by the same mechanism. Complement activation and fixation by endothelial cells provides another possibility for rapid endothelial cell-dependent adherence of leukocytes via their type 3 complement receptor[224].

Once adherent to the endothelial cells, leukocytes have to perceive the chemoattractant gradient and migrate across the endothelium and basal membrane in response to it. Though the existence of soluble chemotaxin gradients across the vessel wall can be postulated, the limited rate of the passive diffusion of chemotaxin between endothelial cells and the very rapid dilution of it by blood[225] suggests the involvement of additional mechanisms. These include the transendothelial active transport of chemotaxins as exemplified in the receptor-mediated uptake and subsequent release of formyl peptides by endothelial cells[226] or the possibility of leukocyte haptotaxis in response to endothelial cell membrane-bound chemotaxins such as NAP-1 and PAF[222]. The chemotaxin-induced site-specific, homologous desensitization suggests that chemotaxins can facilitate leukocyte emigration by a receptor-mediated interaction with either endothelial or other resident cells[137].

Acknowledgments

The critical review of the manuscript by Prof. Marco Baggiolini and Dr Stuart Evans is gratefully appreciated.

References

1. Metchnikoff, E. (1891, reprinted 1968). *Lectures on Comparative Pathology of Inflammation* (New York: Dover Press)
2. Leber, T. (1888). Über die Entstehung der Entzüundung und die Wirkung der entzündungserregenden Schädlichkeiten. *Fortschr. Med.*, **6**, 460–4
3. Rebuck, J. W. and Crowley, J. H. (1955). A method of studying leukocytic function in vivo. *Ann. N.Y. Acad. Sci.*, **59**, 757–60
4. Zimmerli, W. and Gallin, J. I. (1987). Monocytes accumulate on Rebuck skin window coverslips but not in skin chamber fluid. *J. Immunol. Methods*, **96**, 11–17
5. Haris, H. (1954). Role of chemotaxis in inflammation. *Physiol. Rev.*, **34**, 529–62
6. Böyum, A. (1968). Isolation of mononuclear cells and granulocytes from human blood. *Scand. J. Clin. Lab. Invest. Suppl.*, **21**, 77–89
7. Boyden, S. (1962). The chemotactic effect of mixtures of antibody and antigen on polymorphonuclear leucocytes. *J. Exp. Med.*, **115**, 453–66
8. Wilkinson, P. C. (1982). The measurement of leukocyte chemotaxis. *J. Immunol. Methods*, **51**, 133–48
9. Nelson, R. D., Quie, P. G. and Simmons, R. L. (1975). Chemotaxis under agarose: A new and simple method for measuring chemotaxis and spontaneous migration of human polymorphonuclear leukocytes and monocytes. *J. Immunol.*, **115**, 1650–6
10. Islam, L. N., McKay, I. C. and Wilkinson, P. C. (1985). The use of collagen of fibrin gels for the assay of human neutrophil chemotaxis. *J. Immunol. Methods*, **85**, 137–151

11. Zigmond, S. H. (1977). Ability of polymorphonuclear leukocytes to orient in gradients of chemotactic factors. *J. Cell Biol.*, **75**, 606–16
12. Ramsey, W. S. (1972). Analysis of individual leukocyte behavior during chemotaxis. *Exp. Cell. Res.*, **70**, 129–39
13. Allan, R. B. and Wilkinson, P. C. (1978). A visual analysis of chemotactic and chemokinetic locomotion of human neutrophil leucocytes, *Exp. Cell Res.*, **111**, 191–203
14. Horwitz, D. A. and Garrett, M. A. (1971). Use of leukocyte chemotaxis in vitro to assay mediators generated by immune reactions. *J. Immunol.*, **106**, 649–55
15. Swanson, M. J. and Becker, E. L. (1976). Measurement of chemotaxis of human polymorphonuclear leukocytes in filters by counting the number of cells in a single plane and comparison with leading front method. *J. Immunol. Methods*, **13**, 191–7
16. Maderazo, E. G. and Woronick, C. L. (1979). Micropore filter assay of human granulocyte locomotion: problems and solutions. *Clin. Immunol. Immunopathol.*, **11**, 196–211
17. Zigmond, S. H. and Hirsch, J. G. (1973). Leukocyte locomotion and chemotaxis. New methods for evaluation and demonstration of a cell-derived chemotactic factor. *J. Exp. Med.*, **137**, 387–410
18. Galin, J. I., Clark, R. A. and Kimball, H. R. (1973). Granulocyte chemotaxis: An improved in vitro assay employing ^{51}Cr-labeled granulocytes. *J. Immunol.*, **110**, 233–40
19. Watanabe, K., Kinoshita, S. and Nakagawa, H. (1989). Very rapid assay of polymorphonuclear leukocyte chemotaxis in vitro. *J. Pharmacol. Methods*, **22**, 13–18
20. Creamer, H. R., Gabler, W. L. and Bullock, W. W. (1983). Endogenous component chemotactic assay (ECCA). *Inflammation*, **7**, 321-9
21. Falk, W., Goodwin, R. H. and Leonard, E. J. (1980). A 48 well micro chemotaxis assembly for rapid and accurate measurement of leukocyte migration. *J. Immunol. Methods*, **33**, 239–47
22. Rot, A., Henderson, L. E. and Leonard, E. J. (1986). *Staphylococcus aureus*-derived chemoattractant activity for human monocytes. *J. Leukocyte Biol.*, **40**, 43–53
23. Richards, K. L. and McCullough, J. (1984). A modified microchamber method for chemotaxis and chemokinesis. *Immunol. Commun.*, **13**, 49–62
24. Harvath, L., Falk, W. and Leonard, E. J. (1980). Rapid quantitation of neutrophil chemotaxis: use of polyvinylpyrrolidone-free polycarbonate membrane in a multiwell assembly. *J. Immunol. Methods*, **37**, 39–45
25. Leonard, E. J., Skeel, A., Yoshimura, T., Noer, K., Kutvirt, S. and Van Epps, D. (1990). Leukocyte specificity and binding of human neutrophil attractant/activation protein-1. *J. Immunol.*, **144**, 1323–30
26. Gnessi, L., Ruff, M. R., Fraioli, F. and Pert, C. B. (1985). Demonstration of receptor-mediated chemotaxis by human spermatozoa. *Exp. Cell. Res.*, **161**, 219–30
27. Thorgeirsson, U. P., Liotta, L. A., Kalebic, T., Margulies, I. M., Thomas, K., Rios-Candelore, M. and Russo, R. G. (1982). Effect of natural protease inhibitors and a chemoattractant on tumor cell invasion in vitro. *J. Natl. Cancer Inst.*, **69**, 1049–54
28. Bignold, L. P. (1988). Measurement of chemotaxis of polymorphonuclear leukocytes in vitro. *J. Immunol. Methods*, **108**, 1–18
29. Schiffmann, E., Corcoran, B. A. and Wahl, S. M. (1975). N-formylmethionyl peptides as chemoattractants for leucocytes. *Proc. Natl. Acad. Sci. USA*, **72**, 1059–62
30. Ward, P. A., Cochrane, C. G. and Müller-Eberhard, H. J. (1965). The role of serum complement in chemotaxis of leukocytes in vitro. *J. Exp. Med.*, **122**, 327–47
31. Bar-Shavit, R., Kahn, A., Fenton II, J. W. and Wilner, G. D. (1983). Chemotactic response of monocytes to thrombin. *J. Cell Biol.*, **96**, 282–5
32. Senior, R. M., Skogen, W. F., Griffin, G. L. and Wilner, G. D. (1986). Effects of fibrinogen derivatives upon the inflammatory response: Studies with human fibrinopeptide B. *J. Clin. Invest.*, **77**, 1014–19
33. Palmblad, J., Malmsten, C. L., Udèn, A-M., Radmark, O., Engstedt, L. and Samuelsson, B. (1981). Leukotriene B_4 is a potent and stereospecific stimulator of neutrophil chemotaxis and adherence. *Blood*, **58**, 658–61
34. Shaw, J. O., Pinckard, R. N., Ferrigni, K. S., McManus, L. M. and Hanahan, D. J. (1981). Activation of human neutrophils with 1-*O*-hexadecyl/octadecyl-2-acetyl-sn-glyceryl-3-phosphorylcholine (platelet activating factor). *J. Immunol.*, **127**, 1250–5
35. Spilberg, I., Gallacher, A., Mehta, J. M. and Mandell, B. (1976). Urate crystal-induced chemotactic factor. Isolation and partial characterization. *J. Clin. Invest.*, **58**, 815–19

36. Goetzl, E. J. and Austen, K. F. (1975). Purification and synthesis of eosinophilotactic tetrapeptides of human lung tissue: identification as eosinophil chemotactic factor of anaphylaxis. *Proc. Natl. Acad. Sci. USA*, **72**, 4123–7
37. Kownatzki, E., Kapp, A. and Uhrich, S. (1986). Novel neutrophil chemotactic factor derived from human peripheral blood mononuclear leucocytes. *Clin. Exp. Immunol.*, **64**, 214–22
38. Yoshimura, T., Matsushima, K., Tanaka, S., Robinson, E. A., Appella, E., Oppenheim, J. J. and Leonard, E. J. (1987). Purification of a human monocyte-derived neutrophil chemotactic factor that has peptide sequence similarity to other host defense cytokines. *Proc. Natl. Acad. Sci. USA*, **84**, 9233–7
39. Schröder, J-M., Mrowietz, U., Morita, E. and Christophers, E. (1987). Purification and partial biochemical characterization of a human monocyte-derived, neutrophil-activating peptide that lacks interleukin 1 activity. *J. Immunol.*, **139**, 3474–83
40. Walz, A., Peveri, P., Aschauer, H. and Baggiolini, M. (1987). Purification and amino acid sequencing of NAF, a novel neutrophil-activating factor produced by monocytes. *Biochem. Biophys Res. Commun.*, **149**, 755–61
41. Van Damme, J., Van Beeumen, J., Opdenakker, G. and Billiau, A. (1988). A novel NH_2-terminal sequence-characterized human monokine possessing neutrophil chemotactic, skin-reactive, and granulocytosis-promoting activity. *J. Exp. Med.*, **167**, 1364–76
42. Leonard, E. J. and Yoshimura, T. (1990). Human monocyte chemoattractant protein-1 (MCP-1) *Immunol. Today*, **11**, 97–101
43. Wahl, S. M., Hunt, D. A., Wakefield, L. M., McCartney-Francis, N., Wahl, L. M., Roberts, A. B. and Sporn, M. B. (1987). Transforming growth factor type β induces monocyte chemotaxis and growth factor production. *Proc. Natl. Acad. Sci. USA*, **84**, 5788–92
44. Postlethwaite, A. E. and Kang, A. H. (1976). Collagen- and collagen peptide-induced chemotaxis of human blood monocytes. *J. Exp. Med.*, **143**, 1299–1300
45. Senior, R. M., Griffin, G. L. and Mecham, R. P. (1980). Chemotactic activity of elastin-derived peptides. *J. Clin. Invest.*, **66**, 859–62
46. Norris, D. A., Clark, R. A. F., Swigart, L. M., Huff, J. C., Weston, W. L. and Howell, S. E. (1982). Fibronectin fragment(s) are chemotactic for human peripheral blood monocytes. *J. Immunol.*, **129**, 1612–18
47. Terranova, V. P., DiFlorio, R., Hujanen, E. S., Lyall, R. M., Liotta, L. A., Thorgeirsson, U., Siegal, G. P. and Schiffmann, E. (1986). Laminin promotes rabbit neutrophil motility and attachment. *J. Clin. Invest.*, **77**, 1180–6
48. Van Epps, D. E. and Saland, L. (1984). β-Endorphin and met-enkephalin stimulate human peripheral blood mononuclear cell chemotaxis. *J. Immunol.*, **132**, 3046–53
49. Ruff, M., Schiffmann, E., Terranova, V. and Pert, C. B. (1985). Neuropeptides are chemoattractants for human tumor cells and monocytes: A possible mechanism for metastasis. *Clin. Immunol. Immunopathol.*, **37**, 387–96
50. Ruff, M., Pert, C. B., Weber, R. J., Wahl, L. M., Wahl, S. M. and Paul, S. M. (1985). Benzodiazepine receptor-mediated chemotaxis of human monocytes. *Science*, **229**, 1281–3
51. Ruff, M. R., Wahl, S. M. and Pert, C. B. (1985). Substance P receptor mediated chemotaxis of human monocytes. *Peptides*, **6** (Suppl. 2), 107–11
52. Thornhill, M. H., Kyan-Aung, U., Lee, T. H. and Haskard, D. O. (1990). T cells and neutrophils exhibit differential adhesion to cytokine-stimulated endothelial cells. *Immunology*, **69**, 287–92
53. Berman, J. S., Cruikshank, W. W., Beer, D. J., Kornfeld, H., Bernardo, J., Theodore, A. C. and Center, D. M. (1988). Lymphocyte motility and lymphocyte chemoattractant factors. *Immunol. Invest.*, **17**, 625–77
54. Morita, E., Schröder, J-M. and Christophers, E. (1990). Identification of a novel and highly potent eosinophil chemotactic lipid in human eosinophils treated with arachidonic acid. *J. Immunol.*, **144**, 1893–1900
55. Clark, R. A. (1982). Chemotactic factors trigger their own oxidative inctivation by human neutrophils. *J. Immunol.*, **129**, 2725–8
56. Yuli, I. and Snyderman, R. (1986). Extensive hydrolysis of N-formyl-L-methionyl-L-leucyl-L-^{3}H phenylalanine by human polymorphonuclear leukocytes. *J. Biol. Chem.*, **261**, 4902–8
57. Carter, S. B. (1965). Principles of cell motility: the direction of cell movement and cancer invasion. *Nature*, **208**, 1183–7
58. McCarthy, J. B. and Furcht, L. T. (1984). Laminin and fibronectin promote the haptotactic

migration of B16 mouse melanoma cells in vitro. *J. Cell Biol.*, **98**, 1474–80

59. Dierich, M. P., Wilhelmi, D. and Till, G. (1977). Essential role of surface-bound chemoattractant in leukocyte migration. *Nature*, **270**, 351–2
60. Webster, R. O., Zanolari, B. and Henson, P. M. (1980). Neutrophil chemotaxis in response to surface-bound C5a. *Exp. Cell Res.*, **129**, 55–62
61. Wilkinson, P. C. and Allan, R. B. (1978). Chemotaxis of neutrophil leukocytes towards substratum-bound protein attractants. *Exp. Cell Res.*, **117**, 403–12
62. Goldstein, I., Hoffstein, S., Gallin, J. and Weissmann, G. (1973). Mechanism of lysosomal enzyme release from human leukocytes: Microtubule assembly and membrane fusion induced by a component of complement. *Proc. Natl. Acad. Sci. USA*, **70**, 2916–20
63. Showell, H. J., Freer, R. J., Zizmond, S. H., Schiffmann, E., Aswanikumar, S., Corcoran, B. and Becker, E. L. (1976). The structure-activity relations of synthetic peptides as chemotactic factors and inducers of lysosomal enzyme secretion for neutrophils. *J. Exp. Med.*, **143**, 1154–69
64. Boxer, L. A., Yoder, M., Bonsib, S., Schmidt, M., Ho, P., Jersild, R. and Baehner, R. L. (1979). Effects of chemotctic factor, N-formylmethionyl peptide, on adherence, superoxide anion generation, phagocytosis, and microtubule assembly of human polymorphonuclear leukocytes. *J. Lab. Clin. Med.*, **93**, 506–14
65. Hatch, G. E., Gardner, D. E. and Menzel, D. B. (1978). Chemiluminescence of phagocytic cells caused by N-formylmethionyl peptides. *J. Exp. Med.*, **147**, 182–95
66. Cronstein, B. N., Daguma, L., Nichols, D., Hutchinson, A. J. and Williams, M. (1990). The adenosine/neutrophil paradox resolved: Human neutrophils possess both A_1 and A_2 receptors that promote chemotaxis and inhibit O_2-generation, respectively. *J. Clin. Invest.*, **85**, 1150–7
67. Palmblad, J., Gyllenhammar, H., Lindgren, J. A. and Malmsten, C. L. (1984). Effects of leukotrienes and f-met-leu-phe on oxidative metabolism of neutrophils and eosinophils. *J. Immunol.*, **132**, 3041–5
68. Rot, A., Henderson, L. E., Copeland, T. D. and Leonard, E. J. (1987). A series of six ligands for the human formyl peptide receptor: Tetrapeptides with high chemotactic potency and efficacy. *Proc. Natl. Acad. Sci. USA*, **84**, 7967–71
69. Williams, L. T., Snyderman, R., Pike, M. C. and Lefkowitz, R. J. (1977). Specific receptor sites for chemotactic peptides on human polymorphonuclear leukocytes. *Proc. Natl. Acad. Sci. USA*, **74**, 1204–8
70. Chenoweth, D. E. and Hugli, T. E. (1978). Demonstration of specific C5a receptor on intact human polymorphonuclear leukocytes. *Proc. Natl. Acad. Sci. USA*, **75**, 3943–7
71. Goldman, D. W. and Goetzl, E. J. (1982). Specific binding of leukotriene B4 to receptors on human polymorphonuclear leukocytes. *J. Immunol.*, **129**, 160–4
72. Samantha, A. K., Oppenheim, J. J. and Matsushima, K. (1989). Identification and characterization of specific receptors for monocyte-derived neutrophil chemotactic factor (MDNCF) on human neutrophils. *J. Exp. Med.*, **169**, 1185–89
73. Snyderman, R. and Pike, M. C. (1984). Chemoattractant receptors on phagocytic cells. *Ann. Rev. Immunol.*, **2**, 257–81
74. Sklar, L. A. (1986). Ligand-receptor dynamics and signal amplification in the neutrophil. *Adv. Immunol.*, **39**, 95–143
75. Niedel, J. E., Kahane, I. and Cuatrecasas, P. (1979). Receptor-mediated internalization of fluorescent chemotactic peptide by human neutrophils. *Science*, **205**, 1412–14
76. Sullivan, S. J. and Zigmond, S. H. (1980). Chemotactic peptide receptor modulation in polymorphonuclear leukocytes. *J. Cell Biol.*, **85**, 703–11
77. Vitkauskas, G., Showell, H. J. and Becker, E. L. (1980). Specific binding of synthetic chemotactic peptides to rabbit peritoneal neutrophils: Effects on dissociability of bound peptide, receptor activity and subsequent biologic responsiveness (deactivation). *Molecular Immunol.*, **17**, 171–80
78. Galin, J. I. and Seligmann, B. E. (1984). Mobilization and adaptation of human neutrophil chemoattractant fMet-Leu-Phe receptors. *Fed. Proc.*, **43**, 2732–6
79. Borregaard, N., Miller, L. J. and Springer, T. A. (1987). Chemoattractant-regulated mobilization of novel intracellular compartment in human neutrophils. *Science*, **237**, 1204–6
80. Van Epps, D. E., Simpson, S., Bender, J. G. and Chenoweth, D. E. (1990). Regulation of C5a and formyl peptide receptor expression on human polymorphonuclear leukocytes. *J.*

Immunol., **144**, 1062–8

81. O'Flaherty, J. T., Redman, J. F. and Jacobson, D. P. (1990). Cyclical binding, processing, and functional interactions of neutrophils with leukotriene B_4. *J. Cell. Physiol.*, **142**, 299–308
82. Painter, R. G., Zahler-Bentz, K. and Dukes, R. E. (1987). Regulation of the affinity state of the N-formylated peptide receptor of neutrophils: Role of guanine nucleotide-binding proteins and the cytoskeleton. *J. Cell Biol.*, **105**, 2959–71
83. Koo, C., Lefkowitz, R. J. and Snyderman, R. (1983). Guanine nucleotides modulate the binding affinity of the oligopeptide chemoattractant receptor on human polymorphonuclear leukocytes. *J. Clin. Invest.*, **72**, 748–53
84. Zigmond, S. H. and Sullivan, S. J. (1979). Sensory adaptation of leukocytes to chemotactic peptides. *J. Cell Biol.*, **82**, 517–27
85. Seligman, B. E., Fletcher, M. P. and Gallin, J. I. (1982). Adaptation of human neutrophil responsiveness to chemoattractant N-formylmethionylleucylphenylalanin. Heterogeneity and/or negative cooperative interaction of receptors. *J. Biol. Chem.*, **257**, 6280–6
86. Howard, T. H., Wang, D. and Berkow, R. L. (1990). Lipopolysaccharide modulates chemotactic peptide-induced actin polymerization in neutrophils. *J. Leukocyte Biol.*, **47**, 13–24
87. Tennenberg, S. D., Zemlan, F. P. and Solomkin, J. S. (1988). Characterization of N-formyl-methionyl-leucyl-phenylalanine receptors on human neutrophils. *J. Immunol.*, **141**, 3937–44
88. Koo, C., Lefkowitz, R. J. and Snyderman, R. (1982). The oligopeptide chemotactic factor receptor on human polymorphonuclear leukocyte membranes exists in two affinity states. *Biochem. Biophys. Res. Commun.*, **106**, 442–9
89. Goldman, D. W. and Goetzl, E. J. (1984). Heterogeneity of human polymorphonuclear leukocyte receptors for leukotriene B_4. *J. Exp. Med.*, **159**, 1027–41
90. Besemer, J., Hujber, A. and Kuhn, B. (1989). Specific binding, internalization, and degradation of human neutrophil activating factor by human polymorphonuclear leukocytes. *J. Biol. Chem.*, **264**, 17409–15
91. Omann, G. M., Allen, R. A., Bokoch, G. M., Painter, R. G., Traynor, A. E. and Sklar, L. A. (1987). Signal transduction and cytoskeletal activation in the neutrophil. *Phys. Rev.*, **67**, 285–322
92. Snyderman, R., Smith, C. D. and Verghese, M. W. (1986). Model for leukocyte regulation by chemoattractant receptors: roles of a guanine nucleotide regulatory protein and polyphosphoinositide metabolism. *J. Leukocyte Biol.*, **40**, 785–800
93. Snyderman, R. and Verghese, M. W. (1987). Leukocyte activation by chemoattractant receptors: Role of guanine nucleotide regulatory protein and polyphosphoinositide metabolism. *Rev. Infect. Dis.*, **9**, S562–9
94. McLeish, K. R., Gierschik, P., Schepers, T., Sidiropoulos, D. and Jakobs, K. H. (1989). Evidence that activation of a common G-protein by receptors for leukotriene B_4 and N-formylmethionyl-leucyl-phenylalanine in HL-60 cells occurs by different mechanisms. *Biochem. J.*, **260**, 427–34
95. Von Tscharner, V., Prod'hom, B., Baggiolini, M. and Reuter, H. (1986). Ion channels in human neutrophils activated by a rise in free cytosolic calcium concentration. *Nature*, **324**, 369–72
96. Truett III, A. P., Verghese, M. W., Dillon, S. B. and Snyderman, R. (1988). Calcium influx stimulates a second pathway for sustained diacylglycerol production in leukocytes activated by chemoattractants. *Proc. Natl. Acad. Sci. USA*, **85**, 1549–53
97. Berridge, M. J. and Irvine, R. F. (1989). Inositol phosphates and cell signalling. *Nature*, **341**, 197–205
98. Hirata, F. and Axelrod, J. (1980). Phospholipid methylation and biological signal transmission. *Science*, **209**, 1082–90
99. O'Dea, R. F., Viveros, O. H., Axelrod, J., Aswanikumar, S., Schiffmann, E. and Corcoran, B. A. (1978). Rapid stimulation of protein carboxymethylation in leukocytes by a chemotactic peptide. *Nature*, **272**, 462–4
100. Bomalaski, J. S., Dundee, D., Brophy, L. and Clark, M. A. (1990). Leukotriene B_4 modulates phospholipid methylation and chemotaxis in human polymorphonuclear leukocytes. *J. Leuk. Biol.*, **47**, 1–12
101. Reinhold, S. L., Prescott, S. M., Zimmerman, G. A. and McIntyre, T. M. (1990). Activation of human neutrophil phospholipase D by three separable mechanisms. *FASEB J.*, **4**, 208–14

102. Lackie, J. M. (1988). The behavioural repertoire of neutrophils requires multiple signal transduction pathways. *J. Cell Sci.*, **89**, 449–52
103. O'Flaherty, J. T. and Jackobson, D. (1989). Protein kinase C blockers and neutrophil receptors for leukotriene B_4. *Biochem. Biophys. Res. Commun.*, **163**, 1456–60
104. Smith, C. D. and Snyderman, R. (1986). Nucleotide regulatory protein-mediated activation of polyphosphoinositide-specific phospholipase C is inhibited by protein kinase C. *Fed. Proc.*, **45**, 1552
105. Rhee, S. G., Suh, P-G., Ryu, S-H. and Lee, S. Y. (1989). Studies of inositol phospholipid-specific phospholipase C. *Science*, **244**, 546–50
106. Howard, T. H. and Meyer, W. H. (1984). Chemotactic peptide modulation of actin assembly and locomotion in neutrophils. *J. Cell Biol.*, **98**, 1265–71
107. Howard, T. H. and Oresajo, C. O. (1985). The kinetics of chemotactic peptide-induced change in F-actin content, F-actin distribution, and the shape of neutropeptides. *J. Cell Biol.*, **101**, 1078–85
108. Naccache, P. H., Therrien, S., Caon, A. C., Liao, N., Gilbert, C. and McColl, S. R. (1989). Chemoattractant-induced cytoplasmic pH changes and cytoskeletal reorganization in human neutrophils. *J. Immunol.*, **142**, 2438–44
109. Lassing, I. and Lindberg, U. (1988). Evidence that the phosphatidylinositol cycle is linked to cell motility. *Exp. Cell Res.*, **174**, 1–15
110. Lassing, I. and Lindberg, U. (1985). Specific interaction between phosphatidylinositol 4,5-biphosphate and profilactin, *Nature*, **314**, 472–4
111. Janmey, P. A. and Stossel, T. P. (1987). Modulation of gelsolin function by phosphatidylinositol 4,5-biphosphate. *Nature*, **325**, 362–4
112. Pike, M. C., Bruck, M. E., Arndt, C. and Lee, C-S. (1990). Chemoattractants stimulate phosphatidylinositol-4-phosphate kinase in human polymorphonuclear leukocytes. *J. Biol. Chem.*, **265**, 1866–73
113. Harvath, L., McCall, C. E., Bass, D. A. and McPhail, L. C. (1987). Inhibition of human neutrophil chemotaxis by the protein kinase inhibitor, 1-(5-isoquinolinesulfonyl) piperazine. *J. Immunol.*, **139**, 3055–61
114. Wright, T. M., Hoffman, R. D., Nishijima, J., Jakoi, L., Snyderman, R. and Shin, H., S. (1988). Leukocyte chemoattraction by 1,2-diacylglycerol. *Proc. Natl. Acad. Sci. USA*, **85**, 1869–73
115. Bray, D. and White, J. G. (1988). Cortical flow in animal cells. *Science*, **239**, 883–8
116. Kucik, D. F., Elson, E. L. and Sheetz, M. P. (1989). Forward transport of glycoproteins on leading lamellipodia in locomoting cells. *Nature*, **340**, 315–17
117. Bretscher, M. S. (1984). Endocytosis: Relation to capping and cell locomotion. *Science*, **224**, 681–6
118. Sheetz, M. P., Turney, S., Qian, H. and Elson, E. L. (1989). Nanometre-level analysis demonstrates that lipid flow does not drive membrane glycoprotein movements. *Nature*, **340**, 284–8
119. Lee, J., Gustafsson, M., Magnusson, K-E. and Jacobson, K. (1990). The direction of membrane lipid flow in locomoting polymorphonuclear leukocytes. *Science*, **247**, 1229–33
120. Oster, G. F. and Perelson, A. S. (1987). The physics of cell motility. *J. Cell Sci. Suppl.*, **8**, 35–54
121. Malech, H. L., Root, R. K. and Gallin, J. I. (1977). Structural analysis of human neutrophil migration. Centriole, microtubule, and microfilament orientation and function during chemotaxis. *J. Cell Biol.*, **75**, 666–93
122. Gerisch, G. and Keller, H. U. (1981). Chemotactic reorientation of granualocytes stimulated with micropipettes containing fMet-Leu-Phe. *J. Cell Sci.*, **52**, 1–10
123. Zigmond, S. H., Levitsky, H. I. and Kreel, B. J. (1981). Cell polarity: An examination of its behavioral expression and its consequences for polymorphonuclear leukocyte chemotaxis. *J. Cell Biol.*, **89**, 585–92
124. Zigmond, S. H. (1974). Mechanisms of sensing chemical gradients by polymorphonuclear leukocytes. *Nature*, **249**, 450–2
125. Macnab, R. M. and Koshland, D. E. Jr (1972). The gradient-sensing mechanism in bacterial chemotaxis. *Proc. Natl. Acad. Sci. USA*, **69**, 2509–12
126. Vicker, M. G., Lackie, J. M. and Schill, W. (1986). Neutrophil leukocyte chemotaxis is not induced by a spatial gradient of chemoattractant. *J. Cell Sci.*, **84**, 263–80
127. Van Epps, D. E. and Chenoweth, D. E. (1984). Analysis of the binding of fluorescent C5a

and C3a to human peripheral blood leukocytes. *J. Immunol.*, **132**, 2862–7

128. Leonard, E. J., Noer, K. and Skeel, A. (1985). Analysis of human monocyte chemoattractant binding by flow cytometry. *J. Leukocyte Biol.*, **38**, 403–13
129. Falk, W. and Leonard, E. J. (1980). Human monocyte chemotaxis: Migrating cells are a subpopulation with multiple chemotaxin specificities on each cell. *Infect. Immun.*, **29**, 953–9
130. Cianciolo, G. J. and Snyderman, R. (1981). Monocyte responsiveness to chemotactic stimuli is a property of a subpopulation of cells that can respond to multiple chemoattractants. *J. Clin. Invest.*, **67**, 60–68
131. Ohura, K., Katona, I. M., Wahl, L. M., Chenoweth, D. E. and Wahl, S. M. (1987). Co-expression of chemotactic ligand receptors on human peripheral blood monocytes. *J. Immunol.*, **138**, 2633–9
132. Harvath, L. and Leonard, E. J. (1982). Two neutrophil populations in human blood with different chemotactic activities: Separation and chemoattractant binding. *Infect. Immun.*, **36**, 443–9
133. Snyderman, R. and Pike, M. C. (1980). N-formylmethionyl peptide receptors on equine leukocytes initiate secretion but not chemotaxis. *Science*, **209**, 493–5
134. Kreisle, R. A., Parker, C. W., Griffin, G. L., Senior, R. M. and Stenson, W. F. (1985). Studies of leukotriene B_4-specific binding and function in rat polymorphonuclear leukocytes: Absence of a chemotactic response. *J. Immunol.*, **134**, 3356–63
135. Styrt, B. (1989). Species variation in neutrophil biochemistry and function. *J. Leukocyte Biol.*, **46**, 63–74
136. Colditz, I. G. and Movat, H. Z. (1984). Desensitization of acute inflammatory lesions to chemotaxins and endotoxin. *J. Immunol.*, **133**, 2163–8
137. Colditz, I. G. (1985). Margination and emigration of leucocytes. *Surv. Synth. Pathol. Res.*, **4**, 44–68
138. Colditz, I. G. and Movat, H. Z. (1984). Chemotactic factor-specific desensitization of skin to infiltration by polymorphonuclear leukocytes. *Immun. Lett.*, **8**, 83–7
139. Bokisch, V. A. and Müller-Eberhard, H. J. (1970). Anaphylatoxin inactivator of human plasma: Its isolation and characterization as a carboxypeptidase. *J. Clin. Invest.*, **49**, 2427–36
140. Robbins, R. A. and Hamel, F. G. (1990). Chemotactic factor inactivator interaction with Gc-globulin (vitamin D-binding protein). *J. Immunol.*, **144**, 2371–6
141. Cianciolo, G., Hunter, J., Silva, J., Haskill, J. S. and Snyderman, R. (1981). Inhibitors of monocyte responses to chemotaxins are present in human cancerous effusions and react with monoclonal antibodies to the P_{15}(E) structural protein of retroviruses. *J. Clin. Invest.*, **68**, 831–44
142. Wang, J. M., Chen, Z. G., Cianciolo, G. J., Snyderman, R., Breviario, F., Dejana, E. and Mantovani, A. (1989). Production of retroviral P15E-related chemotaxis inhibitor by IL-1 treated endothelial cells. *J. Immunol.*, **142**, 2012–17
143. Weiser, W. Y., Temple, P. A., Witek-Giannotti, J. S., Remold, H. G., Clark, S. C. and David, J. R. (1989). Molecular cloning of a cDNA encoding a human macrophage migration inhibitory factor. *Proc. Natl. Acad. Sci. USA*, **86**, 7522–26
144. Thurman, G. B., Braude, I. A., Gray, P. W., Oldham, R. K. and Stevenson, H. C. (1985). MIF-like activity of natural and recombinant human interferon-γ and their neutralization by monoclonal antibody. *J. Immunol.*, **134**, 305–9
145. McInnes, A. and Rennick, D. M. (1988). Interleukin 4 induces cultured monocytes/macrophages to form giant multinucleated cells. *J. Exp. Med.*, **167**, 598–611
146. Bignold, L. P., Ferante, A. and Haynes, D. R. (1990). Studies of chemotactic, chemotactic movement-inhibiting and random movement-inhibiting effects of interleukin-1 alfa and beta, tumour necrosis factors alfa and beta and interferon gamma on human neutrophils in assays using 'sparse-pore' polycarbonate (nucleopore) membranes in the Boyden chamber. *Int. Arch. Allergy Appl. Immunol.*, **91**, 1–7
147. Kownatzki, E., Liehl, E., Aschauer, H. and Uhrich, S. (1990). Inhibition of chemotactic migration of human neutrophilic granulocytes by recombinant human granulocyte–macrophage colony-stimulating factor. *Immunopharmacology*, **19**, 139–43
148. Harvath, L. (1989). Regulation of neutrophil chemotaxis. *Ann. Rep. Med. Chem.*, **24**, 233–41
149. Keller, H. U. and Sorkin, E. (1967). Studies on chemotaxis. V. On the chemotactic effect of bacteria. *Int. Arch. Allergy*, **31**, 505–17
150. Ward, P. A., Lepow, I. H. and Newman, L. J. (1968). Bacterial factors chemotactic for

polymorphonuclear leukocytes. *Am. J. Pathol.*, **52**, 725–36
151. Schiffmann, E., Showell, H. V., Corcoran, B. A., Ward, P. A., Smith, E. and Becker, E. L. (1975). The isolation and partial characterization of neutrophil chemotactic factors from *Escherichia coli*. *J. Immunol.*, **114**, 1831–7
152. Becker, E. L. (1987). The formylpeptide receptor of the neutrophil. A search and conserve operation. *Am. J. Pathol.*, **129**, 16–24
153. Miyake, Y., Yasuhara, T., Fukui, K., Suginaka, H., Nakajima, T. and Moriyama, T. (1983). Purification and characterization of neutrophil chemotactic factors of *Streptococcus sanguis*. *Biochim. Biophys. Acta*, **758**, 181–6
154. Marasco, W. A., Phan, S. H., Krutzsch, H., Showell, H. J., Feltner, D. E., Nairn, R., Becker, E. L. and Ward, P. A. (1984). Purification and identification of formyl-methionyl-leucyl-phenylalanine as a major peptide neutrophil chemotactic factor produced by *Escherichia coli*. *J. Biol. Chem.*, **259**, 5430–9
155. Rot, A., Henderson, L. E., Sowder, R. and Leonard, E. J. (1989). *Staphylococcus aureus* tetrapeptide with high chemotactic potency and efficacy for human leukocytes. *J. Leukocyte Biol.*, **45**, 114–20
156. Sannomiya, P., Craig, R. A., Clewell, D. B., Suzuki, A., Fukino, M., Till, G. O. and Marasco, W. A. (1990). Characterization of a class of nonformylated *Enterococcus faecalis*-derived neutrophil chemotactic peptides: The sex pheromones. *Proc. Natl. Acad. Sci. USA*, **87**, 66–70
157. Loos, M. (1985). The complement system: activation and control. *Curr. Top. Microbiol. Immunol.*, **121**, 7–18
158. Henricks, P. A. J., Van der Tol, M. E., Engels, F., Nijkamp, F. P. and Verhoef, J. (1986). Human polymorphonuclear leukocytes release leukotriene B_4 during phagocytosis of *Staphylococcus aureus*. *Inflammation*, **10**, 37–47
159. Scheffer, J., König, W., Hacker, J. and Goebel, W. (1985). Bacterial adherence and hemolysin production from *Escherichia coli* induces histamine and leukotriene release from various cells. *Infect. Immun.*, **50**, 271–8
160. Leonard, E. J. and Yoshimura, T. (1990). Human monocyte chemoattractant protein-1 (MCP-1). *Immunol. Today*, **11**, 97–101
161. Leonard, E. J. and Yoshimura, T. (1990). Neutrophil attractant/activation protein-1 [NAP-1 (IL-8)]. *Am. J. Resp. Cell Mol. Biol.*, **2**, 479–86
162. Cutler, J. E. (1977). Chemotactic factor produced by *Candida albicans*. *Infect. Immun.*, **18**, 568–73
163. Czop, J. K. and Austen, K. F. (1985). Generation of leukotrienes by human monocytes upon stimulation of their β-glucan receptor during phagocytosis. *Proc. Natl. Acad. Sci. USA*, **82**, 2751–5
164. Fernandez, H. N., Henson, P. M., Otani, A. and Hugli, T. E. (1978). Chemotactic response to human C3a and C5a anaphylatoxins. *J. Immunol.*, **120**, 109–15
165. Ward, P. A. and Hill, J. H. (1970). C5 chemotactic fragments produced by an enzyme in lysosomal granules of neutrophils. *J. Immunol.*, **104**, 535–43
166. Kaplan, A. P., Kay, A. B. and Austen, K. F. (1972). A prealbumin activator of prekallikrein III. Appearance of chemotactic activity for human neutrophils by the conversion of human prekallikrein to kallikrein. *J. Exp. Med.*, **135**, 81–97
167. Kaplan, A. P., Goetzl, E. J. and Austen, K. F. (1973). The fibrinolytic pathway of human plasma II. The generation of chemotactic activity of activation of plasminogen proactivator. *J. Clin. Invest.*, **52**, 2591–5
168. Wiggins, R. C., Giclas, P. C. and Henson, P. M. (1981). Chemotactic activity generated from the fifth component of complement by plasma kallikrein of the rabbit. *J. Exp. Med.*, **153**, 1391–1404
169. Wetsel, R. A. and Kolb, W. P. (1982). Complement-independent activation of the fifth component (C5) of human complement: limited trypsin digestion resulting in the expression of biologic activity. *J. Immunol.*, **128**, 2209–16
170. Leonard, E. J. and Skeel, A. (1983). A high molecular weight chemoattractant generated from C5 by ultracentrifugation of mouse serum without activation of complement. *Mol. Immunol.*, **20**, 589–95
171. Hugli, R. E. and Müller-Eberhard, H. J. (1978). Anaphylatoxins: C3a and C5a. *Adv. Immunol.*, **26**, 1–53
172. Marder, S. R., Chenoweth, D. E., Goldstein, I. M. and Perez, H. D. (1985). Chemotactic responses of human peripheral blood monocytes to the complement-derived peptides C5a

and C5a des Arg. *J. Immunol.*, **134**, 3325–31
173. Perez, H. D., Goldstein, I. M., Webster, R. O. and Henson, P. M. (1981). Enhancement of the chemotactic activity of human C5a des Arg by an anionic polypeptide ('cochemotaxin') in normal serum and plasma. *J. Immunol.*, **126**, 800–4
174. Perez, H. D., Kelly, E., Chenoweth, D. and Elfman, F. (1988). Identification of the C5a des Arg cochemotaxin. Homology with vitamin D-binding protein (group-specific component globulin). *J. Clin. Invest.*, **82**, 360–3
175. Kew, R. R. and Webster, R. O. (1988). Gc-globulin (vitamin D-binding protein) enhances the neutrophil chemotactic activity of C5a and C5a des Arg. *J. Clin. Invest.*, **82**, 364–9
176. Berenberg, J. L. and Ward, P. A. (1973). Chemotactic factor inactivator in normal human serum. *J. Clin. Invest.*, **52**, 1200–6
177. Ward, P. A. and Ozols, J. (1976). Characterization of the protease activity in the chemotactic factor inactivator. *J. Clin. Invest.*, **58**, 123–9
178. Ford-Hutchinson, A. W., Bray, M. A., Doing, M. V., Shipley, M. E. and Smith, J. H. (1980). Leukotriene B_4 a potent chemokinetic and aggregating substance released from polymorphonuclear leukocytes. *Nature*, **286**, 264–5
179. Malmsten, C. L., Palmblad, J., Udèn, A.-M., Radmark, O., Engstedt, L., Samuelsson, B. (1980). A highly potent and stereospecific factor stimulating migration of polymorphonuclear leukocytes. *Acta Physiol. Scand.*, **110**, 449–51
180. Benveniste, J., Henson, P. M. and Cochrane, C. G. (1972). Leukocyte-dependent histamine release from rabbit platelets. The role of IgE, basophils, and a platelet-activating factor. *J. Exp. Med.*, **136**, 1356–77
181. Hanahan, D. J., Demopoulos, C. A., Liehr, J. and Pinckard, R. N. (1980). Identification of platelet activating factor isolated from rabbit basophils as acetyl glyceryl ether phosphorylcholine. *J. Biol. Chem.*, **255**, 5514–16
182. Clark, P. O., Hanahan, D. J. and Pinckard, R. N. (1980). Physical and chemical properties of platelet-activating factor obtained from human neutrophils and monocytes and rabbit neutrophils and basophils. *Biochim. Biophys. Acta*, **628**, 69–75
183. Camussi, G., Aglietta, M., Malavasi, F., Tetta, C., Piacibello, W., Sanavio, F. and Bussolino, F. (1983). The release of platelet-activating factor from human endothelial cells in culture. *J. Immunol.*, **131**, 2397–403
184. Snyder, F. (ed.) (1988). *Platelet-activating Factor and Related Lipid Mediators* (New York: Plenum Press)
185. Czarnetzki, B. (1983). Increased monocyte chemotaxis towards leukotriene B_4 and platelet activating factor in patients with inflammatory dermatoses. *Clin. Exp. Immunol.*, **54**, 486–92
186. Wardlaw, A. J., Moqbel, R., Cromwell, O. and Kay, A. B. (1986). Platelet-activating factor. A potent chemotactic and chemokinetic factor for human eosinophils. *J. Clin. Invest.*, **78**, 1701–6
187. Morita, E., Schröder, J-M. and Christophers, E. (1989). Differential sensitivities of purified human eosinophils and neutrophils to defined chemotaxins. *Scand. J. Immunol.*, **29**, 709–16
188. Sigal, C. E., Valone, F. H., Holtzman, M. J. and Goetzl, E. J. (1987). Preferential human eosinophil chemotactic activity of the platelet-activating factor (PAF)1-*O*-hexadecyl-2-acetyl-sn-glyceryl-3-phosphocholine (AGEPC). *J. Clin. Immunol.*, **7**, 179–84
189. Altman, L. C., Snyderman, R., Opcnheim, J. J. and Mergenhagen, S. E. (1973). A human mononuclear leukocyte chemotactic factor: Characterization, specificity and kinetics of production by homologous leukocytes. *J. Immunol.*, **110**, 801–10
190. Oppenheim, J. J., Zachariae, O. C., Mukaida, N. and Matsushima, K. (1991). Properties of the novel proinflammatory supergene 'intercrine' cytokine family. *Annu. Rev. Immunol.*, **9**, 617–48
191. Baggiolini, M., Walz, A. and Kunkel, S. L. (1989). Neutrophil activating peptide-1/interleukin 8, a novel cytokine that activates neutrophils. *J. Clin. Invest.*, **84**, 1045–9
192. Matsushima, K. and Oppenheim, J. J. (1989). Interleukin 8 and MCAF: Novel inflammatory cytokines inducble by IL-1 and TNF. *Cytokine*, **1**, 2–13
193. Wolpe, S. D. and Cerami, A. (1989). Macrophage inflammatory proteins 1 and 2: members of a novel superfamily of cytokines. *FASEB J.*, **3**, 2565–73
194. Schröder, J.-M., Persoon, N. L. M. and Christophers, E. (1990). Lipopolysaccharide-stimulated human monocytes secrete, apart from neutrophil-activating peptide 1/interleukin 8, a second neutrophil-activating protein. *J. Exp. Med.*, **171**, 1091–100
195. Walz, A., Dewald, B., Tscharner, V. and Baggiolini, M. (1989). Effects of the neutrophil-activating

peptide NAP-2, platelet basic protein, connective tissue-activating peptide III, and platelet factor 4 on human neutrophils. *J. Exp. Med.*, **170**, 1745–50

196. Leonard, E. J., Yoshimura, T., Rot, A., Noer, K., Walz, A., Baggiolini, M., Walz, D., Goetzl, E. J. and Castor, C. W. (1991). Chemotactic activity and receptor binding of neutrophil attractant/activation protein-1 (NAP-1) and structurally related host defense cytokines: Interaction of NAP-2 with the NAP-1 receptor. *J. Leukocyte Biol.* (In press)
197. Schröder, J.-M., Sticherling, M., Henneicke, H. H., Preissner, W. C., and Christophers, E. (1990). IL-1α or tumor necrosis factor-α stimulate release of three NAP-1/IL-8-related neutrophil chemotactic proteins in human dermal fibroblasts. *J. Immunol.*, **144**, 2223–32
198. Gimbrone, M. A., Jr., Obin, M. S., Brock, A. F., Luis, E. A., Hass, P. E., Hébert, C. A., Yip, Y. K., Leung, D. W., Lowe, D. G., Kohr, W. J., Darbonne, W. C., Bechtol, K. B. and Baker, J. B. (1989). Endothelial interleukin-8: a novel inhibitor of leukocyte–endothelial interactions. *Science*, **246**, 1601–3
199. Sylvester, I., Rankin, J. A., Yoshimura, T., Tanaka, S. and Leonard, E. J. (1990). Secretion of neutrophil attractant/activation protein (NAP-1) by lipopolysaccharide-stimulated lung macrophages, determined by both enzyme-linked immunosorbent assay and N-terminal sequence analysis. *Am. Rev. Respir. Dis.*, **141**, 683–8
200. Van Damme, J., Bunning, R. A. D., Conings, R., Russell, R. G. G. and Opdenakker, G. (1991). Characterization of granulocyte chemotactic activity from human cytokine-stimulated chondrocytes as interleukin-8. *Cytokine* (In press)
201. Larsen, C. G., Anderson, A. O., Appella, E., Oppenheim, J. J. and Matsushima, K. (1989). The neutrophil-activating protein (NAP-1) is also chemotactic for T lymphocytes. *Science*, **243**, 1464–6
202. Van Damme, J., Decock, B., Conings, R., Lenmaerts, J-P., Opdenakker, G. and Billiau, A. (1989). The chemotactic activity for granulocytes produced by virally infected fibroblasts is identical to monocyte-derived interleukin 8. *Eur. J. Immunol.*, **19**, 1189–94
203. Van Damme, J., Decock, B., Lenaerts, J-P., Conings, R., Bertini, R., Mantovani, A. and Billiau, A. (1989). Identification by sequence analysis of chemotactic factors for monocytes produced by normal and transformed cells stimulated with virus, double-stranded RNA or cytokine. *Eur. J. Immunol.*, **19**, 2367–73
204. Carp, H. (1982). Mitochondrial *N*-formylmethionyl proteins as chemoattractants for neutrophils. *J. Exp. Med.*, **155**, 264–75
205. Yoshimura, T., Matsushima, K., Oppenheim, J. J. and Leonard, E. J. (1987). Neutrophil chemotactic factor produced by lipopolysaccharide (LPS)-stimulated human blood mononuclear leukocytes: Partial characterization and separation from interleukin 1 (IL-1). *J. Immunol.*, **139**, 788–93
206. Newman, I. and Wilkinson, P. C. (1989). Chemotactic activity of lymphotoxin and tumour necrosis factor alpha for human neutrophils. *Immunology*, **66**, 318–20
207. Sayers, T. J., Wiltrout, T. A., Bull, C. A., Denn III, A. C., Pilaro, A. M. and Lokesh, B. (1988). Effect of cytokines on polymorphonuclear neutrophil infiltration in the mouse. *J. Immunol.*, **141**, 1670–7
208. Graves, D. T., Grotendorst, G. R., Antoniades, H. N., Schwartz, C. J. and Valente, A. J. (1989). Platelet-derived growth factor is not chemotactic for human peripheral blood monocytes. *Exp. Cell Res.*, **180**, 497–503
209. Migliorisi, G., Folkes, E. and Cramer, E. B. (1988). Differences in the ability of neutrophils and monocytes to traverse epithelial occluding junctions. *J. Leukocyte Biol.*, **44**, 485–92
210. Territo, M. C., Ganz, T., Selsted, M. E. and Lehrer, R. (1989). Monocyte-chemotactic activity of defensins from human neutrophils. *J. Clin. Invest.*, **84**, 2017–20
211. Banda, M. J., Rice, A. G., Griffin, G. L. and Senior, R. M. (1988). The inhibitory complex of human α1-proteinase inhibitor and human leukocyte elastase is a neutrophil chemoattractant. *J. Exp. Med.*, **167**, 1608–15
212. Petrone, W. F., English, D. E., Wong, K. and McCord, J. M. (1980). Free radicals and inflammation: Superoxide-dependent activation of a neutrophil chemotactic factor in plasma. *Proc. Natl. Acad. Sci. USA*, **77**, 1159–63
213. Godfrey, H. P., Frenz, D. A., Canfield, L. S., Akiyama, S. K. and Newman, S. A. (1989). Non-chemotactic translocation of phagocytic cells mediated by fibronectin-related human lymphokine. *J. Immunol.*, **143**, 3691–6
214. Smith, C. W., Kishimoto, T. K., Abbass, O., Hughes, B., Rothlein, R., McIntire, L. V.,

Butcher, E. and Anderson, D. C. (1991). Chemotactic factors regulate lectin adhesion molecule 1 (LECAM-1)-dependent neutrophil adhesion to cytokine-stimulated endothelial cells in vitro. *J. Clin. Invest.*, **87**, 609–18

215. Tonnesen, M. G., Smedley, L. A. and Henson, P. M. (1984). Neutrophil-endothelial cell interactions. Modulation of neutrophil adhesiveness induced by complement fragments C5a and C5a des arg and formyl-methionyl-leucyl-phenylalanine *in vitro*. *J. Clin. Invest.*, **74**, 1581–92
216. Lo, S. K., Detmers, P. A., Levin, S. M. and Wright, S. D. (1989). Transient adhesion of neutrophils to endothelium. *J. Exp. Med.*, **169**, 1779–93
217. Anderson, D. C. and Springer, T. A. (1987). Leukocyte adhesion deficiency: an inherited defect in the Mac-1, LFA-1, and p150,95 glycoproteins. *Ann. Rev. Med.*, **38**, 175–94
218. Lawrence, M. B., Smith, C. W., Eskin, S. G. and McIntyre, L. V. (1990). Effect of venous shear stress on CD18-mediated neutrophil adhesion to cultured endothelium. *Blood*, **75**, 227–37
219. Lawrence, M. B. and Springer, T. A. (1991). Leukocytes roll on a selectin at physiologic flow rates: distinction from and prerequisite for adhesion through integrins. *Cell.*, **65**, 859–73
220. Dustin, M. L., Rothlein, R., Bhan, A. K., Dinarello, C. A. and Springer, T. A. (1986). Induction by IL-1 and interferon-gamma: tissue distribution, biochemistry, and function of natural adherence molecule (ICAM-1). *J. Immunol.*, **137**, 245–54
221. Bevilacqua, M. P., Stengelin, S., Gimbrone, M. A., Jr. and Seed, B. (1989). Endothelial leukocyte adhesion molecule 1: an inducible receptor for neutrophils related to complement regulatory proteins and lectins. *Science*, **243**, 1160–5
222. Zimmerman, G. A., McIntyre, T. M., Mehra, M. and Prescott, S. M. (1990). Endothelial cell-associated platelet-activating factor: a novel mechanism for signaling intercellular adhesion. *J. Cell Biol.*, **110**, 529–40
223. Geng, J-G., Bevilacqua, M. P., Moore, K. L., McIntyre, T. M., Prescott, S. M., Kim, J. M., Bliss, G. A., Zimmerman, G. A. and McEver, R. P. (1990). Rapid neutrophil adhesion to activated endothelium by GMP-140. *Nature*, **343**, 757–60
224. Marks, R. M., Todd III, R. F. and Ward, P. A. (1989). Rapid induction of neutrophil endothelial adhesion by endothelial complement fixation. *Nature*, **339**, 314–17
225. Wilkinson, P. C., Haston, W. S. and Shields, J. M. (1982). Some determinants of the locomotory behaviour of phagocytes and lymphocytes in vitro. *Clin. exp. Immunol.*, **50**, 461–73
226. Rotrosen, D., Malech, H. L. and Gallin, J. I. (1987). Formyl peptide leukocyte chemoattractant uptake and release by cultured human umbilical vein endothelial cells. *J. Immunol.*, **139**, 3034–40

Index